AF400832

Mathematics and Visualization

Series editors
Hans-Christian Hege
David Hoffman
Christopher R. Johnson
Konrad Polthier
Martin Rumpf

More information about this series at http://www.springer.com/series/4562

Andrea Fuster • Aurobrata Ghosh • Enrico Kaden •
Yogesh Rathi • Marco Reisert

Editors

Computational Diffusion MRI

MICCAI Workshop, Athens, Greece, October 2016

With 73 Figures, 69 in color

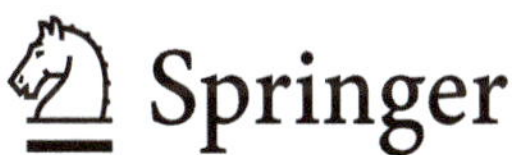

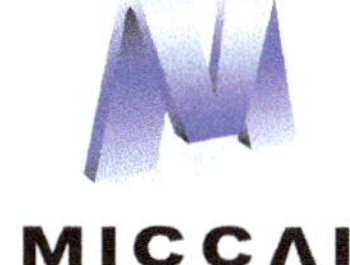

Editors

Andrea Fuster
Department of Mathematics
  and Computer Science
Eindhoven University of Technology
Eindhoven, The Netherlands

Aurobrata Ghosh
Centre for Medical Image Computing
University College London
London, United Kingdom

Enrico Kaden
Centre for Medical Image Computing
University College London
London, United Kingdom

Yogesh Rathi
Department of Psychiatry
Brigham & Womens Hospital
Boston, MA, USA

Marco Reisert
Medical Physics
University Medical Center
Freiburg, Germany

ISSN 1612-3786   ISSN 2197-666X   (electronic)
Mathematics and Visualization
ISBN 978-3-319-54129-7   ISBN 978-3-319-54130-3   (eBook)
DOI 10.1007/978-3-319-54130-3

Library of Congress Control Number: 2017936142

Mathematics Subject Classification (2010): 92BXX, 62P10, 65Z99, 00A66, 65CXX, 65DXX

Cover illustration: Guillermo Gallardo (taken from "Groupwise Structural Parcellation of the Cortex: A Sound Approach Based on Logistic Models" by Guillermo Gallardo, Rutger Fick, William Wells III, Rachid Deriche, and Demian Wassermann)

Printed on acid-free paper

This Springer imprint is published by Springer Nature
The registered company is Springer International Publishing AG
The registered company address is: Gewerbestrasse 11, 6330 Cham, Switzerland

Preface

This volume offers a valuable starting point for anyone interested in learning computational diffusion MRI and mathematical methods for brain connectivity while also sharing new perspectives and insights on the latest research challenges for those currently working in the field.

Over the last decade, interest in diffusion MRI has virtually exploded. The technique provides unique insights into the microstructure of living tissue and enables in vivo connectivity mapping of the brain. Computational techniques are key to the continued success and development of diffusion MRI and to its widespread transfer into the clinic, while new processing methods are essential to addressing issues at each stage of the diffusion MRI pipeline: acquisition, reconstruction, modeling and model fitting, image processing, fiber tracking, connectivity mapping, visualization, group studies, and inference.

These papers from the 2016 MICCAI Workshop "Computational Diffusion MRI" which was intended to provide a snapshot of the latest developments within the highly active and growing field of diffusion MRI cover a wide range of topics, from fundamental theoretical work on mathematical modeling to the development and evaluation of robust algorithms and applications in neuroscientific studies and clinical practice. The contributions include rigorous mathematical derivations; a wealth of rich, full-color visualizations; and biologically or clinically relevant results. As such, they will be of interest to researchers and practitioners in the fields of computer science, MR physics, and applied mathematics.

Eindhoven, The Netherlands
London, UK
London, UK
Boston, MA, USA
Freiburg, Germany Andrea Fuster
Aurobrata Ghosh
Enrico Kaden
Yogesh Rathi
Marco Reisert

Contents

Program Committee

The MR Physics of Advanced Diffusion Imaging

Matt G. Hall

Abstract Over the last decade, the number of models used to analyse and interpret diffusion MRI data has increased dramatically. Exponentials and biexponentials have been joined by stretched exponentials, HARDI methods, compartment-based microstructure models and effective medium theories. At the same time, the field has experienced a cultural shift away from MR physics and towards computer science, emphasising Bayesian statistics and Machine Learning. This has meant that understanding imaging methodology whilst still keeping in mind the underlying physical assumptions can be challenging.

This chapter reviews the Diffusion MR modelling literature from the point of view of the underlying physics. We show how the Bloch-Torrey equation can be derived, and then how different physical assumptions and formulations lead to different models. The intention is to show the different assumptions made in different models, to aid understanding and model selection.

1 Introduction

The manipulation of spin magnetic moments is central to NMR and MRI. Via a wide variety of mechanisms, it is possible to excite signals of various kinds from samples placed in the scanner's magnetic field by applying controlled RF pulses and magnetic field gradients. Since the behaviour of spins is affected by the chemical and physical environment they experience, NMR and MRI measurements provide a vector for analysing the chemical make-up and physical structure of objects or living organisms.

The Bloch equation describes the change in magnetisation of a continuum of spins in a field $\mathbf{B}$, assuming that spins are stationary. It is an effective theory which captures smaller-scale effects like spin-spin and spin-lattice interaction via decay constants. In many situations, however, it is useful to consider the effects of diffusive motion on spin magnetisation, which can have an important effect on NMR

M.G. Hall, Ph.D (✉)
Developmental Imaging and Biophysics, UCL GOS Institute of Child Health,
University College London, London, UK
e-mail: matt.hall@ucl.ac.uk

© Springer International Publishing AG 2017
A. Fuster et al. (eds.), *Computational Diffusion MRI*, Mathematics
and Visualization, DOI 10.1007/978-3-319-54130-3_1

measurements. Spin diffusion was first incorporated by Torrey [40], who included an additional additive diffusion term.

Torrey's derivation assumes that spins have only a very small drift velocity, but in more recent literature it is common to also include a linear flow term. The full form is

$$\frac{d\mathbf{M}}{dt} = \gamma\mathbf{M} \times \mathbf{B} - \frac{M_x\hat{\mathbf{i}} + M_y\hat{\mathbf{j}}}{T_2} - \frac{M_z - M_0}{T_1}\hat{\mathbf{k}} - \nabla \cdot (D\nabla\mathbf{M}) - \nabla \cdot \mathbf{u}\mathbf{M} \qquad (1)$$

where $\mathbf{M} = (M_x, M_y, M_z)^T$ is the local magnetisation, M_0 is the equilibrium magnetisation, $\hat{\mathbf{i}}$, $\hat{\mathbf{j}}$, $\hat{\mathbf{k}}$ are unit vectors defining the lab frame, $\mathbf{B}$ is the static scanner field, T_1 and T_2 are relaxation constants related to spin-lattice and spin-spin interactions respectively, and γ is the gyromagnetic constant for the medium, D describes the local diffusivity, and $\mathbf{u}$ is a vector describing coherent flow.

The Bloch-Torrey equation led to the development of various pulse sequences which allow the diffusive term to be quantified (see, e.g. [11, 39]), which in turn has lead to the development of diffusion-weighted imaging (DWI).

Diffusive motion encodes information about the environment experienced by diffusing particles. This encoding, however, is non-trivial and extracting environmental information from measurements of diffusion, particularly when it happens in the presence of microstructure, is hugely challenging. Nevertheless, the fact that the length scales of diffusive motion over the timescale of a typical MR pulse sequence are orders of magnitude smaller than a typical scan voxel has led to considerable research effort into how best to analyse diffusion-weighted measurements. This in turn has lead to a large number of models and approaches to diffusion imaging which can be confusing to someone new to the field.

All of diffusion imaging is ultimately grounded in the Bloch-Torrey equation—different solutions provide the models used to analyse diffusion-weighted data. This chapter reviews how the Bloch-Torrey equation is derived, and shows how a minor and straightforward generalisation of the transport term provides a useful unifying principle which we can use to reveal the relationships between different models.

The Bloch-Torrey equation treats magnetisation as a continuum. The presence of the spatial derivative requires that $\mathbf{M}$ be smoothly varying in space. Similarly, the time derivative assumes that the continuum is changing smoothly with time. This is compatible with the concept of magnetisation as a vector field rather than being defined discretely on separate, point-like particles. We can think of this as a "local magnetisation"—the magnetisation per unit volume—given by

$$\mathbf{M}_{\text{net}} = \sum_{i=1}^{N} \boldsymbol{\mu}_i \simeq \iiint_V \mathbf{M}dV \qquad (2)$$

where $\boldsymbol{\mu}_i$ are individual magnetisation vectors due to point charges in the applied field $\mathbf{B}$, V is a small control volume over which the derivatives are smooth, and $\mathbf{M}$ is a smooth continuum approximating the underlying discrete magnetisation distribution. This can be derived by considering the conservation of mass as applied to a vector quantity via the continuity equation. Note that V is not typically associated with a scan voxel—it is a theoretical volume over which the continuum approximation holds. For experimental purposes it may be regarded as vanishingly small.

We will review diffusion MRI models starting with a derivation of the continuity equation for a vector quantity, showing how this leads to the Bloch-Torrey equation. We then show how different models can be seen as choices of transport mechanism, and then explore generalisations to multiple continua and models with boundary conditions. The aim is to give a comprehensive overview of the diffusion MRI modelling literature whilst also providing a physical basis for the assumptions made in each one.

2 The Continuity Equation for Vector-Valued Quantities

Conservation laws and conserved quantities are familiar concepts to every physicist. The idea is that the total amount of a particular quantity is constant. Whilst conservation is very general and useful, in many situations it is helpful to require that the distribution of the conserved quantity is smooth. The presence of jumps means that derivatives are not defined, and hence approaches to studying dynamics that rely on differential equations, such as the Bloch-Torrey equation, will fail. This extension of conservation to include local smoothness is called Continuity. Continuity is a widespread approach in physics. The first usage was probably by Euler who used the idea as early as 1757 [3]. This section describes how continuity is formalised for the vector-valued quantities of interest in MR physics.

We can think about this by considering the amount of a quantity in a particular control volume V. Let $\mathbf{M}(\mathbf{r})$ be the density of some vector quantity at a point $\mathbf{r}$ in space. The total amount in an arbitrary volume V at time t is then

$$\mathbf{M}_{\mathrm{net}}(t) = \iiint_V \mathbf{M}(\mathbf{r}, t) dV. \tag{3}$$

Unlike a global conservation law, this quantity is not guaranteed to be constant. In fact, its rate of change can be readily defined as

$$\frac{d\mathbf{M}_{\mathrm{net}}(t)}{dt} = \frac{d}{dt} \iiint_V \mathbf{M}(\mathbf{r}, t) dV = \iiint_V \frac{\partial \mathbf{M}(\mathbf{r}, t)}{\partial t} dV. \tag{4}$$

This change can also be expressed in terms of the processes that cause it. The change in the total amount of a quantity in the volume V is given by the net amount of the quantity entering and leaving the volume, and also by the intrinsic change in the amount of quantity present due to its creation and destruction. Figure 1 illustrates these two processes—a process transferring a quantity into (or out of) a region is

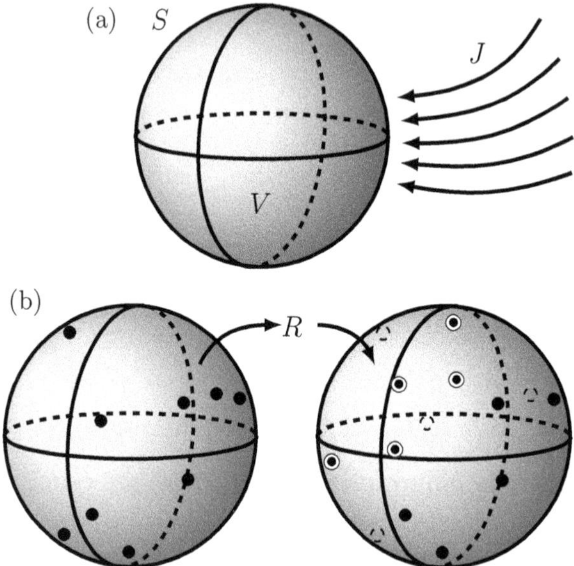

Fig. 1 The two mechanisms by which the amount of a quantity of interest in a region V can change. (**a**) Transport in or out via a flux process J, or (**b**) intrinsic changes in the quantity itself via a source/sink process R. Black particles decay away (*dotted circles*), and new particles emerge (*ringed circles*)

known as a flux (a). A quantity may also change in the absence of movement (b) for example chemical reactions can occur or radioactive decay may transform one quantity into another. Let $J(\mathbf{r}, t)$ be the net flux of $\mathbf{M}$ in to/out of a point $\mathbf{r}$ and time t, and define the net intrinsic change in the quantity in the volume at time t as $\boldsymbol{\Sigma}(t)$. This means we can write the net change in $\mathbf{M_{net}}(t)$ as

$$\frac{d\mathbf{M}_{\mathrm{net}}(t)}{dt} = \oiint_S J(\mathbf{r}, t)dS - \boldsymbol{\Sigma}(t) \tag{5}$$

where S is the surface that bounds V. The source and sink process is described by a net additive vector, but the flux term is more subtle. In the scalar case the flux is a vector, but here we need to describe the transport of a vector quantity in a vector direction, necessitating a rank-two object. We will write this as $J(\mathbf{M})$, giving

$$\frac{d\mathbf{M}_{\mathrm{net}}(t)}{dt} = \oiint_S J(\mathbf{M})dS - \boldsymbol{\Sigma}(t) \tag{6}$$

Equating Eqs. (4) and (6) we have

$$\iiint_V \frac{\partial \mathbf{M}(\mathbf{r}, t)}{\partial t}dV = \oiint_S J(\mathbf{M})dS - \boldsymbol{\Sigma}(t). \tag{7}$$

With a small amount of manipulation we can put this in a more convenient form. A generalisation of the divergence theorem using tensor contraction [4] gives

$$\oiint_S J(\mathbf{M})dS = \iiint_V \nabla \cdot J(\mathbf{M})dV \tag{8}$$

and the source term can be written in terms of a local density

$$\Sigma(t) = \iiint_V \sigma(\mathbf{r}, t)dV. \tag{9}$$

Substituting these into Eq. (7) gives

$$\iiint_V \frac{\partial \mathbf{M}(\mathbf{r}, t)}{\partial t}dV = \iiint_V \nabla \cdot J(\mathbf{M})dV - \iiint_V \sigma(\mathbf{r}, t)dV. \tag{10}$$

Notice now that all three terms now contain volume integrals over V. Since V is arbitrary, the only way in which Eq. (10) can hold is if the integrands are equal, i.e.

$$\frac{\partial \mathbf{M}}{\partial t} = \nabla \cdot J(\mathbf{M}) - \sigma(\mathbf{r}, t) \tag{11}$$

This is the *continuity equation* for a vector quantity. It captures the changes in a conserved quantity in the presence of a flux, $\mathbf{J}$ and a source and sink process σ. This is a very general equation, describing local conservation of a continuum tagged with a vector quantity which is not strongly coupled to the flux motion. As yet, we have made no assumptions about the nature of this quantity other than the fact that it is a vector. In MR physics we are interested in particles tagged with a vector quantity: Magnetisation. We shall see that looking at diffusion MRI through the lens of continuity is a powerful unifying principle which reveals different assumptions made in different models.

3 Continuity of Magnetisation: The Bloch-Torrey Equation

We will now show that the Bloch and Bloch-Torrey equations, which are fundamental to NMR and MRI experiments may be derived from the continuity of a vector quantity, and are in fact both particular cases of the continuity of magnetisation in the presence of a strong applied field.

3.1 The Bloch Terms as Sources and Sinks

The source and sink terms of the continuity equation describe the evolution of the quantity of interest that occurs independently of transport in the medium. A vector quantity may change not only magnitude but also orientation. In the present context, they capture the interaction between a spin's magnetisation and the local magnetic field—exactly the role of the terms of the Bloch equation. We may therefore consider the Bloch equation as a set of source and sink terms for our vector continuity equation and write Eq. (11) as

$$\frac{d\mathbf{M}}{dt} = \gamma \mathbf{M} \times \mathbf{B} - \frac{M_x\hat{\mathbf{i}} + M_y\hat{\mathbf{j}}}{T_2} - \frac{M_z - M_0}{T_1}\hat{\mathbf{k}} - \nabla \cdot J(\mathbf{M}). \tag{12}$$

We can immediately see the similarity between Eq. (12) and the traditional form of the Bloch-Torrey equation. Equation (12) describes the change in magnetisation of a continuous quantity in an applied magnetic field with an arbitrary transport process given by $J(\mathbf{M})$. This is, of course, the same approach used by Torrey in deriving his equation in the first place. The difference being that Torrey does not start from the general form with an unspecified $J(\mathbf{M})$ but instead proceeds directly to the drift-diffusion case [40].

We note that Eq. (12) employs unit vector notation. This is perfectly valid, but obscures the essentially simple nature of the equation. We can re-write the T_1 and T_2 terms in matrix form as

$$\frac{M_x\hat{\mathbf{i}} + M_y\hat{\mathbf{j}}}{T_2} - \frac{M_z - M_0}{T_1}\hat{\mathbf{k}} \rightarrow \begin{pmatrix} -\frac{1}{T_2} & 0 & 0 & 0 \\ 0 & -\frac{1}{T_2} & 0 & 0 \\ 0 & 0 & -\frac{1}{T_1} & \frac{M_0}{T_1} \\ 0 & 0 & 0 & 1 \end{pmatrix} \begin{pmatrix} M_x \\ M_y \\ M_z \\ 1 \end{pmatrix}. \tag{13}$$

The Bloch terms also contain a precessional term, which takes the form of a cross product with the applied field. A cross product can also be written in matrix form. Adding this to Eq. (13) gives

$$\begin{pmatrix} \frac{dM_x}{dt} \\ \frac{dM_y}{dt} \\ \frac{dM_z}{dt} \\ 1 \end{pmatrix} = \begin{pmatrix} -\frac{1}{T_2} & -\gamma B_z & \gamma B_y & 0 \\ \gamma B_z & -\frac{1}{T_2} & -\gamma B_x & 0 \\ -\gamma B_y & \gamma B_z & -\frac{1}{T_1} & \frac{M_0}{T_1} \\ 0 & 0 & 0 & 1 \end{pmatrix} \begin{pmatrix} M_x \\ M_y \\ M_z \\ 1 \end{pmatrix} = R\mathbf{M}. \tag{14}$$

Thus the Bloch equation can be expressed as a single matrix multiplication. This notation also allows us a layer of abstraction with regards coordinate system. The matrix R can be written in the lab frame, as here, or can be transformed into the rotating frame. By writing our systems (and solutions) in terms of R we are free to specify what coordinate frame we use separately. Equation (12) then becomes

$$\frac{\partial \mathbf{M}}{\partial t} = R\mathbf{M} - \nabla \cdot J(\mathbf{M}). \tag{15}$$

Table 1 Flux term choices and corresponding diffusion models

Flux	Form	Technique
0	$\cdot$	T_1 and T_2 weighting
$\mathbf{u}\mathbf{M}$	$R_{\mathbf{z}}(\mathbf{u} \cdot \mathbf{q}t)$	Velocity-weighted phase contrast
$-D\nabla\mathbf{M}$	$e^{-\mathbf{q}D\mathbf{q}t}$	Diffusion tensor imaging
$-D\frac{\partial^{\beta}}{\partial|x|^{\beta}}\mathbf{M}$	$e^{-D|q|^{\beta+1}t}$	Stretched exponential
$D\nabla\mathbf{M}-\frac{1}{3}D\nabla K\nabla\cdot D\nabla\mathbf{M}t$	$e^{-\mathbf{q}D\mathbf{q}t}e^{-\frac{1}{6}\mathbf{q}D\mathbf{q}K\mathbf{q}D\mathbf{q}t^2}$	Diffusion Kurtosis Imaging

3.2 The Flux Terms: Transport Processes

Different choices of flux lead to different solutions of Eq. (15), and in many cases to different specific MR imaging techniques. We will give solutions in terms of the q-space approximation, assuming a Fourier relationship between spatial variables $\mathbf{x}$ and displacement spatial frequencies $\mathbf{q} = \gamma\delta\mathbf{G}$. In most cases solutions are found via the Fourier-Laplace method applied to the Bloch-Torrey equation in question.

This section reviews the diffusion MRI modelling literature in the context of the theoretic framework developed above. We will show how many existing techniques stem from choices of flux terms of generalised Bloch-Torrey equations and demonstrates that the framework acts as a unifying principle across what can otherwise appear a bewildering maze of different models. We will also see that the common assumption that the phase information is not important is only valid in particular special cases (The different combinations are summarised in Table 1).

3.3 T_1- and T_2-Weighted Imaging

The simplest example is one where there is no flux present in the system, and only the Bloch terms contribute. In this case the equation reduces to the Bloch equation. In the vector form developed above, this is

$$\frac{\partial\mathbf{M}}{\partial t} = R\mathbf{M}. \tag{16}$$

The solution is a the matrix exponential in R. This can be written as

$$\mathbf{M}(t) = \mathbf{M}_0 \begin{pmatrix} e^{-\frac{t}{T_2}} & 0 & 0 & 0 \\ 0 & e^{-\frac{t}{T_2}} & 0 & 0 \\ 0 & 0 & \left(1 - e^{-\frac{t}{T_1}}\right) & 0 \\ 0 & 0 & 0 & 1 \end{pmatrix} \tag{17}$$

which contains the familiar expressions describing T_1 and T_2 decay.

3.4 Diffusion Tensor Imaging

The next simplest case is Diffusion Tensor Imaging [7]. DTI is directly related to the canonical form of the Bloch-Torrey equation, which has a flux defined by the tensor version of Fick's law for the local magnetisation i.e.

$$J(\mathbf{M}) = -D\nabla\mathbf{M}. \tag{18}$$

where D is the diffusion tensor.

The solution of the Bloch-Torrey equation with a tensorial Fickian flux is

$$\mathbf{m}(t) = \mathbf{m}_0 e^{Rt} e^{-\mathbf{q}D\mathbf{q}t}. \tag{19}$$

It is common not to write the decay term explicitly and simply call the Bloch equation pre-factor S_0 and the measured signal S. S is related to $\mathbf{M}$ via an integral over the local spin phase distribution, which is also implicit in the q-space approximation [33]. Determining the elements of D requires several measurements of this attenuation term. This is usually performed by formulating and inverting a linear system, the structure of which is derived from this solution (see, e.g. [30]).

From this we can see that the diffusion tensor follows simply from the flux. The form of the expression is the result of this assumption and the q-space approximation—an inverse Fourier Transform leads us back to a Gaussian spin displacement and time dependence. We also note that diffusion terms enter this equation entirely via the magnitude of the signal. Diffusion attenuates via a scalar term, rather than as an additional transformation on its orientation.

3.5 Velocity-Weighted Phase Contrast

Another straightforward case is coherent flow. This is equivalent to velocity-weighted imaging. Although a drift term was originally considered by Torrey [40], coherent flow effects are not traditionally considered alongside diffusion-weighted methods.

Coherent flow is described locally by a vector $\mathbf{u}$, giving us

$$J(\mathbf{M}) = \mathbf{u}\mathbf{M}. \tag{20}$$

where the $\mathbf{u}\mathbf{M}$ is the dyadic product of the two vectors. Substituting this into Eq. (15) yields the following solution

$$\mathbf{m}(t) = \mathbf{m}_0 R_{\mathbf{x}}(\mathbf{q} \cdot \mathbf{u}t) e^{Rt}. \tag{21}$$

where $R_z(\theta)$ is a rotation in the transverse plane by an angle θ. The angle of rotation is given by the dot product of the local flow and the $\mathbf{q}$ vector, manifesting as a phase shift without a change in magnitude.

The combination of coherent flow and diffusion is equivalent to an advection-diffusion equation where spins both flow and diffuse but the two processes are essentially uncoupled.

3.6 Stretched-Exponentials and Space-Fractional Super-Diffusion

The physical interpretation of the stretched-exponential is sometimes a little mysterious. This section will show that they can be seen as modelling a particular form of transport process: the Lévy walk. Particles executing Lévy walks make many short steps with occasional much longer displacements. They are characterised by random walk-like processes with a power-law distribution of step lengths. i.e. step length ℓ follows

$$p(\ell) \propto \ell^{-\beta}. \tag{22}$$

Just as a Brownian random walk leads to a Fickian flux, a similar calculation shows that a Lévy walk leads to a flux with a fractional-order derivative (see Appendix for derivation). Fractional derivatives are derivatives of non-integer order. They have been extensively applied to transport theory. Whilst not providing a unique link to the microstructural details of the system, fractional approaches nonetheless provide access to systems in which diffusion-like transport it not well-described by Gaussian diffusion processes derived from the usual form of Fick's law.

For mathematical simplicity, we will assume an isotropic process and treat diffusion in one dimension. In this case the flux is written as

$$J(\mathbf{M}) = -D\frac{\partial^\beta}{\partial|x|^\beta}\mathbf{M} \tag{23}$$

where D is a constant and $0 < \beta < 1$ is the order of the derivative and step distribution and $\frac{\partial^\beta}{\partial|x|^\beta}$ is the Reisz fractional derivative [29]. The derivation of the fractional form of Fick's law is given in the appendix.

The solution of the Bloch-Torrey equation with a fractional flux is

$$\mathbf{m} = \mathbf{m}_0 e^{Rt} e^{-D|q|^{\beta+1}t}. \tag{24}$$

This form of spin transport is known as super-diffusion, so-called because the mean squared-displacement of particles increases faster than linear with time. The stretched exponential in this form is thus a model of super-diffusion.

Stretched exponentials have been employed by several authors [9, 12, 16], although the form chosen varies. The form derived here has the stretching exponent on the q terms only, although authors often apply the stretching exponent to both q and t. The model has been criticised on the grounds that the exponent is difficult to interpret physically, but the derivation here illustrates that it can be directly associated with the statistics of the underlying random walk: the fitted exponent is related to transport, not structure.

3.7 Diffusion Kurtosis Imaging

Diffusion Kurtosis Imaging (DKI) seeks to provide a better approximation of non-Gaussian spin displacements by expanding the expression to the fourth-order moment of the distribution, Kurtosis (odd orders are assumed to be zero in the absence of net coherent transport) [24]. This approach has the advantage that it makes no strong assumptions about what is causing the non-Gaussianity, but nonetheless quantifies it in a well-understood way. Indeed, non-zero excess Kurtosis is often described as being a signature of restriction [44] but is has also been shown to be special case of fractional diffusion models [20]

DKI can be derived from both physical and statistical arguments, but we will concentrate on the former. Here the Fickian flux from DTI is extended to include a fourth-order term which adds additional degrees of freedom. The fourth order flux is

$$J(\mathbf{M}) = -D\nabla\mathbf{M} - \frac{1}{3}D\nabla K\nabla \cdot D\nabla\mathbf{M}t \tag{25}$$

where K is the fourth order Kurtosis tensor which modifies the Gaussian flux process. The factor of t is required to correct the dimensionality of the kurtosis term. Substituting this into Eq. (15) and solving yields the following solution

$$\mathbf{m}(t) = \mathbf{m}_0 e^{R\mathbf{M}} e^{-\mathbf{q}D\mathbf{q}t} e^{-\frac{1}{6}\mathbf{q}D\mathbf{q}K\mathbf{q}D\mathbf{q}t^2} \tag{26}$$

which is the 3D form of the usual diffusion kurtosis solution. As with DTI, this can be used to construct a linear system over several measurements that can be inverted to find the elements of the diffusion and kurtosis tensors.

3.8 Multiple Continua

So far we have considered models with only a single, well-mixed continuum present in the sample. There is still a large class of models in the diffusion MR literature which we have not covered. To go beyond this we need to introduce the idea of multiple continua. The idea is that instead of a single Bloch-Torrey equation, we have a system of two or more. Here we have equations with their own relaxation process, their own fluxes, and potentially also exchange between them. A two-continuum system might be written as

$$\frac{\partial \mathbf{M}_1(t)}{\partial t} = R_1 \mathbf{M}_1 + \nabla \cdot J_1(\mathbf{M}_1) - E_{12}\mathbf{M}_1 + E_{21}\mathbf{M}_2 \tag{27a}$$

$$\frac{\partial \mathbf{M}_2(t)}{\partial t} = R_2 \mathbf{M}_2 + \nabla \cdot J_2(\mathbf{M}_2) - E_{21}\mathbf{M}_1 + E_{12}\mathbf{M}_2 \tag{27b}$$

where $\mathbf{M}_i$ is the magnetisation in compartment i, J_i and R_i describe the flux and relaxation processes in each one and E_{ik} defines the rate of exchange between compartments. Conservation of total number of spins also means we have that

$$\mathrm{Trace}(E) = 1. \tag{28}$$

The overall magnetisation of the system is the sum of the two components

$$\mathbf{M} = f_1 \mathbf{M}_1 + (1 - f_1)\mathbf{M}_2. \tag{29}$$

where f_i defines the relative sizes of the compartments. This formulation can be readily extended to three or more compartments. This version of the system is quite general, but the solutions can be difficult to work with in practice. For example, there is a degeneracy between the different relaxation constants and the volume fractions which prevent unique fitting without fixing one or the other.

The simplest assumption is zero flux and zero exchange. This leads to a bi- or multi-exponential model of T1 and T2 decay, which is often applied in T2 imaging when more than one tissue type in present in a voxel. A more common approach in diffusion imaging, however, is to assume a common relaxation process in all compartments and to concentrate on flux.

Assuming zero exchange, (i.e. E is diagonal) we can immediately construct the two-tensor model in which we have a common relaxation process, separate Fickian fluxes and no exchange.

$$\frac{\partial \mathbf{M}_1(t)}{\partial t} = R\mathbf{M}_1 + \nabla \cdot D_1 \nabla \mathbf{M}_1 \tag{30a}$$

$$\frac{\partial \mathbf{M}_2(t)}{\partial t} = R\mathbf{M}_2 + \nabla \cdot D_2 \nabla \mathbf{M}_2, \tag{30b}$$

The solution of which is a superposition of two exponentials of tensors. This was a common model in the early days of HARDI methods, and also covers Behrens' Ball and Stick model [8], in which we restrict the eigenvalues of the tensors such that one has all three equal and the other has only one non-zero.

The most general version of this model with a closed-form solution is two Fickian compartments with non-zero exchange. This is the Kärger model [28], which models a pair of well-mixed fluids with a Poisson exchange process. The Kärger model can

Table 2 Relaxation, flux, and exchange choices

R	J	E	Model
Compartmental	0	N	Multicomp. T_2
Uniform	Fickian	N	Multiexp./multitensor
Uniform	Fickian	Y	Kärger
Uniform	Fractional	N	Multi-stretched exp.

be shown to be equivalent to a bi-exponential model with diffusivities transformed by the exchange process [15].

Assuming no exchange and the same relaxation terms in all compartments, multiple continua models allow descriptions of the diffusion signal to be built up additively from different components. Since we are free to choose any flux terms we like we can potentially describe multiple exponentials (or tensors), or potentially less common choices such as mixtures of stretched exponentials [17]. We summarise which choices lead to which models in Table 2.

3.9 Models with Boundary Conditions

The idea of multiple, non-exchanging continua can be extended to include assumptions about geometry. By imposing boundary conditions on the fluxes in each compartment it is possible to impose hard boundaries with certain shapes and orientations. Solutions for Fickian fluxes can be constructed over a unit interval, from which we can construct expressions for geometries such as cylinders, spherical shells, and parallel planes. These can be combined together with models such as the tensor in multi-compartment models which can then be fitted to the signal [36].

These models are solutions of multiple Bloch-Torrey equations with uniform relaxation and without exchange. Each compartment has a chosen boundary condition which is expressed parametrically in the expression for the signal. Superpositions of expressions for diffusion in multiple compartments with different geometries provides expressions for the signal which can be fitted to diffusion-weighted measurements. Of course, there is no guarantee that the combination of geometries chosen is appropriate for the tissue being measured, so care is required in both construction and interpretation of results.

Distributions as Compartments If we fix the relaxation terms across all the system, it is mathematically possible to add more and more compartments without limit—provided there is enough data to support all the parameters. In this case the signal can be written as

$$S = S_0 \sum_{k=1}^{K} f_k S_k \tag{31}$$

where f_k is the volume fraction of the kth compartment, with signal S_k and subject to the constraint that $\sum_{k=1}^{K} f_k = 1$. This represents K non-exchanging compartments with any chosen geometry, all with the same T_2. This approach can be extended to give access to a new class of compartment: one with a continuous distribution of compartments. The approach is to let $K \rightarrow \infty$ and change the sum to an integral,

$$S = S_0 \int f(\mathbf{x}, \mathbf{y}) R(\mathbf{y}) d\mathbf{y}. \tag{32}$$

In this case the signal has a contribution from a continuous set of compartments with a weight function describing the contribution from each member of the set. Here $R(\mathbf{y})$ is the response function of an individual component compartment and $f(\mathbf{x}, \mathbf{y})$ is an unknown function describing their distribution. Different approaches make different assumptions about the form of this integral, although in some cases this is not immediately obvious.

Spherical Deconvolution

The first approach of this type in the literature was Tournier's Spherical Deconvolution [25, 41, 42], used to infer the orientations of multiple populations of white matter fibres—part of a class of methods known as High Angular Resolution Diffusion Imaging (HARDI). Here the signal is modelled by assuming that the measured signal is a convolution of the single fibre response function and an unknown fibre orientation distribution (FOD) function. This is equivalent to assuming that $f(\mathbf{x}, \mathbf{y}) = f(\mathbf{x} - \mathbf{y})$, i.e. a function of displacement only, and explicitly integrating out the radial direction. The approach deconvolves the unknown FOD, assuming or measuring some form for the single fibre response function. Spherical deconvolution approaches have been highly successful in multi-fibre tractography, largely because the technique provides very sharp and informative FOD estimates using fast, linear formulations for the deconvolution process itself. An interesting extension of this approach is by Kaden et al. [27] who allow parameters of the kernel to be fitted alongside the FOD.

Interestingly, it has been shown that other HARDI methods such as PAS-MRI [21] and Q-ball imaging [1, 43] can be shown to be forms of deconvolution, illustrating the power of the convolution formulation of the signal.

Continuous Parametric Compartments The convolution methods assume the form of the fibre response kernel, but nothing about the FOD. Other approaches make different and stronger assumptions, however, leading to a parametric representation. Given an assumption for the form of a particular compartment, a continuous version can be constructed by assuming a distribution over one or more parameters. The result is a distributed compartment with distribution parameters which can be fitted to the data.

A simple example of this approach is Jbabdi's model of distributed diffusivities [22]. Here we assume that rather than a single free diffusion compartment, there is a continuum of non-exchanging compartments with diffusivities given by a gamma distribution. The resulting model has a closed form, with the shape and scale parameters of the gamma distribution taking the place of the single diffusivity in the single compartment version. This is similar to an argument made by Bennett [9] in relation to the stretched exponential, although the final form is quite different.

A related assumption is made in the CHARMED model [5], and other similar approaches such as AxCalibre [6] and ActiveAx [2], in which compartments are constructed from cylinders with gamma-distributed radii. In this case care must be taken to weight the cylinders' contributions by volume fraction in the distributed compartment: larger cylinders take up more space than smaller ones and hence each one has a larger volume fraction and a larger contribution to the signal.

Another common variant of this approach is to assume a distribution of orientations on some directed geometry. Models such as VERDICT [37] assume a uniform distribution of orientation in cylinders or sticks. Between the limiting cases of completely parallel orientation and uniform orientation distribution lies orientation distributions with some finite width distribution. NODDI [45] makes use of a compartment in which the orientations of a continuum of sticks is described by a Watson distribution, which provides directional analogues to a mean and standard deviation. NODDI interprets the standard deviation as an estimate of fibre dispersion in the voxel.

The above makes it clear that NODDI is a combination of continuous and non-continuous compartments without exchange, making strong assumptions on the form of each of them. In the current context, it is worth emphasising that it is therefore a solution of a quite artificial set of Bloch-Torrey equations. It also fixes intrinsic diffusivity and requires it to be equal across all compartments. Recent work has pointed out that this set of assumptions is flawed [26], and that the resulting model can lead to misleading conclusions [34], and well as highly biased parameter estimates [23].

Both NODDI and VERDICT combine continuous compartments with other compartments without distributions, such as spherical shells or tensors. They also restrict the parameters describing different compartments to have the same values. Table 3 summarises compartment choices in different microstructure models.

One difficulty with constructing compartment-based models is the sheer number of possible combinations to choose from. Ten to twelve possible compartments with various different constraints lead to hundreds of potential two compartment

Table 3 Compartment combinations in microstructure models

Compartments	Model
Tensor, gamma-cylinders, ball	CHARMED [5]
Ball, astrosticks, sphere	VERDICT [37]
Tensor, cylinder, dot	ActiveAx [2]
Tensor, Watson-sticks, dot	NODDI [45]

models and thousands of possible three compartment models. Comparing these combinations is a significant and time-consuming undertaking, and although such comparisons have been undertaken [13, 37], strictly a model selection step is necessary in each individual application. Making a priori choices about tissue geometry also requires prior information, for example from histology, and intuition about how to relate underlying biological complexity to the very simple geometries for which explicit expressions for compartments are possible.

Another important caveat is packing. Multi-compartment models make no explicit assumption about how geometric compartments are arranged in space. Packing is captured indirectly via volume fractions and a tortuosity assumption in the extra cellular space. This can be important since these approximations may be more or less valid in different volume fraction regimes.

3.10 Other Models

This section describes models which take a slightly different approach to that considered so far. The continuity and Bloch-Torrey approach is fundamental to diffusion MRI, but can be formulated under slightly different assumptions than those so far. Here we consider two further cases.

Random Permeable Barriers

This model assumes a single, effective medium-level description of a population of diffusing spins in a compartment containing randomly oriented permeable barriers [35]. This description is on a length scale long enough that the contributions of the barriers can be treated as an spatial average, and that the central limit theorem applies locally, but still much shorter than the size of a typical scan voxel. This means that care is required during the derivation of he Bloch-Torrey equations to step upwards in scale from the microscopic, disordered regime to the intermediate, ensemble average. The authors employ a renormalisation group approach, and show that diffusion at this scale is described by a diffusivity with a power-law time dependence, specifically

$$D_{\text{inst}}(t) \simeq D_{\infty} + A \cdot t^{-\theta} \tag{33}$$

where D_{∞} is the asymptotic, long time diffusivity, A is a constant, and θ is an exponent defining the time dependence.

This approach is powerful, identifying different universality classes in temporal scaling which contain information about environmental disorder. The exponent value differentiates between disorder classes. $\theta = 0.5$ corresponding to long-range order and $\theta = \frac{d}{2}$ for the short-range order case of dimension d. The short time limit is also related to the surface area to volume ratio experienced by spins and has been used to estimate surface area to volume ratio in tissue [38].

The approach requires measurements over a wide range of diffusion times to infer critical exponents, and is often used in conjunction with oscillating gradient acquisitions, which provide access to shorter diffusion times than the more common PGSE. Fitting is typically performed in the frequency domain. This model has been applied to imaging in brain [10] and muscle [14].

Fractional Diffusion

We have already seen that the stretched exponential can be derived from the assumption of a space-fractional process. A more general form of this approach is to consider time-fractional transport as well. Here, the transport process makes use of a Continuous-time Random Walk (CTRW) model, in which spins have a waiting time associated with successive steps in their random walks. This model describes a more general class of transport processes than conventional Fickian approaches, including subdiffusion, in which mean squared-displacement of diffusing spins increases more slowly than linearly with time. The CTRW model predicts a signal curve described by the Mittag-Leffler function

$$S(q, \Delta) = S(0) \sum_{k=0}^{\infty} \frac{\left(-D_{\alpha,\beta} q^{\beta} \Delta^{\alpha}\right)^k}{\Gamma(\alpha k + 1)} \tag{34}$$

where $\Gamma(\cdot)$ is the gamma function and α and β are temporal and spatial scaling exponents respectively. Note that when $\alpha = 1$ this reduces to the series expression for the exponential.

Again, this model assumes a single continuum and make no strong assumptions about tissue geometry. The continuous time random walk provides a very flexible model of an effective diffusion process and describes the observed signal in very few parameters, but making microstructural inferences from the model is more difficult. Strictly speaking, this model requires measurements over a range of diffusion times, although additional assumptions make it possible to apply to multiple b-values at a single diffusion time. This model has been applied to rat and human brain [19, 31, 46] and also in muscle [18].

4   Discussion

The Bloch-Torrey equation is a lens through which different models in the diffusion MRI literature can be compared. We have attempted here to lay out the relationships between different approaches in terms of the underlying physics, avoiding discussion of inverse problems, machine learning, and other technical aspects which are commonly the focus elsewhere in the literature.

We can see that models assume different numbers of compartments and (often implicitly) different transport processes. We can also see that it is not possible to identify one particular approach as being superior to all others. In some cases we may wish to approach the signal with as few assumptions as possible, in others we may have extensive prior knowledge that it may be helpful to include in our models. Clinical constraints may enforce very short acquisition times or preclude more advanced acquisitions or processing and therefore require simpler methods.

In choosing a model or developing a new one it may be helpful to consider how natural a set of assumptions is. Although features such as direction anisotropy can be readily extracted from measurements, diffusion decay curves are extremely featureless. Although diffraction patterns are an exception to this, these patterns are only visible under very specific circumstances in which tissue geometry is highly regular. In more realistic situations tissue heterogeneity means that decay curves are very smooth, and we are faced with a problem of model degeneracy: given a sufficiently dense sampling of data we can, in principle, fit any (reasonably well-posed) model we choose. This makes model selection all the more important. We hope that looking at different models in terms of the physical assumptions is a useful aid.

Appendix: Fractional Fick's Law

We assume a Lèvy walk-type process, which is fractional in space but not time. We start with the distribution of step lengths

$$P(|x - x_0| \geq \Delta X) = \frac{1}{\Gamma(1 - \beta)} |x - x_0|^{-\beta} \tag{35}$$

The derivative with respect to x gives the probability density function,

$$p(|x - x_0|) = \frac{\beta}{\Gamma(1 - \beta)} |x - x_0|^{-\beta - 1}. \tag{36}$$

where in both cases the gamma function is a necessary normalising factor [32]. We assume that spins are displaced in either direction with equal probability, which gives the total flux through a point x as

$$J(\mathbf{M}) = \frac{1}{2} D \left[\int_{-\infty}^{x} P(x - x_0) \mathbf{M}(x_0) dx_0 + \int_{x}^{\infty} P(x_0 - x) \mathbf{M}(x_0) dx_0 \right]. \tag{37}$$

By substitution from Eq. (35), the first term in the above becomes

$$\int_{-\infty}^{x} P(x - x_0)\mathbf{M}(x_0)dx_0 = \frac{1}{\Gamma(1-\beta)} \int_{-\infty}^{x} (x - x_0)^{-\beta}\mathbf{M}(x_0)dx_0. \qquad (38)$$

which is the definition of the RHS (or positive-x) Weyl fractional derivative of $\mathbf{M}$ of order β with respect to x [29]. We denote this operator $^{W}\mathcal{D}_{x+}^{\beta}$.

Similarly, substituting Eq. (35) into Eq. (37) gives

$$\int_{x}^{\infty} P(x_0 - x)\mathbf{M}(x_0)dx_0 = \frac{1}{\Gamma(1-\beta)} \int_{x}^{\infty} (x_0 - x)^{-\beta}\mathbf{M}(x_0)dx_0, \qquad (39)$$

which is the definition of the LHS Weyl derivative, $^{W}\mathcal{D}_{x-}^{\beta}$. Equation (37) then becomes

$$J(\mathbf{M}) = -\frac{1}{2}D\left[^{W}\mathcal{D}_{x+}^{\beta} + {}^{W}\mathcal{D}_{x-}^{\beta}\right]\mathbf{M}. \qquad (40)$$

Finally, the Reisz-Weyl fractional derivative is defined as

$$\frac{\partial^{\beta}}{\partial|x|^{\beta}} = -\frac{1}{2}\left[^{W}\mathcal{D}_{x+}^{\beta} + {}^{W}\mathcal{D}_{x-}^{\beta}\right] \qquad (41)$$

which means Eq. (40) becomes

$$J(\mathbf{M}) = -D\frac{\partial^{\beta}}{\partial|x|^{\beta}}\mathbf{M}. \qquad (42)$$

References

1. Aganj, I., Lenget, C., Sapiro, G., Yacoub, E., Ugurbil, K., Haref, N.: Reconstruction of the orientation distribution function in single- and multiple-shell q-ball imaging with constant solid angle. Magn. Reson. Med. **64**, 544–566 (2010)
2. Alexander, D.C., Hubbard, P.L., Hall, M.G., Moore, F.A., Ptito, M., Parker, G.J., Dyrby, T.B.: Orientationally invariant indices of axon diameter and density from diffusion MRI. NeuroImage **52**(4), 1374–1389 (2010)
3. Anderson, J.D.: Compuational Fluid Dynamics. McGraw-Hill Higher Education, New York (1995)
4. Arfken, G.: Mathematical Methods for Physicists, 7th edn. Academic, New York (2012)
5. Assaf, Y., Basser, P.J.: Composite hindered and restricted model of diffusion (CHARMED) MR imaging of the human brain. NeuroImage **27**(1), 48–58 (2008)
6. Assaf, Y., Blumenfeld-Katzir, T., Yovel, Y., Basser, P.J.: Axcaliber: a method for measuring axon diameter distribution from diffusion MRI. Magn. Reson. Med. **59**(6), 1347–1354 (2008)
7. Basser, P.J., Mattiello, J., LeBihan, D.: MR diffusion tensor spectroscopy and imaging. Biophys. J. **66**(1), 259–267 (1994)

8. Behrens, T.E.J., Johansen-Berg, H., Woolrich, M.W., Smith, S.M., Wheeler-Kingshott, C.A.M., Boulby, P.A., Barker, G.J., Sillery, E.L., Sheehan, K., Ciccarelli, O., Thompson, A.J., Brady, J.M., Matthews, P.M.: Non-invasive mapping of connections between human thalamus and cortex using diffusion imaging. Nat. Neurosci. **6**, 750–757 (2003)
9. Bennett, K.M., Schmainder, K.M., Bennett, R.T., Rowe, D.B., Lu, H., Hyde, J.S.: Characterization of continuously distributed cortical water diffusion rates with a stretched exponential model. Magn. Reson. Med. **50**(4), 727–734 (2003)
10. Burcaw, L.M., Fieremans, E., Novikov, D.S.: Mesoscopic structure of neuronal tracts from time-dependent diffusion. NeuroImage **114**, 18–37 (2015)
11. Carr, H.Y., Purcell, E.M.: Effects of diffusion on free precession in nuclear magnetic resonance experiments. Phys. Rev. **94**(3), 630–638 (1954)
12. De Santis, S., Gabrielli, A., Bozzali, M., Maraviglia, B., Macaluso, E., Capuani, S.: Anisotropic anomalous diffusion assessed int he human brain by scalar invariant indices. Magn. Reson. Med. **65**(4), 1043–1052 (2011)
13. Ferizi, U., Schneider, T., Panagiotaki, E., Nedjati-Gilani, G., Zhang, H., Wheeler-Kingshott, C.A.M., Alexander, D.C.: A ranking of diffusion MRI compartment models with in vivo human brain data. Magn. Reson. Med. **72**(6), 1785–1792 (2014)
14. Fieremans, E., Lemberskiy, G., Varaart, J., Sigmund, E.E., Gyftopoulos, S., Novikov, D.S.: In vivo measurement of membrane permeability and myofiber size in human muscle using time-dependent diffusion tensor imaging and the random permeable barrier model. NMR Biomed. **30**(3) (2016). http://onlinelibrary.wiley.com/doi/10.1002/nbm.3612/pdf
15. Fieremans, E., Novikov, D.S., Jensen, J.H., Helpern, J.A.: Monte-carlo study of a two-compartment model of diffusion. NMR Biomed. **23**(7), 711–724 (2010)
16. Hall, M.G., Barrick, T.R.: From diffusion-weighted MRI to anomalous diffusion imaging. Magn. Reson. Med. **59**(3), 447–455 (2008)
17. Hall, M.G., Bongers, A., Sved, P., Watson, G., Bourne, R.M.: Assessment of non-gaussian diffusion with singly and doubly stretched biexponential models of diffusion-weighted MRI (DWI) signal attenuation in prostate tissue. NMR Biomed. **28**(4), 486–495 (2015)
18. Hall, M.G., Porcari, P., Blamire, A., Clark, C.A.: Fractional diffusion as a probe of microstructural change in a mouse model of duchenne muscular dystrophy. In: Proceedings of the 24th meeting of the International Society for Magnetic Resonance in Medicine, p. 1981 (2016)
19. Ingo, C., Magin, R.L., Colon-Perez, L., Triplett, W., Mareci, T.H.: On random walks and entropy in diffusion-weighted magnetic resonance imaging studies of neural tissue. Magn. Reson. Med. **71**(2), 617–627 (2014)
20. Ingo, C., Magin, R.L., Parrish, T.B.: New insights into the fractional order diffusion equation using entropy and kurtosis. Entropy **16**(11), 5838–5852 (2014)
21. Jansons, K.M., ALexander, D.C.: Persistent angular structure: new insights from diffusion magnetic resonance imaging. Inverse Prob. **19**(5), 1031–1046 (2003)
22. Jbabdi, S., Sotiropoulos, S.N., Savio, A.M., Graña, M., Behrens, T.E.J.: Model-based analysis of multishell diffusion MR data for tractography: how to get over fitting problems. Magn. Reson. Med. **68**(6), 1846–1855 (2012)
23. Jelescu, I.O., Veraart, J., Fieremans, E., Novikov, D.S.: Degeneracy in model parameter estimation for multi-compartmental diffusion in neuronal tissue. NMR Biomed. **29**(1), 33–47 (2016)
24. Jensen, J.H., Helpern, J.A., Lu, H., Kaczynski, K.: Diffusional kurtosis imaging: the quantification of non-gaussian water diffusion by means of magnetic resonance imaging. Magn. Reson. Med. **53**(6), 1432–1440 (2005)
25. Jeurissen, B., Tournier, J.-D., Dhollander, T., Connelly, A., Sijbers, J.: Multi-tissue constrained spherical deconvolution for improved analysis of multi-shell diffusion MRI data. NeuroImage **103**, 441–426 (2014)
26. Kaden, E., Kelm, N.D., Carson, R.P., Does, M.D., Alexander, D.C.: Multi-compartment microscopic diffusion imaging. NeuroImage **139**, 346–359 (2016)

27. Kaden, E., Kruggel, F., Alexander, D.C.: Quantitative mapping of the per-axon diffusion coefficients in brain white matter. Magn. Reson. Med. **75**, 1752–1763 (2016)
28. Karger, J., Pfiefer, H., Heinik, W.: Principles and application of self-diffusion measurements by nuclear magnetic resonance. Adv. Magn. Reson. **12**, 1–89 (1988)
29. Klages, R., Radons, G., Sokolov, I.M. (eds.): Anomalous Transport: Foundations and Applications. Wiley, New York (2008)
30. Le Bihan, D., Mangin, J.-F., Poupon, C., Clark, C.A., Pappata, S., Molko, N., Chabriat, H.: Diffusion tensor imaging: concepts and applications. J. Magn. Reson. Imaging **13**(4), 534–546 (2001)
31. Magin, R.L., Adbullah, O., Baleanu, D., Zhou, X.J.: Anomalous diffusion expressed through fractional order differential operators in the bloch-torrey equation. J. Magn. Reson. **190**(2), 255–270 (2008)
32. Meerschaert, M.M.: Fractional calculus, anomalous diffusion, and probability, Chap. 11. In: Klafter, J., Lim, S.C., Metler, R. (eds.) Recent Advances in Fractional Dynamics. World Scientific, Singapore (2003)
33. Neuman, C.H.: Spin echo of spins diffusing in a bounded medium. J. Chem. Phys. **60**(11), 4508–4511 (1974)
34. Nilsson, M.: Diffusion tensor distributions and fat b-tensors. In: Proceedings of the ISMRM Workshop on Breaking the Barriers of Diffusion Lisbon (2016)
35. Novikov, D.S., Kiselev, V.G.: Effective medium theory of a diffusion-weighted signal. NMR in Biomed. **23**(7), 682–697 (2010)
36. Panagiotaki, E., Schneider, T., Siow, B., Hall, M.G., Lythgoe, M.F., Alexander, D.C.: Compartment models of the diffusion MR signal in brain white matter: a taxonomy and comparison. NeuroImage **59**(3), 2241–2254 (2012)
37. Panagiotaki, E., Walker-Samuel, S., Siow, B., Johnson, S.P., Rajkumar, V., Pedley, R.B., Lythgoe, M.F., Alexander, D.C.: Noninvasive quantification of solid tumor microstructure using verdict MRI. Cancer Res. **74**(7), 1902–1912 (2014)
38. Reynaud, O., Winters, K.V., Hoang, D.M., Wadghiri, Y.Z., Novikov, D.S., Sungheon, G.K.: Surface-to-volume ratio mapping of tumor microstructure using oscillating gradient diffusion weighted imaging. Magn. Reson. Med. **76**(1), 237–247 (2016)
39. Stejskal, E.O., Tanner, J.E.: Spin diffusion measurements: spin echoes in the presence of a time-dependent field gradient. J. Chem. Phys. **42**(1), 288–292 (1965)
40. Torrey, H.C.: Bloch equations with diffusion terms. Phys. Rev. **104**(3), 563 (1956)
41. Tournier, J-D., Calamante, F., Connelly, A.: Robust determination of the fibre orientation in diffusion MRI: non-negativity constrained super-resolved spherical deconvolution. NeuroImage **35**(4), 1459–1472 (2007)
42. Tournier, J-D., Calamante, F., Gadian, D., Connelly, A.: Direct estimation of the fiber orientation density function from diffusion-weighted MRI data using spherical deconvolution. NeuroImage **23**(3), 1176–1185 (2010)
43. Tuch, D.S.: Q-ball imaging. Magn. Reson. Med. **52**(6), 1358–1372 (2004)
44. Wu, E.X., Cheung, M.M.: MR diffusion kurtosis for neural tissue characterisation. NMR Biomed. **23**(7), 836–848 (2010)
45. Zhang, H., Schneider, T., Wheeler-Kingshott, C.A., Alexander, D.C.: NODDI: practical *in vivo* neurite orientation dispersion and density imaging of the human brain. NeuroImage **61**(4), 1000–1016 (2012)
46. Zhou, X.J., Gao, Q., Abdullah, O., Magin, R.L.: Studies of anomalous diffusion in the human brain using fractional order calculus. Magn. Reson. Med. **63**(3), 562–569 (2010)

Noise Floor Removal via Phase Correction of Complex Diffusion-Weighted Images: Influence on DTI and q-Space Metrics

Marco Pizzolato, Rutger Fick, Timothé Boutelier, and Rachid Deriche

Abstract The non-Gaussian noise distribution in magnitude Diffusion-Weighted Images (DWIs) can severely affect the estimation and reconstruction of the true diffusion signal. As a consequence, also the estimated diffusion metrics can be biased. We study the effect of phase correction, a procedure that re-establishes the Gaussianity of the noise distribution in DWIs by taking into account the corresponding phase images. We quantify the debiasing effects of phase correction in terms of diffusion signal estimation and calculated metrics. We perform in silico experiments based on a MGH Human Connectome Project dataset and on a digital phantom, accounting for different acquisition schemes, diffusion-weightings, signal to noise ratios, and for metrics based on Diffusion Tensor Imaging and on Mean Apparent Propagator Magnetic Resonance Imaging, i.e. q-space metrics. We show that phase correction is still a challenge, but also an effective tool to debias the estimation of diffusion signal and metrics from DWIs, especially at high b-values.

1 Introduction

Diffusion-Weighted Magnetic Resonance Imaging (DW-MRI) is inherently a low Signal to Noise Ratio (SNR) technique [1]. More diffusion weighting—globally encoded by a larger b-value—leads to lower signal intensities and consequently to a poorer SNR. In such a low SNR regime, the magnitude of the complex DW signal can be dominated by a bias, namely noise floor, which is due to the non-Gaussian distribution of the noise. This generally falls within the non-central χ^2 family, depending on the adopted MR acquisition strategy (number of coils, multi-coil reconstruction, acceleration, etc.) [2]. However, some diffusion MRI techniques require the acquisition of Diffusion-Weighted Images (DWIs) at relatively high b-values [3–5], where the Noise Floor affects the signal estimation and consequent

M. Pizzolato (✉) • R. Fick • R. Deriche
Université Côte d'Azur, Inria, France
e-mail: marco.pizzolato@inria.fr; pizzolato.marco@gmail.com

T. Boutelier
Olea Medical, La Ciotat, France

© Springer International Publishing AG 2017
A. Fuster et al. (eds.), *Computational Diffusion MRI*, Mathematics and Visualization, DOI 10.1007/978-3-319-54130-3_2

parameter calculations. A strategy for removing the Noise Floor from the magnitude DWIs, is *phase correction* [6]. This method consists on estimating the true phase from the complex DWIs to transfer the image content—which is split between real (rDWI) and imaginary (iDWI) parts—into the real part only, such that the rDWIs contain the signal corrupted by Gaussian distributed noise. In this work, we quantify the influence of phase correction in terms of unbiased signal estimation and reconstruction. In the latter case, we focus on two popular signal-driven representations of the diffusion process, such as Diffusion Tensor Imaging (DTI) [7] and Mean Apparent Propagator Magnetic Resonance Imaging (MAP) [3], and we quantify the effects of phase correction on the corresponding scalar parameters. We present in silico experiments based on a MGH Human Connectome Project (HCP) dataset and on a digital phantom.

The noise floor causes a signal overestimation that is more important at high b-values and when diffusion is less restricted, i.e. when the signal is low. This introduces a bias that leads to the distortion of the estimated quantitative diffusion metrics, such as the underestimation of the Apparent Diffusion Coefficient (ADC) in DTI [1]. This affects the principal diffusivity (PD), i.e. the amplitude of the tensor's eigenvector aligned to the least restricted direction, which is underestimated. Similar considerations hold for other DTI metrics, such as the fractional anisotropy (FA). Moreover, since MAP signal reconstruction typically requires high b-values, we also expect some of the derived q-space metrics to be biased. In this scenario, phase correction is a promising tool to calculate unbiased metrics.

Phase correction exploits the phase images associated with the magnitude DWIs. Some advantages of using the phase of the DW signal, to perform a reconstruction directly in the complex domain, have been previously reported [8], while assuming phase coherence among q-space samples. However, in actual DW-MRI acquisitions the phase images are subject shot-wise variations that are mainly dominated by movements, cardiac pulsation, blood circulation or field inhomogeneity. Thus, coherent phase contributions related to the diffusion process, e.g. asymmetries due to tissue configurations or experimental setups [9–11], are hardly observable and are not explicitly accounted in noise floor removal via phase correction.

Recent phase corrections for noise floor removal consist on filtering the real and imaginary images, i.e. the rDWI and iDWI, to obtain a low-frequency version of the DWI's phase, which is used to complex-rotate the rDWI and iDWI such that the former contains signal plus Gaussian distributed noise, and the latter only noise (which will be discarded). The filtering is typically performed via a convolution procedure [12, 13] or complex total variation [14]. However, the correct estimation of the low-frequency phase depends on the correct choice of the convolution kernel (and its size) or regularization parameter. Therefore, the effectiveness of phase correction on signal debiasing and diffusion parameters estimation, such as DTI and MAP metrics, needs to be assessed.

In this work, we implement a phase correction procedure based on total variation [14]. We first apply it to in silico complex DWIs, created by processing a HCP dataset, in order to assess the effectiveness of the phase correction in a realistic scenario, for different diffusion weightings, i.e. b-values, and SNRs. At the same time, we assess the amount of noise floor bias in typical magnitude DWIs ($|$DWI$|$)—based on signal probability distribution metrics—and the corresponding improvement after phase correction. In second place, we assess the influence of phase correction on DTI and q-space metrics. Particularly, we apply phase correction to complex DWIs produced by using a modified version of Phantomαs [15], while accounting for different total variation regularizations and for typical acquisition setups, i.e. single-shell at $b \in \{1000, 2000, 3000\}\,\mathrm{s/mm^2}$ (DTI), and multi-shell (DTI, MAP).

2 Methods

In this section we describe the implemented phase correction procedure, and illustrate the generation of the data used for the experiments, such as the acquisition setup, the generation of a synthetic phase, and the SNR convention.

The phase correction takes into account a complex DWI

$$\mathrm{DWI}_{xy} = \mathrm{rDWI}_{xy} + j \cdot \mathrm{iDWI}_{xy} \tag{1}$$

where x and y represent the pixel coordinates, r and i indicate the real and imaginary parts, and j is the imaginary unit. If $\widehat{\angle DWI}_{xy}$ is a good estimation of the phase, then the phase-corrected image is obtained via complex rotation

$$\mathrm{DWI}^{pc}_{xy} = |\mathrm{DWI}|_{xy} e^{j\left(\angle\mathrm{DWI}_{xy} - \widehat{\angle\mathrm{DWI}}_{xy}\right)} \tag{2}$$

where $\angle\mathrm{DWI}_{xy}$ and $|\mathrm{DWI}|_{xy}$ are the original noisy phase and magnitude. The real part of the phase-corrected complex DWI, $\Re(\mathrm{DWI}^{pc}_{xy})$, contains the signal (tissue contrast) plus Gaussian distributed noise, whereas the imaginary part, $\Im(\mathrm{DWI}^{pc}_{xy})$, only contains noise. Henceforth, any classical diffusion modeling and reconstruction taking into account additive Gaussian noise can be performed on $\Re(\mathrm{DWI}^{pc}_{xy})$, where the noise floor is absent.

The effectiveness of phase correction clearly depends on the quality of the phase estimation. In this work we implement a total variation method, known to better preserve discontinuities in the images [14]. Particularly, for each complex DWI image $u_0 \in \mathrm{rDWI}_{xy}, \mathrm{iDWI}_{xy}$ defined on coordinates $x \in X, y \in Y$, we find the image u such that it is the minimizer of

$$\inf_{u\in\mathbb{C}} \lambda \int_{X,Y} (u_0 - u)^2 dxdy + \int_{X,Y} |\nabla u| dxdy \tag{3}$$

where λ is the regularization parameter expressing the attachment to data. The estimates of rDWI_{xy} and iDWI_{xy} obtained with Eq. (3) are then used to compute $\widehat{\angle\mathrm{DWI}}_{xy}$ and perform the complex rotation in Eq. (2).

2.1 Simulation and Diffusion Signal Reconstruction

The complex DWIs have in all cases been created by generating a synthetic phase image, Φ_{xy}, associated with a magnitude image, M_{xy}. The phase images are created in order to mimic the outcome of subject movements. We assume a bi-dimensional sinusoidal wave oriented along the direction $\mathbf{v} = (v_x, v_y)$ with frequencies f_x, f_y and initial shifts ϕ_x, ϕ_y

$$\Phi(x, y) = \pi \cdot sin\left(2\pi \frac{v_x}{||\mathbf{v}||} f_x \frac{x}{w_x} + \phi_x + 2\pi \frac{v_y}{||\mathbf{v}||} f_y \frac{y}{w_y} + \phi_y\right) \tag{4}$$

where w_x, w_y are scale parameters: in this case they correspond to the width of the image along the corresponding direction ($w_x = card(X)$, $w_y = card(Y)$). Eventually, constant phase patches are added. Assuming to have the ground-truth images of magnitude M_{xy} and phase Φ_{xy}, the latter resulting from Eq. (4), then

$$rDWI_{xy} = M_{xy} \cdot cos(\Phi_{xy}) + \eta^r_{xy}$$
$$iDWI_{xy} = M_{xy} \cdot sin(\Phi_{xy}) + \eta^i_{xy} \tag{5}$$

where $\eta^r_{xy}, \eta^i_{xy} \in N(0, \sigma^2)$. The noise is added with a value of σ calculated according to the DW-MRI convention $\sigma = \left(card[\rho(X \times Y)]^{-1} \sum_{x,y} \rho(x, y) M^{b=0}_{xy}\right) / SNR_0$, where SNR_0 is defined on the magnitude image without diffusion weighting $M^{b=0}_{xy}$, and $\rho \in \{0, 1\}$ is a mask defined on the pairs (x, y), e.g., a mask of the tissue-related signal like the brain mask. The Rician magnitude $|DWI|_{xy}$ and the phase $\angle DWI_{xy}$ are calculated from the real and imaginary parts in Eq. (5).

The data used for the experiments is a HCP brain dataset corrected for eddy currents where we selected DWIs of interest for $b \in [0, 1000, 3000]\,s/mm^2$. Other experiments use Phantomαs [15] to obtain the ground-truth magnitude images, M_{xy}. This software requires input with a geometrical description of tissue structures and fiber bundles. We used the well known geometry produced for the HARDI reconstruction challenge 2013.[1] We generated DWIs for a 3-shells scheme with $b \in \{1000, 2000, 3000\}\,s/mm^2$, 51 samples *per* shell, with samples uniformly distributed within and among shells [16].

The phase-corrected real DWIs can contain negative values: the noise is zero-mean Gaussian and the noise floor is absent. Therefore, the DTI reconstruction is performed by non-linearly en forcing signal positivity, and MAP is performed with Laplacian regularization imposing positivity on the recovered Ensemble Average Propagator [17].

---

[1]http://hardi.epfl.ch/static/events/2013_ISBI/,https://github.com/ecaruyer/phantomas/blob/master/examples/isbi_challenge_2013.txt.

3 Experiments and Results

We perform three experiments with two objectives: first, quantifying the effect of phase correction on signal debiasing, by processing real data from a HCP dataset; second, assessing the debiasing on diffusion metrics, calculated with DTI and MAP reconstructions, on a digital dataset generated for typical scenarios such as DTI at b-value 1000, 2000, 3000 s/mm^2 and DTI and MAP multi-shell.

In the *first experiment*, we clustered a HCP dataset to obtain typical signal values at b-value 1000 and 3000 s/mm^2. Particularly, for each b-value we applied k-means to divide the signal intensities of the DWIs—accounting for all the gradient directions—into four clusters. We used the centroid of each cluster to define respectively background, low, medium, and high mean signal values. Based on these, we created a ground-truth synthetic magnitude image—M_{xy} in Eq. (5)—composed of three circles each containing, from left to right, low, medium and high signal respectively. Outside the circles we added background signal. A synthetic phase was generated and the noisy complex DWI was created. After calculating the average $b = 0$ signal ($S(0)_{avg} = 758\,a.u.$) in the HCP dataset, noise was added as in Eq. (5) in low SNR regime: $SNR_0 = 10$. Figure 1 shows, for each b-value, the noisy magnitude $|DWI|_{xy}$ and the estimated phase-corrected real part $\Re(DWI_{xy}^{pc})$ (λ set to 0.75 after visual inspection). In addition, an effective SNR map is present along with histograms of the magnitude and phase-corrected real signals for each circle. We conclude that in both cases the phase-corrected real image presents more contrast with the background compared to the magnitude. This is more evident at low SNR values—left circle at $b = 1000$ s/mm^2, left and central circles at $b = 3000$ s/mm^2—that are more likely with high b-values. The $\Re(DWI_{xy}^{pc})$ shows darker colors, i.e. lower signal intensities, as highlighted by the histograms: the magnitude (green line) has a Rician distribution for low SNRs (typically below $SNR = 5$) whereas the estimated real part (blue line) always shows a Gaussian distribution, thus including negative signal intensities. We point out that since this is an experiment grounded on real data, the centroid of the clusters—especially at low signal values—are based on Rician data and might overestimate the actual (noise-free) ones. This means that the Rician bias in histograms (green line) might be an underestimation of the true one.

In the *second experiment*, we use the HCP dataset to create a mean ground-truth magnitude DWI, M_{xy}, in order to quantify the Rician bias, i.e. the distance from Gaussianity. We calculate the mean $b = 0$ image $S(0)_{xy}$, for a slice of interest, by averaging the 40 non-diffusion-weighted images in the dataset. Since the SNR is very high, the averaging procedure is not biased. Then, we select all the DWIs corresponding to $b = 1000$ s/mm^2 and perform DTI to obtain the mean diffusivity map, MD_{xy}. At this point, we obtain a ground-truth magnitude DWI at any b-value by extrapolating with $M_{xy} = S(b)_{xy} = S(0)_{xy} \exp(-b \cdot MD_{xy})$. Although we assume Gaussian isotropic diffusion, this phantom represents an average description of a

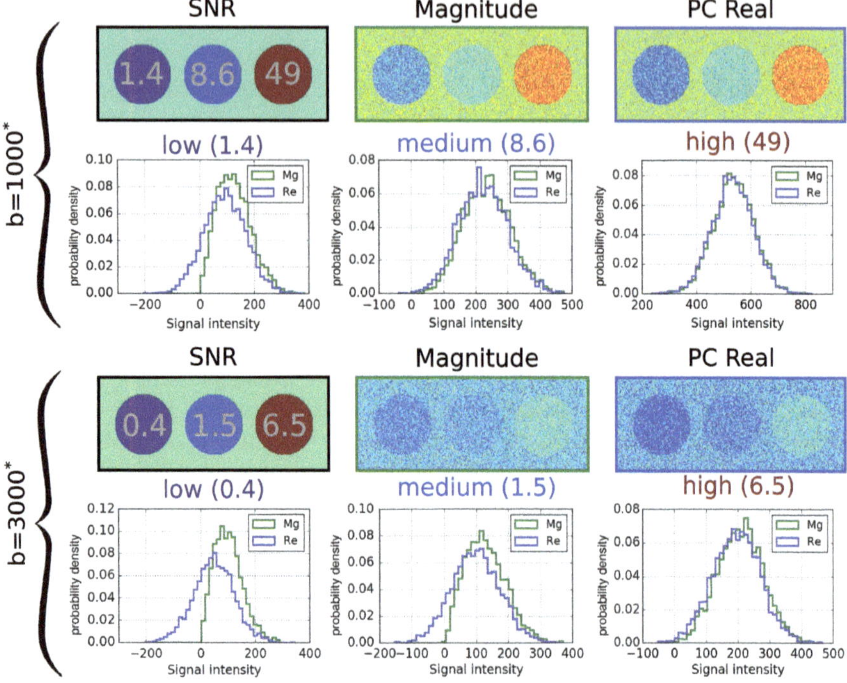

Fig. 1 The signal contrast and distributions for synthetic complex DWIs, at $b = 1000$, $3000 \, \text{s/mm}^2$, created from clustering a real HCP dataset ($\text{SNR}_0 = 10$). In the rectangular frames from *left* to *right*: the SNR map, the Rician magnitude (Mg) and the phase-corrected estimated real image (Re). Below, the histograms of the signal intensities corresponding to the circles with low, medium, and high signal/SNR, for Mg (*green*) and Re (*blue*). Background SNR: 21.5 for $b = 1000 \, \text{s/mm}^2$ and 3.2 for $b = 1000 \, \text{s/mm}^2$. *: s/mm^2

magnitude DWI. After generating a synthetic phase image, as described in Sect. 2, we calculate the noisy complex DWI for each b-value, as in Eq. (5). Figure 2 shows the $b = 0$ magnitude and the phase used for the phantom (left column). We then calculate the Rician magnitude $|\text{DWI}|_{xy}$ and the phase-corrected real part $\Re(\text{DWI}^{pc}_{xy})$ ($\lambda = 0.75$). Additionally, we calculate a magnitude image with Gaussian distributed noise $|\text{DWI}|^{G}_{xy}$, by adding Gaussian noise (with the same SNR_0) to M_{xy}. This will be used as reference for Gaussianity measures. We generate 1000 noise occurrences and calculate, for each pixel of the images, the signal intensities histogram (as in Fig. 1). For each pixel we generate three histograms: one for the Rician $|\text{DWI}|_{xy}$, one for the phase-corrected $\Re(\text{DWI}^{pc}_{xy})$, and one for the Gaussian $|\text{DWI}|^{G}_{xy}$. The hypothesis is that, for each pixel, the phase-corrected signal distribution should be closer to that of the Gaussian magnitude image than the Rician magnitude one. As

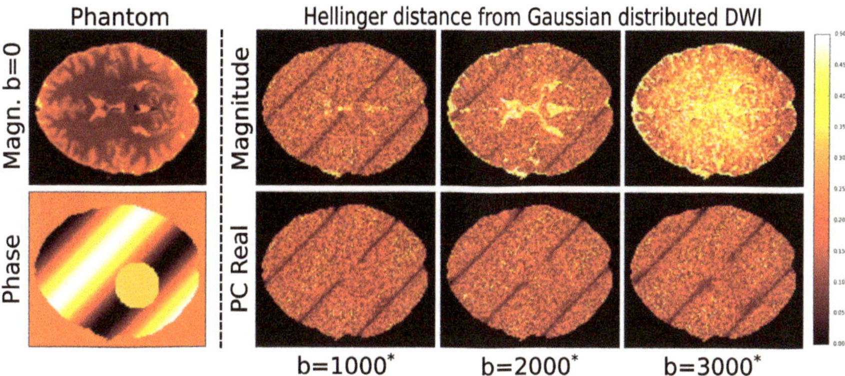

Fig. 2 The distance from Gaussianity of complex DWIs obtained by processing a HCP dataset and a synthetic phase image. In the *first column* the $b = 0$ magnitude image obtained from real data, and the generated phase. In the *columns* from the *second to the fourth*, the distance from the Gaussianity measured with Eq. (6) for the Rician magnitude (*first row*) and the phase-corrected real part (*second row*), at different b-values (*columns*). Contrarily to the case of the Rician magnitude, the distance from Gaussianity remains visually unchanged as the diffusion-weighting increases. *: s/mm^2

a distance from Gaussianity, we use the discrete Hellinger distance [18]

$$H(P,Q) = \frac{1}{\sqrt{2}}||\sqrt{P} - \sqrt{Q}||_2 \tag{6}$$

where P and Q are two discrete probability distributions, and $0 \leq H(P,Q) \leq 1$ where 1 means maximum distance. In columns 2–4, Fig. 2 shows the maps of Hellinger distance from the Gaussian magnitude, for the Rician magnitude (first row) and the phase-corrected real part (second row), at b-value 1000, 2000 and 3000 s/mm^2.

We see that the Rician magnitude shows more bias (higher H), especially in regions where MD is high. As expected, at higher b-values (from left to right) the signal intensity is lower and the bias occurs in a larger number of pixels. Conversely, the phase-corrected real part does not show a clear change.

In the *third experiment*, we quantify the bias on the estimated DTI and MAP metrics for the Rician magnitude, and we quantify the debiasing power of phase correction by looking at the change in the distributions of such metrics compared to the Gaussian noise case. We generate complex DWIs with Phantomαs [15] as described in Sect. 2. For each gradient direction $\mathbf{g} = (g_x, g_y, g_z)$, the synthetic phase image is oriented towards $\mathbf{v} = (g_x, g_y)$ [see Eq. (4)] with constant phase shifts between slices (along the z direction). Figure 3 shows the original noisy data (Rician magnitude, phase, real and imaginary parts) and the one after phase correction for a reference slice ($b = 1000$ s/mm^2). For each SNR$_0 \in \{10, 20, 30\}$

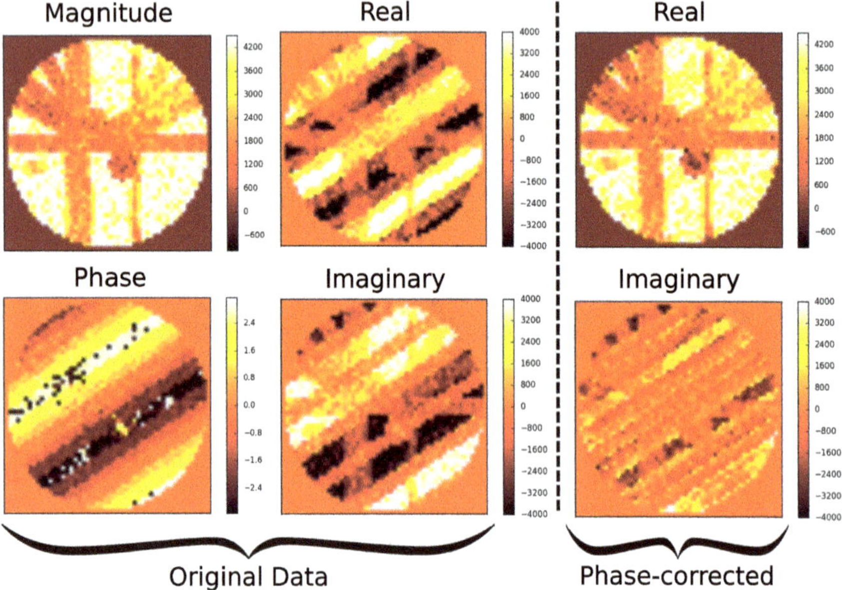

Fig. 3 A slice of data generated with the digital phantom for $SNR_0 = 10$, $b = 1000\,s/mm^2$. *On the left*: the original noisy data calculated with a ground-truth magnitude image obtained with Phantomαs [15] and a synthetic phase. *On the right*: the phase-corrected real and imaginary parts ($\lambda = 0.75$); the signal information is almost entirely contained in the real part, whereas the imaginary part mainly contains Gaussian noise

we generate the Rician magnitude data and, as for the second experiment, the Gaussian DWI image to be used as reference. In this experiment we also investigate the effect of the regularization parameter λ of the total variation filtering in Eq. (3). Therefore, for each SNR_0 we generate six phase-corrected datasets, for $\lambda \in \{0.25, 0.5, 0.75, 1, 2, 5\}$. For each combination of SNR_0 and type of data— Rician, Gaussian and the six phase corrections—we fit DTI with single-shell scheme at b-value 1000, 2000 and $3000\,s/mm^2$, and DTI and MAP with multi-shell scheme. For DTI, we calculate the mean diffusivity (MD), the principal diffusivity (PD), and the fractional anisotropy (FA). We calculate q-space metrics based on closed formulas derived for MAP. These are the return to origin (RTOP), axis (RTAP) and plane (RTPP) probabilities [3], the mean squared displacement (MSD) and the q-space inverse variance (QIV) [17]. We create a mask of voxels within fibers, based on the noise-free dataset, by considering only the voxels where $RTOP \in [0.5e6, 0.7e6]$ (range chosen based on visual inspection). For each value of λ and for each calculated DTI and q-space metric, we compute the probability distribution inside the mask. So we do for the Rician and Gaussian data. Figure 4 illustrates the influence of the regularization parameter λ (decreasing along the

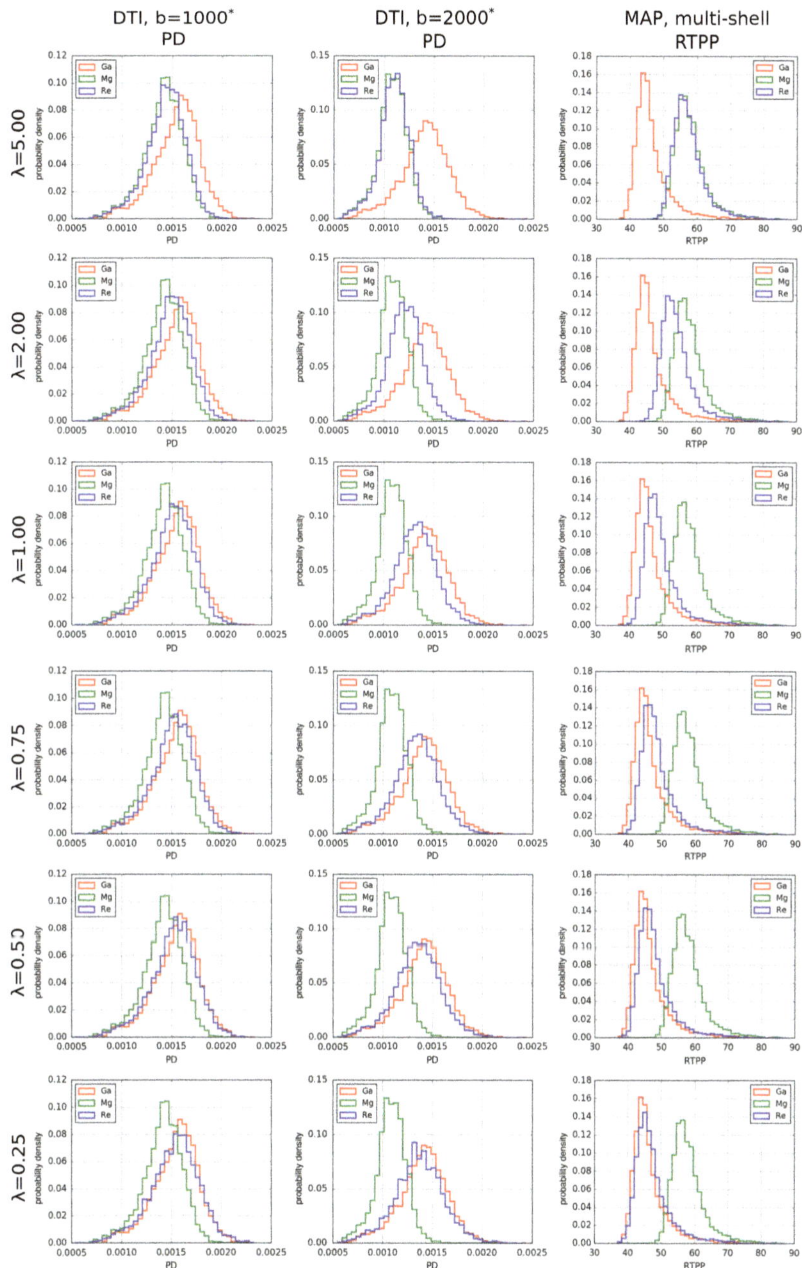

Fig. 4 Histograms of the principal diffusivity (PD)—for DTI at 1000, 2000 s/mm² —and return to plane probability (RTPP)—for MAP—estimated on Gaussian DWI ("Ga", *red*), Rician magnitude ("Mg", *green*), and phase-corrected real part ("Re", *blue*), $SNR_0 = 10$. While the *red* and *green histograms* remain unchanged along the *rows*, the *blue histograms* change as function of the regularization parameter λ [see Eq. (3)]. As the attachment to data decreases (from *top to bottom*) the phase-corrected histograms overlap more with the *red* Gaussian ones. *: s/mm²

rows) on the recovered metric's probability distribution. The figure shows the Gaussian (red line), Rician (green line), and phase-corrected (blue line) probability distributions ($SNR_0 = 10$) of PD (DTI at 1000, 2000 s/mm^2) and RTPP (MAP). The results confirm the underestimation of PD that increases with the b-value, i.e. the green histograms are left to the red ones. Consequently, also MD (see Sect. 1) is underestimated [1]. Inverse analogous considerations hold for RTPP. We observe that λ has a great influence on the phase correction results. Particularly, a large λ implies strong attachment to data, resulting in a poor phase-correction since the estimated low-frequency phase is very similar to the original noisy one, $\widehat{\angle DWI}_{xy} \approx \angle DWI_{xy}$ in Eq. (2). Indeed, the blue histograms (phase-corrected) in the first row of Fig. 4 almost entirely overlap the green ones (Rician magnitude data). As the attachment to the data decreases (from top to bottom), the blue phase-corrected histograms move towards the (red) Gaussian based distributions, visually reducing the distance from Gaussianity. As in the second experiment, we quantify the distance from Gaussian metrics by using Hellinger's formula in Eq. (6). Figure 5 illustrates the variation of the H distance for the phase-corrected data as function of λ, for each acquisition setup, reconstruction method (DTI, MAP), and diffusion metric. In each image, the dashed lines represent the distance of the metric calculated on Rician magnitude data from the corresponding Gaussian one, whereas the solid lines report the distance from Gaussianity for metrics calculated on phase-corrected data, which varies with λ (abscissa). Color codes indicate the SNR_0 value. We observe that phase correction leads to metric distributions that are closer to the Gaussianity (H distance close to 0) than the Rician magnitude ones, for specific ranges of λ. In general, phase correction debiases the metric distributions up to a great extent. The improvement over the Rician magnitude is clearly correlated with the combination of acquisition scheme—especially the maximum b-value—and SNR_0 as also indicated by the signal intensities experiments illustrated in Figs. 1 and 2. Indeed, at high b-values the signal is low—especially along the less restricted diffusion direction—which, in combination with a poor SNR_0, causes the effective SNR to fall well below 5 where a Rician distribution diverges from a Gaussian one. Therefore, the best λ value (highlighted with a dot in Fig. 5) also depends on these factors. We point out that in some cases, as for DTI at $b = 1000$ s/mm^2, too much filtering (small λ) causes the phase-corrected metric distributions to be more distant from Gaussianity compared to those based on the Rician magnitude (dashed lines). The best λ also seems to have a dependence on the considered metric. For instance, at $SNR_0 = 30$ the best λ for RTPP is 0.75 whereas for RTAP is 2. This can be associated to the fact that metrics that are highly related to signal measured along the less restricted diffusion direction (low intensity signal), such as PD and RTPP, benefit more than others of phase correction. See Table 1 for a comprehensive summary.

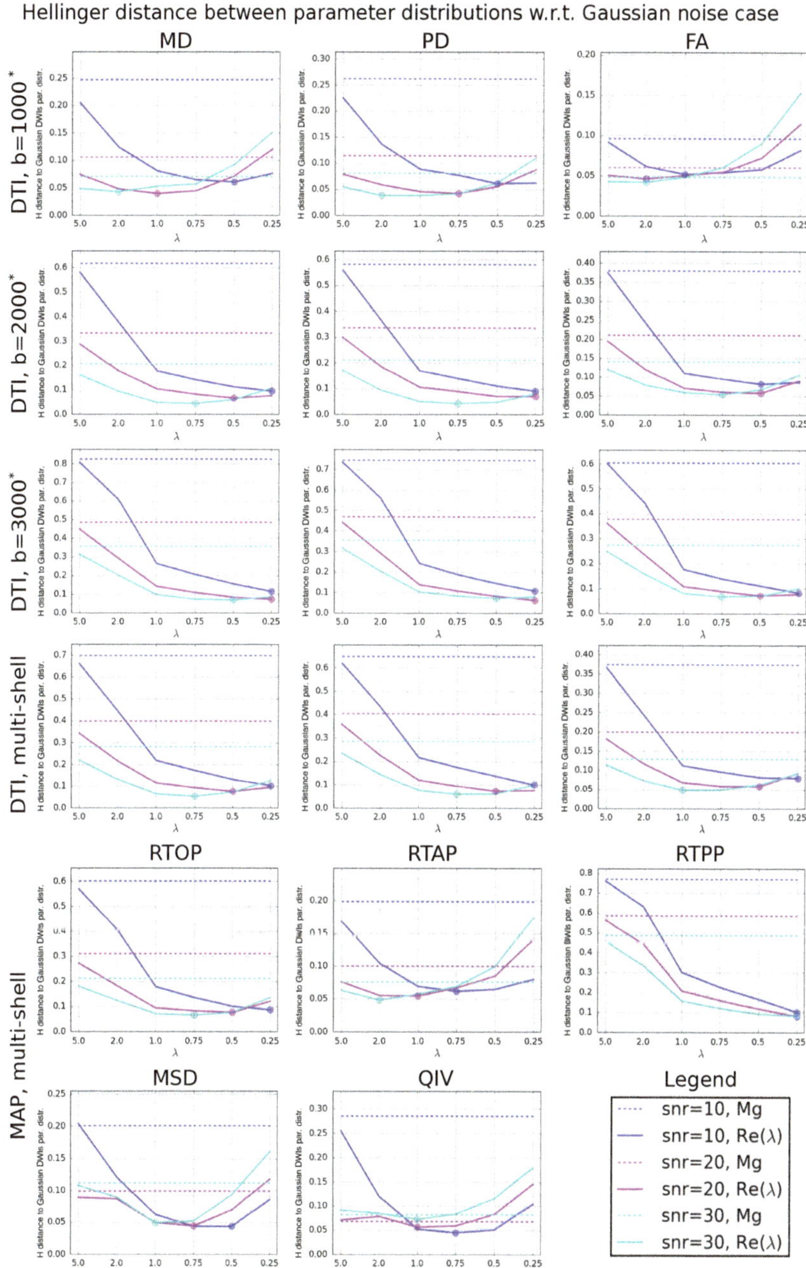

Fig. 5 Distance from Gaussianity [see Eq. (6)] for DTI and q-space metrics calculated on Rician magnitude data ("Mg", *dashed lines*) and on phase-corrected real data ("Re", *solid lines*) as function of λ. The acquisition scheme changes for DTI in the *first four rows*. Each image reports *color-encoded lines* for different values of $SNR_0 \in \{10, 20, 30\}$. The minimum distance for each *solid line* is highlighted by a *dot*. A lower value signifies more closeness to Gaussianity. *: s/mm^2

Table 1 Maximum relative reduction [0, 1] in H distance after phase correction compared to Rician magnitude (bias reduction)

SNR_0	MD	PD	FA	RTOP	RTAP	RTPP	MSD	QIV
	(1K,2K,3K,ms)	(1K,2K,3K,ms)	(1K,2K,3K,ms)	ms	ms	ms	ms	ms
10	(0.75,0.84,0.85,0.85)	(0.76,0.84,0.85,0.84)	(0.45,0.78,0.86,0.78)	0.85	0.68	0.86	0.78	0.84
20	(0.62,0.80,0.84,0.81)	(0.63,0.79,0.86,0.82)	(0.24,0.72,0.86,0.70)	0.75	0.45	0.85	0.55	0.16
30	(0.39,0.78,0.80,0.80)	(0.52,0.80,0.79,0.79)	(0.13,0.61,0.75,0.62)	0.68	0.36	0.82	0.56	0.11

Values are reported for each acquisition type—$b = 1000, 2000, 3000$ s/mm^2 (1K,2K,3K), and multi-shell (ms)—and SNR_0

4   Conclusion

We investigated the effects of phase correction of DWIs in terms of signal debiasing and Noise Floor removal. We quantitatively assess that phase correction has the potential of rendering nearly unbiased DTI and q-space metrics. Indeed, the noise distribution transformation, from Rician to Gaussian, allows compliance with the assumptions required to use standard least squares methods for signal estimation, thus avoiding noise floor related signal overestimation. In this work, we illustrate the importance of accurate phase estimation of complex DWIs, necessary condition for a good phase correction. We plan to extend this work to other diffusion signal metrics, such as those derived from NODDI [5]. We believe that phase correction is a still challenging but promising tool for boosting the estimation of diffusion metrics.

Acknowledgements Data for this project was provided by the MGH-USC Human Connectome Project. This work has received funding from the European Research Council (ERC) under the European Union's Horizon 2020 research and innovation program (ERC Advanced Grant agreement No 694665 : CoBCoM).

Marco Pizzolato expresses his thanks to Olea Medical and the Provence-Alpes-Côte d'Azur (PACA) Regional Council for providing grant and support for this work.

References

1. Jones, D.K., Basser, P.J.: Squashing peanuts and smashing pumpkins: how noise distorts diffusion-weighted MR data. Magn. Reson. Med. **52**(5), 979–993 (2004)
2. Aja-Fernández, S., Tristán-Vega, A.: A review on statistical noise models for magnetic resonance imaging. LPI, ETSI Telecomunicacion, Universidad de Valladolid, Technical Report (2013)
3. Özarslan, E., Koay, C.G., Shepherd, T.M., Komlosh, M.E., İrfanoğlu, M.O., Pierpaoli, C., Basser, P.J.: Mean apparent propagator (MAP) MRI: a novel diffusion imaging method for mapping tissue microstructure. NeuroImage **78**, 16–32 (2013)
4. Alexander, D.C.: A general framework for experiment design in diffusion MRI and its application in measuring direct tissue-microstructure features. Magn. Reson. Med. **60**(2), 439–448 (2008)
5. Zhang, H., Schneider, T., Wheeler-Kingshott, C.A., Alexander, D.C.: NODDI: practical in vivo neurite orientation dispersion and density imaging of the human brain. Neuroimage **61**(4), 1000–1016 (2012)
6. Bernstein, M.A., Thomasson, D.M., Perman, W.H.: Improved detectability in low signal-to-noise ratio magnetic resonance images by means of a phase-corrected real reconstruction. Med. Phys. **16**(5), 813–817 (1989)
7. Basser, P.J., Mattiello, J., LeBihan, D.: MR diffusion tensor spectroscopy and imaging. Biophys. J. **66**(1), 259–267 (1994)
8. Pizzolato, M., Ghosh, A., Boutelier, T., Deriche, R.: Magnitude and complex based diffusion signal reconstruction. In: CDMRI, pp. 127–140 (2014)
9. Liu, C., Bammer, R., Acar, B., Moseley, M.E.: Characterizing non-gaussian diffusion by using generalized diffusion tensors. Magn. Reson. Med. **51**(5), 924–937 (2004)

10. Pizzolato, M., Wassermann, D., Boutelier, T., Deriche, R.: Exploiting the phase in diffusion MRI for microstructure recovery: towards axonal tortuosity via asymmetric diffusion processes. In: MICCAI (2015)
11. Pizzolato, M., Wassermann, D., Duval, T., Campbell, J.S., Boutelier, T., Cohen-Adad, J., Deriche, R.: A temperature phantom to probe the ensemble average propagator asymmetry: an in-silico study. In: CDMRI, pp. 183–194 (2016)
12. Prah, D.E., Paulson, E.S., Nencka, A.S., Schmainda, K.M.: A simple method for rectified noise floor suppression: phase-corrected real data reconstruction with application to diffusion-weighted imaging. Magn. Reson. Med. **64**(2), 418–429 (2010)
13. Sprenger, T., Sperl, J.I., Fernandez, B., Haase, A., Menzel, M.I.: Real valued diffusion-weighted imaging using decorrelated phase filtering. Magn. Reson. Med. (2016). doi:10.1002/mrm.26138
14. Eichner, C., Cauley, S.F., Cohen-Adad, J., Möller, H.E., Turner, R., Setsompop, K., Wald, L.L.: Real diffusion-weighted MRI enabling true signal averaging and increased diffusion contrast. NeuroImage **122**, 373–384 (2015)
15. Caruyer, E., Daducci, A., Descoteaux, M., Houde, J.-C., Thiran J.-P., Verma, R.: Phantomas: a flexible software library to simulate diffusion MR phantoms. In: ISMRM14 (2014)
16. Caruyer, E., Lenglet, C., Sapiro, G., Deriche, R.: Design of multishell sampling schemes with uniform coverage in diffusion MRI. Magn. Reson. Med. **69**(6), 1534–1540 (2013)
17. Fick, R.H., Wassermann, D., Caruyer, E., Deriche, R.: MAPL: tissue microstructure estimation using Laplacian-regularized MAP-MRI and its application to HCP data. NeuroImage **134**, 365–385 (2016)
18. Hellinger, E.: Neue Begründung der Theorie quadratischer Formen von unendlichvielen Veränderlichen. J Reine Angew. Math. **136**, 210–271 (1909)

Regularized Dictionary Learning with Robust Sparsity Fitting for Compressed Sensing Multishell HARDI

Kratika Gupta, Deepali Adlakha, Vishal Agarwal, and Suyash P. Awate

Abstract This paper presents a new compressed sensing framework for multishell HARDI. Unlike methods that model diffusion signals using analytical bases, we *learn a dictionary of multishell diffusion signals*, with a proposed *regularization* term to handle low signal-to-noise ratios at high b values. We combine the dictionary model for diffusion signals together with a multiscale (wavelet-based) spatial model on images for compressed sensing. To control overfitting of the dictionary to tracts with unknown orientations, we use a *strong non-sparsity penalty* that behaves close to the desirable L^0 pseudo-norm. Our framework allows undersampling gradient directions, shells, and k-space. The results show improved reconstructions from our framework, over the state of the art.

1 Introduction and Related Work

Multishell high angular resolution diffusion imaging (HARDI) [1, 20] acquires diffusion weighted (DW) magnetic resonance (MR) images using a large number of gradient directions over multiple shells (i.e., b values). Multishell HARDI combines (1) higher signal-to-noise ratio (SNR) at lower b values with (2) the greater ability to resolve tract directions and narrow-angle crossings at larger b values [19], at the cost of scan time.

We propose a novel compressed sensing framework that allows undersampling gradient directions, shells, and k-space. The key approach for speeding up HARDI scans is, indeed, undersampling the set of gradient directions and the results in

---

Suyash P. Awate thanks funding via IIT Bombay Seed Grant 14IRCCSG010. All work done at IIT Bombay.

K. Gupta • V. Agarwal • S.P. Awate (✉)
Computer Science and Engineering Department, Indian Institute of Technology (IIT) Bombay, Mumbai, India
e-mail: suyash@cse.iitb.ac.in

D. Adlakha
Ads Team, Facebook, London, UK

© Springer International Publishing AG 2017
A. Fuster et al. (eds.), *Computational Diffusion MRI*, Mathematics and Visualization, DOI 10.1007/978-3-319-54130-3_3

the paper focus on that practical scenario. Nevertheless, the framework is general and allows to explore reconstructions involving undersampling in shells or k-space. In some DW MRI applications involving a small number of diffusion-encoding directions, k-space undersampling can be preferred, as shown for diffusion tensor MRI in [13]; our framework is applicable, in principle, to such scenarios as well. Unlike methods [6, 7, 10, 15, 18] that model diffusion signals using analytical bases (e.g., spherical harmonics or ridgelets) for each shell independently, we propose to *learn a dictionary of multishell diffusion signals*, exploiting correlations between multiple shells. In addition to the dictionary, we use an *overcomplete wavelet* frame for multiscale spatial regularization; others works use total-variation (TV) regularization [15, 17] or *no* spatial regularization [2, 11]. Our approach is similar to the one in [3] for dynamic MRI.

Some works [2, 4, 11, 14] use dictionaries based on tensor or parametric models to reconstruct diffusion signals from single-shell HARDI with undersampled directions. Some methods [9, 11] use positivity constraints on the dictionary atoms through nonnegative sparse coding, which relates to our approach. To handle unknown tract orientations in practice, while [11] expands the dictionary to include rotated atoms at the risk of overfitting, [2, 4] explicitly optimize each atom's rotation at a high computational cost and the risk of local optima with corrupted data. In contrast, we (1) fit the dictionary to arbitrarily oriented tracts while controlling overfitting at low computational cost by *modifying the non-sparsity penalty to give sparser dictionary fits* and (2) reconstruct multishell HARDI directly from undersampled noisy k-space data.

In this paper, we propose a new method for learning a dictionary of multishell diffusion signals, employing a *spherical-domain regularization on the estimated atoms* to counter the low SNR at higher b values. Our formulation leads to a convex optimization problem in each variable (atoms or coefficients), which can be solved efficiently. We propose a new framework for compressed sensing that employs the learned dictionary together with multiscale spatial regularity using wavelets. While the learned dictionary is expanded to handle arbitrary tract orientations, we control overfitting by a strong non-sparsity penalty that behaves close to the desirable L^0 pseudo-norm [8] and leads to an efficient majorization minimization (MM) algorithm performing convex optimization iteratively. Our compressed sensing framework reconstructs DW MR images directly from undersampled noisy k-space data. In this way, the framework allows exploration of application-specific acquisition optimization regarding the choice of (1) number of shells, (2) gradient directions in each shell, and (3) undersampling in q-space and k-space. Results show the advantages of our framework over the state of the art.

2 Methods

This section describes our methods for regularized dictionary learning, strongly sparse fitting, and compressed sensing multishell HARDI directly from k-space data.

2.1　Dictionary Learning for Multishell HARDI

Using a HARDI image dataset, we collect multishell signals at voxels in regions that have a single tract passing through them, e.g., corpus callosum and lateral corticospinal tract, where the strongly anisotropic diffusion leads to higher contrast-to-noise ratios in the signal. To factor out arbitrary differences in (1) imaging coordinate-frame origins and poses across individuals, (2) orientations of a specific tract across individuals, and (3) orientations of different tracts within an individual, we reorient each diffusion signal to align it with a fixed diffusion signal that models prolate-tensor diffusion along a fixed direction ($[0, 0, 1]^\top$). The alignment entails interpolation, on the spherical domain of the diffusion-signal function, using Barycentric coordinates and geodesic distances on the sphere $\mathbb{S}^2$. We align two real-valued functions, i.e., diffusion signals, defined on the spherical domain of gradient directions. The underlying deformation is rotation. The registration gives aligned signals defined on the same gradient directions (for each shell). We divide each aligned signal by the voxel value in the corresponding $b0$ image.

Because diffusion signal values are modeled as non-negative real [20], we learn atoms with non-negative values from magnitude HARDI images. We constrain coefficients to be non-negative real to ensure that the fits lie in the same space as the data. For multishell diffusion signals, shells with larger b values lead to drastic reductions in SNR. To counter the noise, during dictionary learning, we propose to enforce a *smoothness prior* on the atom over the spherical domain of gradient directions. We use a robust penalty to reduce noise while preserving contrast over the spherical domain.

Let the HARDI acquisition employ S shells, with shell s comprising N_s gradient directions $\{g_{sn} \in \mathbb{R}^3 : \|g_{sn}\|_2 = 1\}_{n=1}^{N_s}$. In a training dataset of I aligned multishell diffusion signals, let the i-th signal be f^i. Let $f_{sn}^i \in \mathbb{R}_{\geq 0}$ be the signal value from shell s for gradient direction g_{sn}. Let the dictionary matrix $\mathcal{D}$ comprise K multishell diffusion signals (atoms) d^k as columns. Let $d_{sn}^k \in \mathbb{R}_{\geq 0}$ be the atom value from shell s for gradient direction g_{sn}. Let c^i be the vector of non-negative coefficients used to represent f^i. We propose the optimal dictionary as the solution to

$$\min_{\mathcal{D},c} \left(\sum_{i=1}^{I} \left[\|f^i - \mathcal{D}c^i\|_2^2 + \alpha\|c^i\|_1 \right] + \sum_{k=1}^{K} \sum_{s=1}^{S} \beta_s \sum_{n=1}^{N_s} \sum_{m=1}^{N_s} w_{smn} H(d_{sn}^k - d_{sm}^k, \delta) \right)$$

$$\text{under the constraints} : \forall (k, s, n) : d_{sn}^k \geq 0, \|d^k\|_2 \leq 1, \text{and} \forall (i, k) : c_k^i \geq 0, \tag{1}$$

where $H(\cdot, \delta)$ is the Huber loss function [12] (a smooth approximation to the L^1 penalty) with parameter δ, $\alpha > 0$ controls the sparsity prior strength, $\beta_s > 0$ controls the strength of the robust smoothness prior $H(\cdot, \cdot)$ for shell s of each atom's diffusion signal, $w_{smn} \in [0, 1]$ weights the roughness penalty for the deviation between atom values between directions g_{sn} and g_{sm}; $w_{smn} := \exp(-0.5|\arccos(g_{sn}, g_{sm})|^2/(\pi/12)^2)$.

We use iterative optimization to alternatingly optimize atoms d^k and coefficient vectors c^i, while fixing the other, in each case solving a convex optimization problem. We use K-means to initialize d^k to the K cluster centers. Fixing atoms $\{d^k\}_{k=1}^K$, the optimization problem for each coefficient vector c^i has a quadratic objective function and a linear (positive) constraint; the global minimum has a closed form. Fixing coefficient vectors $\{c^i\}_{i=1}^I$, because we choose $H(\cdot, \delta)$ as convex, the optimization problem for each atom d^k is convex; we find the global minimum via projected gradient descent with adaptive step size. To the learned dictionary, we add constant atoms d^{K+s}, one for each shell s, to better model isotropic diffusion in the fluid and gray matter.

2.2 Compressed Sensing Multishell HARDI

We formulate the problem of reconstructing multishell HARDI image u from undersampled data z (complex valued vector). Let the anatomical image comprise V voxels. Let the HARDI acquisition employ S shells, with shell s comprising N_s gradient directions. The matrix u is of dimension $V \times (\sum_{s=1}^{S} N_s)$. Let u_{sn} be the spatial image of diffusion signal values for shell s and gradient direction g_{sn}. Let u_v be the multishell diffusion signal at voxel v. Let z_{sn} be the vector of undersampled data for shell s and gradient direction g_{sn}. Let operator $\widehat{\mathcal{F}}_{sn}$ represent the undersampled Fourier transform (vectorized output) related to the k-space data acquisition corresponding to image u_{sn}. $\widehat{\mathcal{F}}_{sn}$ can model undersampling in gradient directions, shells, and k-space; skipping direction g_{sn} corresponds to $\widehat{\mathcal{F}}_{sn}$ *not* sampling any data in k-space. Let $\mathcal{W}$ be an operator representing a wavelet transform (vectorized output) applied on a spatial image. We enforce a prior on uncorrupted images u such that each spatial image u_{sn} has a sparse wavelet representation, by penalizing the L^1 norm of the vector of wavelet coefficients.

We use the dictionary $\mathcal{D}$ learned in Sect. 2.1, using orientation-aligned multishell diffusion signal data, to create another dictionary $\mathcal{D}^\Theta$ for use during compressed sensing. To enable fits to tracts with unknown orientations, we build an expanded dictionary $\mathcal{D}^\Theta$ by using each atom d^k in $\mathcal{D}$ to create multiple copies $\{d^{k\theta_j}\}_{j=1}^J$ by reorienting the diffusion signal d^k along a large set of directions $\{\theta_j\}_{j=1}^J$ spread roughly uniformly over the hemisphere. For simplicity, we model the set of θ_j to be same as the gradient directions g_{sn} for the shell s that acquired the maximum number of directions N_s.

Let $\mathcal{D}^\Theta$ be a dictionary of KJ atoms representing the multishell diffusion signals (real valued, non-negative) at any voxel in the anatomy. Let c_v be the vector of coefficients used for representing the multishell diffusion signal u_v at voxel v. We constrain coefficients c_{vm} to be real non-negative. We design a prior on uncorrupted images u such that, at each voxel v, u_v has a sparse representation in dictionary $\mathcal{D}^\Theta$.

While this multiplicity results in a large increase in the number of atoms ($KJ \gg K$) in $\mathcal{D}^\Theta$, we know that very few of these should be needed for a fit; e.g., a voxel involving a single tract would probably use only 1 of the reoriented atoms (the one matching the tract orientation), a voxel involving two crossing tracts would probably use only 2 of such reoriented atoms (the ones matching the orientations of the two crossing tracts), etc. To ensure such sparse fits, we use a *strong sparsity prior by penalizing the logarithm of the L^1 norm* of each coefficient vector c_v. We choose this logarithm function because it penalizes non-sparsity more strongly compared to the L^p norms for p close to 1; indeed, the log-L^1 penalty behaves similar to the L^p-to-power-p penalty for p close to 0, thereby mimicking the desirable L^0 pseudo-norm [5, 8]. Furthermore, we propose an efficient optimization scheme for sparse coding dealing with this logarithmic form.

The formulation naturally models u as complex valued. We use the corresponding magnitude image for visualization. While the image u is a complex-valued matrix, the proposed dictionary can model only real-valued diffusion signals. Hence, to model the complex phase of the signal u_v, at each voxel v, we introduce a complex-valued vector ϕ_v that is of the same length as u_v and each component of which has unit magnitude.

We propose the optimal reconstruction u^* as the solution to

$$\min_{u,c,\phi} \left(\lambda \sum_{s=1}^{S} \sum_{n=1}^{N_s} \|\mathcal{W}u_{sn}\|_1 + (1-\lambda) \sum_{v=1}^{V} \left[\|u_v - \phi_v \odot \mathcal{D}^\Theta c_v\|_2^2 + \gamma \sum_{i=1}^{K'} \log(|c_{vi}| + \epsilon) \right] \right)$$

$$\text{such that} \forall v, s, n, m : c_{vm} \geq 0, |\phi_{vsn}| = 1, \text{and} \|\widehat{\mathcal{F}}_{sn}u_{sn} - z_{sn}\|_2 \leq \eta_{sn}, \tag{2}$$

where $\lambda \in [0, 1]$ balances the strengths of the priors enforcing wavelet-based and dictionary-based sparsity, $\odot$ represents component-wise multiplication of 2 vectors, $\gamma > 0$ controls the sparsity of coefficients, η_{sn} is the noise norm, and $\epsilon = 10^{-4}$ avoids numerical issues. We propose to alternatingly optimize variables u, c, and ϕ. We initialize $u_{sn} \leftarrow \widehat{\mathcal{F}}_{sn}^\dagger z_{sn}$, where $(\cdot)^\dagger$ is the Moore-Penrose pseudo inverse.

Optimizing Phase ϕ Fixing u, we can optimize ϕ by independently optimizing ϕ_{vsn} at each voxel v, shell s, and gradient direction g_{sn}. The optimization problem reduces to $\phi_{vsn}^* := \arg\min_{\phi_{vsn}} |u_{vsn} - \phi_{vsn}x_{vsn}|^2$, where x_v is any fit given by the dictionary. When $u_{vsn} > 0$, this has a closed-form solution $\phi_{vsn}^* = u_{vsn}/|u_{vsn}|$, independent of x_v. When u_{vsn} equals 0, we set $\phi_{vsn}^* = 1$.

Optimizing Coefficients c Fixing u and ϕ_v, we optimize c_v independently at each voxel v. The optimization problem reduces to $c_v^* := \arg\min_{c_v} \|u_v - \phi_v \odot \mathcal{D}^\Theta c_v\|_2^2 + \gamma \sum_{i=1}^{K'} \log(|c_{vi}| + \epsilon)$ under the positivity constraint on the coefficient values. Having chosen the optimal ϕ_v as the complex phase of u_v, we optimize the coefficient vector c_v so that the dictionary fits to the magnitude vector $\widetilde{u}_v$, where $\widetilde{u}_{vsn} = |u_{vsn}|$. Thus, the objective function reduces to $\|\widetilde{u}_v - \mathcal{D}^\Theta c_v\|_2^2 + \gamma \sum_{i=1}^{K'} \log(|c_{vi}| + \epsilon)$.

We optimize using MM. Within each iteration, we majorize the objective function by exploiting (1) the positivity of the coefficients and (2) the concavity of the log function. We use the first-order Taylor-series approximation to majorize the log function, evaluated only on the positive orthant, by its tangent hyperplane at the current estimate $\widehat{c}_v$. The majorized objective function is $\|\widetilde{u}_v - \mathcal{D}^\Theta c_v\|_2^2 + \gamma \|\omega \odot c_v\|_1$, where the weight vector components are $\omega_m := 1/(\widehat{c}_{vm} + \epsilon)$. Compared to the unweighted case, the weights ω_{sn} promote a sparser fit by increasing (relatively) the penalty on non-zero coefficients c_{vm} for those atoms for which the current coefficient estimate $\widehat{c}_{vm}$ is smaller.

To solve this problem, we substitute $\widetilde{c}_v := \omega \odot c_v = \Omega c_v$, where Ω is a diagonal matrix whose diagonal elements are in the same order as those in the vector ω. This substitution reduces the problem to $\widetilde{c}_v^* := \arg\min_{\widetilde{c}_v} \|\widetilde{u}_v - \mathcal{D}^\Theta \Omega^{-1} \widetilde{c}_v\|_2^2 + \gamma \|\widetilde{c}_v\|_1$, under positivity constraints on $\widetilde{c}_v$. This is a non-negative sparse coding problem using the modified dictionary $\mathcal{D}^\Theta \Omega^{-1}$ that scales each atom d^m in the dictionary $\mathcal{D}^\Theta$ by the current coefficient estimates $\widehat{c}_{vm} + \epsilon$. This reweighting promotes sparser fits because it scales down (relatively) those atoms that correspond to smaller coefficients $\widehat{c}_{vm}$ in the current estimate, thereby effectively increasing (relatively) the penalty on their coefficients in the new optimal estimate c_{vm}, leading to even smaller coefficients. This sparse coding problem, within each iteration of the MM algorithm, has a quadratic objective function and a convex (positive) constraint; we find the global minimum in closed form. The optimal estimate $\widetilde{c}_v^*$ gives the desired optimal estimate $c_v^* := \Omega^{-1} \widetilde{c}_v^*$.

Optimizing Multishell HARDI Image u Fixing c and ϕ, the objective function for u reduces to $\lambda \|\mathcal{W}u\|_1 + (1 - \lambda)\|u - y\|_2^2$, where $y_v := \phi_v \odot x_v$. The constraint set for u comes from the fidelity constraints $\|\widehat{\mathcal{F}}_{sn} u_{sn} - z_{sn}\|_2 \leq \eta_{sn}$. We propose to solve this (large) convex optimization problem for u using an efficient algorithm for non-smooth convex optimization [16] that significantly improves the typical bounds on the number of iterations required for convergence for gradient-based algorithms.

3 Results and Conclusion

We evaluate the proposed framework on simulated and human brain HARDI images. The parameters λ, α, β_s, and γ need to be tuned empirically using cross-validation.

Regularized Dictionary Learning for Brain HARDI While we learn a multishell dictionary for compressed sensing later, we first show the utility of the smoothness prior via single-shell learning. From the brain dataset, we obtained 1000 high-variance diffusion signals for $b = 1000\,\text{s/mm}^2$ as "clean" and learned a dictionary of ten atoms from that (two examples in Fig. 1a); we show the diffusion signal values, colormapped, at the corresponding gradient directions on a unit hemisphere. We then used the corresponding 1000 diffusion signals from the shell with $b = 3000\,\text{s/mm}^2$, corrupted it with noise, and learned two dictionaries, one using the smoothness prior and one without. Atoms learned without the smoothness prior undesirably exhibited more noise/random perturbations (examples in Fig. 1b) than atoms learned with the prior (examples in Fig. 1c). The relative root mean squared error (RRMSE) between the fitted diffusion signals a and the reference signal b is $\|a - b\|/\|b\|$. The regularized atoms, expectedly, produced better fits to noisy data, which were qualitatively smoother (example in Fig. 2c, e) and quantitatively having

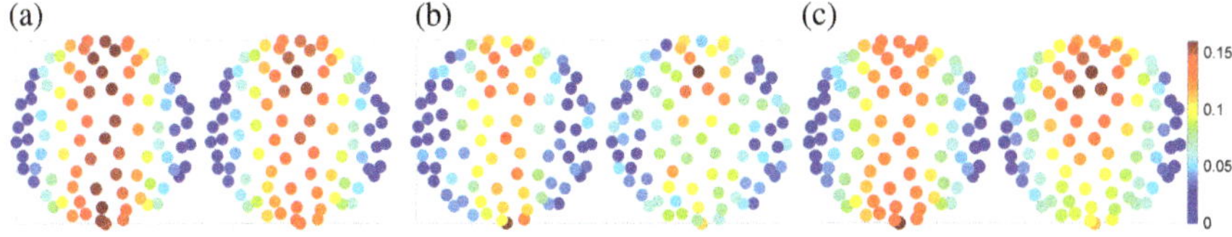

Fig. 1 Regularized dictionary learning. Two example atoms learned: (**a**) using clean data at $b = 1000$ s/mm^2 (considered as baseline), (**b**) using noisy data at $b = 3000$ s/mm^2, *without* smoothness prior ($\beta_s = 0$), and (**c**) using noisy data at $b = 3000$ s/mm^2, *with* smoothness prior ($\beta_s > 0$) (**proposed**). *Dot locations* $\equiv$ gradient direction vectors; *colors* $\equiv$ diffusion signal values

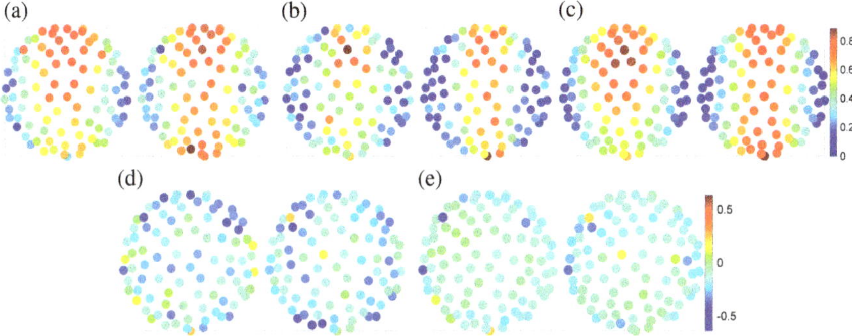

Fig. 2 Regularized dictionary learning. Example *fit* to noisy data at $b = 3000$ s/mm^2 using a dictionary learned: (**a**) using clean data (reference), (**b**) using noisy data, *without* smoothness prior ($\beta_s = 0$), and (**c**) using noisy data, *with* smoothness prior ($\beta_s > 0$) (**proposed**). (**d**)–(**e**) Residuals for (**b**)–(**c**), respectively

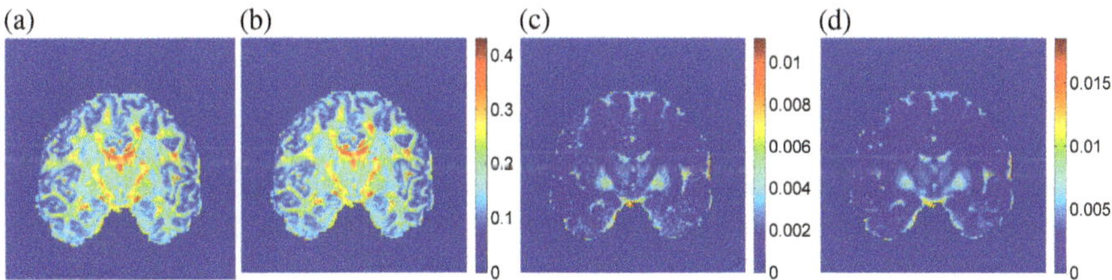

Fig. 3 Dictionary modeling of human brain HARDI. (**a**) Baseline (high quality) GFA image, averaged over shells. (**b**) GFA of the image resulting from fitting the dictionary to the baseline image. (**c**) Magnitude of the difference between per-voxel GFA in image (a) and (b). (**d**) Per voxel RRMSEs between baseline and dictionary-fitted diffusion signals

about half the RRMSE, as compared to the atoms learned without regularization (example in Fig. 2b, d).

Figure 3 evaluates the utility of the proposed dictionary learning framework in modeling brain HARDI. The GFA of the baseline HARDI signals (Fig. 3a) and the GFA of the dictionary-fitted HARDI signal (Fig. 3b) are very similar, with differences (Fig. 3c) almost always being less than half percent or less. The per-

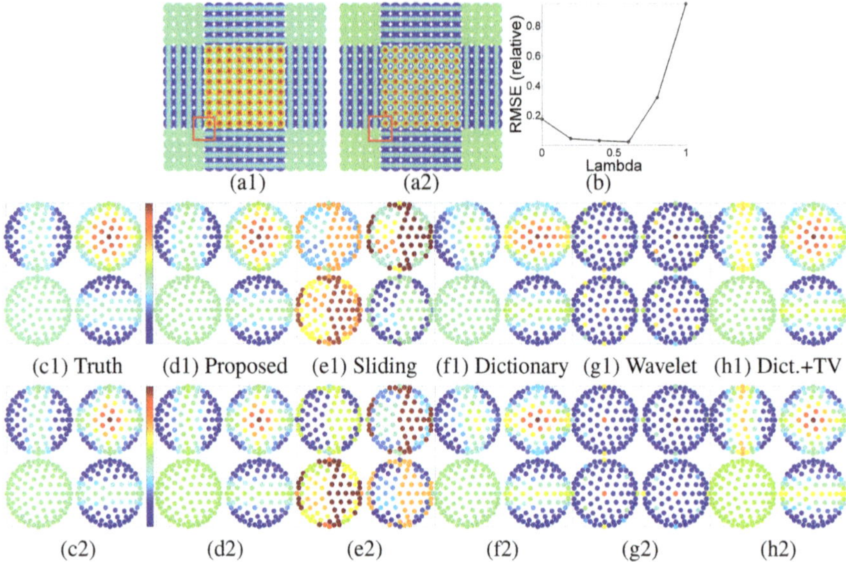

Fig. 4 Compressed sensing simulated HARDI. **(a1)–(a2)** Ground truth diffusion signals, for 2 shells, in simulated phantom. We simulated *16X undersampling in gradient directions* and SNR-7 noise (see text). **(b)** Proposed method's performance with different weights λ for the dictionary and wavelet prior. **(c1)–(c2)** True signal (zoomed in 2×2 patch boxed *red* $\square$ in **(a)**–**(b)**), for both shells. Reconstructions with: **(d1)–(d2)** dictionary and wavelet, $\lambda = 0.6$, RRMSE 0.02 **(proposed)** which is near perfect; **(e1)–(e2)** sliding window, RRMSE 0.44; **(f1)–(f2)** dictionary, $\lambda = 0$, RRMSE 0.17; **(g1)–(g2)** wavelet (3D overcomplete), $\lambda = 1$ (RRMSE 0.94); **(h1)–(h2)** dictionary and TV, optimized λ (RRMSE 0.05)

voxel RRMSEs (Fig. 3d) between the dictionary fit and the baseline image are almost always less than 1%.

Compressed Sensing Simulated HARDI We use a simulated phantom; 16×16 voxel matrix, 81 gradient directions, 2 shells) comprising 2 crossing tracts, 1 horizontal and 1 vertical (Fig. 4(**a1**), (**a2**)). We simulate $16X$ undersampling in gradient directions, acquiring only 5 of the 81 directions, per shell, spread roughly uniformly over the hemisphere that resulted in small magnitudes of the inner-product between pairs of selected directions. We introduce independent and identically distributed zero-mean complex Gaussian noise of variance σ^2 in k-space such that the SNR, defined as the largest signal magnitude among all DW images divided by σ, equals 7 that mimics a realistic clinical acquisition scenario. The proposed framework gives results [Fig. 4(**d1**), (**d2**)] that are near perfect, as compared to other approaches. The best performance occurs when both multishell-dictionary- and wavelet-based models are used, i.e., λ roughly midway between 0 and 1 (Fig. 4c). The simple sliding window reconstruction [Fig. 4(**e1**), (**e2**)], where we replace the missing k-space data by the acquired data for the same location in k-space but in the nearest direction in the same shell, fails to enforce any regularity on the reconstruction in space or directions. The dictionary model alone gives results with poor spatial regularity [Fig. 4(**f1**), (**f2**)]. An analytical wavelet basis jointly for space and directions/shells does poorer because the proposed approach uses a dictionary that is adapted to multishell diffusion signals [Fig. 4(**g1**), (**g2**)]. The dictionary model with a spatial TV prior cannot model multiscale spatial regularity, unlike wavelet transforms [Fig. 4(**h1**), (**h2**)]; a spatial TV prior can be easily incorporated in our framework by replacing the wavelet transform with a linear transform that takes one-sided spatial derivatives along each dimension of the image.

Compressed Sensing Brain HARDI We used ten fully-sampled high-quality 2-shell HARDI images with 90 gradient directions, treated as baselines, and performed retrospective undersampling and noise corruption (mimicking SNR 7). We performed 6X undersampling of directions (15 out of 90 directions acquired roughly uniformly over the hemisphere, for each shell) and 1.3X undersampling of k-space (undersampled frequency encodes), corresponding to a reduction in scan time by a factor slightly larger than 6. The reconstructions (Figs. 5 and 6) from our approach of using the learned multishell dictionary model combined with a spatial regularity model (wavelet or TV) are of significantly higher quality than the other

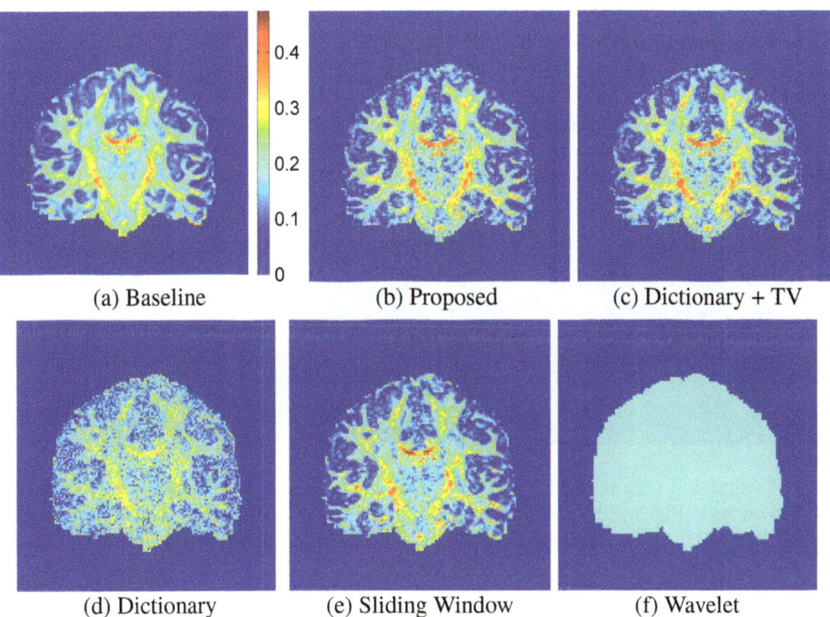

(a) Baseline   (b) Proposed   (c) Dictionary + TV

(d) Dictionary   (e) Sliding Window   (f) Wavelet

Fig. 5 Compressed sensing brain HARDI (slice I). (**a**) Baseline (high quality) GFA images, averaged over shells. We simulated *6X undersampling of directions* and 1.3X undersampling of k-space for each direction acquired, introducing noise to get SNR 7 (see text). GFA images of reconstructions with: (**b**) dictionary and wavelet, $\lambda = 0.7$, RRMSE 0.12 (**proposed**); (**c**) dictionary and TV with optimized λ, RRMSE 0.12; (**d**) dictionary, $\lambda = 0$, RRMSE 0.23; (**e**) sliding window, RRMSE 0.23; (**f**) wavelet (3D overcomplete), $\lambda = 1$, RRMSE 0.91

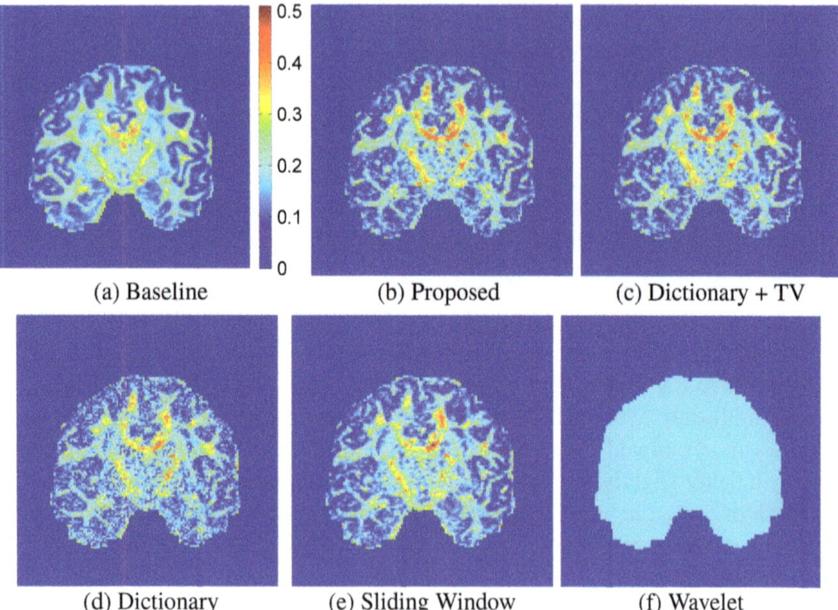

(a) Baseline   (b) Proposed   (c) Dictionary + TV

(d) Dictionary   (e) Sliding Window   (f) Wavelet

Fig. 6 Compressed sensing brain HARDI (slice II). (**a**) Baseline (high quality) GFA images, averaged over shells. We simulated *6X undersampling of directions* and 1.3X undersampling of k-space for each acquired direction, introducing noise to get SNR 7 (see text). GFA images of reconstructions with (**b**) dictionary and wavelet, $\lambda = 0.7$, RRMSE 0.12 (**proposed**); (**c**) dictionary and TV with optimized λ, RRMSE 0.12; (**d**) dictionary, $\lambda = 0$, RRMSE 0.23; (**e**) sliding window, RRMSE 0.22; (**f**) wavelet (3D overcomplete), $\lambda = 1$, RRMSE 0.9

(a)   (b)   (c)   (d)

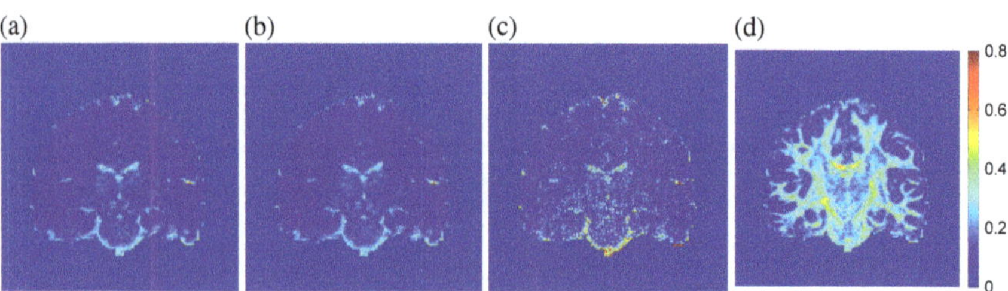

Fig. 7 Compressed sensing brain HARDI (slice I). Images of per-voxel RRMSE (multishell) for reconstructions in Fig. 5 with (**a**) dictionary and wavelet, RRMSE 0.12 (**proposed**); (**b**) dictionary and TV, RRMSE 0.12; (**c**) dictionary, RRMSE 0.23; (**d**) sliding window, RRMSE 0.23

approaches. The approach using the dictionary alone failed to reproduce spatial regularity in the reconstructed image, and instead produced noisy reconstructions with about twice as much RRMSE. The sliding window approach lead to a similar lack of regularity and much larger RRMSE. The approach using the wavelet frame only, coupled in space and directions, performed the worst because, compared to the dictionary, the wavelets are unable to effectively model the regularity for this class of signals. The images of RMS errors (Figs. 7 and 8) clearly show that our coupled

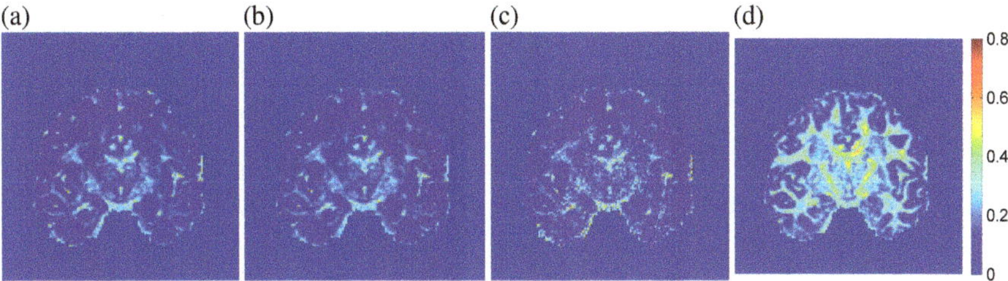

Fig. 8 Compressed sensing brain HARDI (slice II). Images of per-voxel RRMSE (multishell) for reconstructions with (**a**) dictionary and wavelet, RRMSE 0.12 (**proposed**); (**b**) dictionary and TV, RRMSE 0.12; (**c**) dictionary, RRMSE 0.23; (**d**) sliding window, RRMSE 0.22

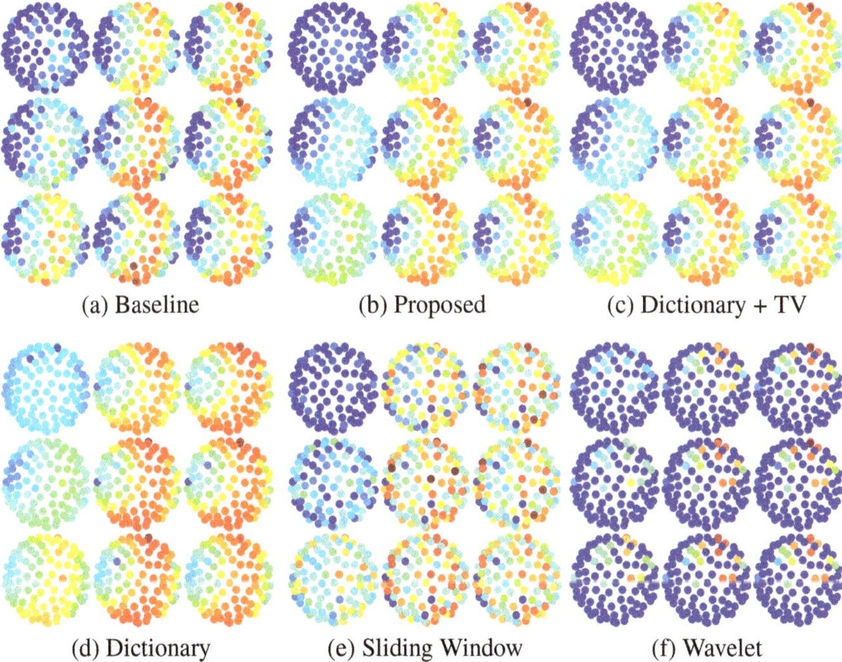

Fig. 9 Compressed sensing brain HARDI (region I: corpus callosum) (**a**) Baseline diffusion signals, for $b = 1000\,\text{s/mm}^2$. Reconstructed diffusion signals with (**b**) dictionary and wavelet, (**c**) dictionary and TV, (**d**) dictionary, (**e**) sliding window, (**f**) wavelet (3D overcomplete)

approach, dictionary in addition to spatial regularization (wavelet or TV), yields the lowest errors.

We now show the reconstruction in two regions: a 3×3 voxel patch in the corpus callosum in Fig. 9, and another 3×3 voxel patch in a fiber-crossing region of the corpus callosum and the lateral corticospinal tract in Fig. 10. In the corpus callosum (Fig. 9), while the dictionary-only reconstruction underfits to the data, the wavelet-only and sliding-window reconstructions are noisy and erroneous. In the crossing

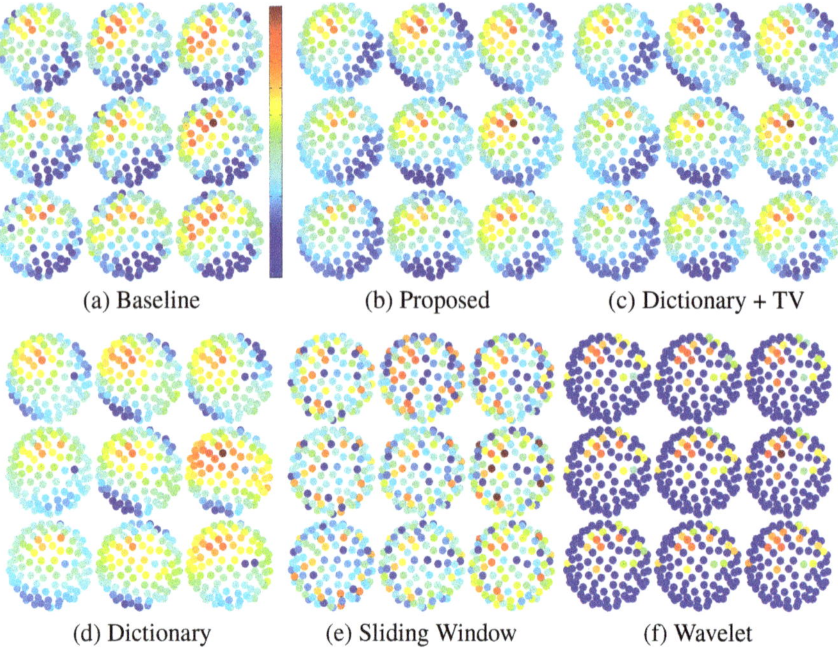

(a) Baseline   (b) Proposed   (c) Dictionary + TV

(d) Dictionary   (e) Sliding Window   (f) Wavelet

Fig. 10 Compressed sensing brain HARDI (region II: fiber crossing) (**a**) Baseline diffusion signals, for $b = 1000\,\text{s/mm}^2$. Reconstructed diffusion signals with (**b**) dictionary and wavelet, (**c**) dictionary and TV, (**d**) dictionary, (**e**) sliding window, (**f**) wavelet (3D overcomplete)

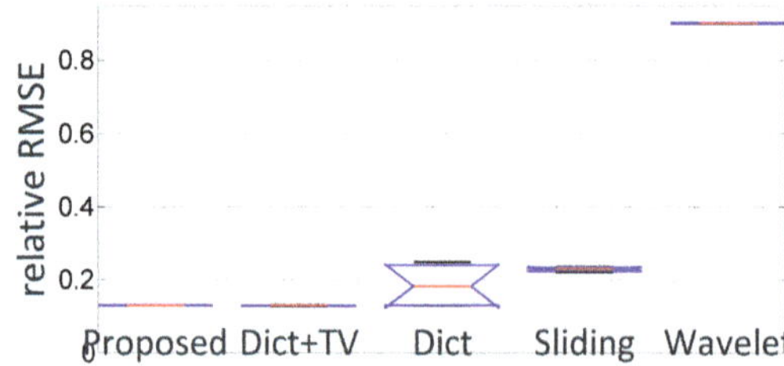

Fig. 11 Box plots of RRMSEs for ten randomly selected coronal brain MRI slices

region (Fig. 10), the dictionary-only reconstruction has modified the directions of the individual tracts; at each voxel, the blue area shifts from the bottom right to the bottom left. Our approach of using the dictionary coupled with spatial regularization (wavelet or TV) gives the best results. We experimented with ten different coronal slices from brain HARDI images and found (Fig. 11) that our approach of using the dictionary along with a spatial prior (wavelet or TV) outperforms other approaches.

Conclusion We present a new compressed sensing framework for multishell HARDI. We propose a regularized dictionary learning method for multishell signals, to handle low SNR at high b values and show its advantages in getting improved fits to human brain HARDI. To control overfitting of the dictionary to tracts with unknown orientations, we propose a strong non-sparsity penalty similar to the L^0 pseudo-norm. Our framework reconstructs images directly from HARDI data undersampled in gradient directions, thereby allowing an acquisition speedup of the same factor as the gradient-direction undersampling factor. We propose efficient optimization schemes and show results that improve the state of the art.

References

1. Alexander, D.: Multiple-fiber reconstruction algorithms for diffusion MRI. Ann. N. Y. Acad Sci. **1064**, 113–33 (2005)
2. Aranda, R., Ramirez-Manzanares, A., Rivera, M.: Sparse and adaptive diffusion dictionary for recovering intra-voxel white matter structure. Med. Image Anal. **26**(1), 243–55 (2015)
3. Awate, S.P., DiBella, E.V.R.: Spatiotemporal dictionary learning for undersampled dynamic MRI reconstruction via joint frame-based and dictionary-based sparsity. In: IEEE Symposium on Biomedical Imaging, pp. 318–321 (2012)
4. Awate, S.P., DiBella, E.V.R.: Compressed sensing HARDI via rotation-invariant concise dictionaries, flexible k-space undersampling, and multiscale spatial regularity. In: IEEE International Symposium on Biomedical Imaging, pp. 9–12 (2013)
5. Candes, E., Wakin, M., Boyd, S.: Enhanced sparsity by reweighted l_1 minimization. J. Fourier Anal. Appl. **14**, 877–905 (2008)
6. Cheng, J., Deriche, R., Jiang, T., Shen, D., Yap, P.T.: Non-negative spherical deconvolution for estimation of fiber orientation distribution function in single-/multi-shell diffusion MRI. NeuroImage **101**, 750–64 (2014)
7. Descoteaux, M., Deriche, R., LeBihan, D., Mangin, J.F., Poupon, C.: Multiple q-shell diffusion propagator imaging. Med. Imag. Anal. **15**, 603–621 (2011)
8. Donoho, D., Elad, M.: Optimally sparse representation in general (nonorthogonal) dictionaries via $l1$ minimization. Proc. Natl. Acad. Sci. **100**(5), 2197–2202 (2003)
9. Gramfort, A., Poupon, C., Descoteaux, M.: Denoising and fast diffusion imaging with physically constrained sparse dictionary learning. Med. Imag. Anal. **18**(1), 36–49 (2014)
10. Jian, B., Vemuri, B.: A unified computational framework for deconvolution to reconstruct multiple fibers from diffusion weighted MRI. IEEE Trans. Med. Imag. **26**, 1464–1471 (2007)
11. Landman, B., Bogovic, J., Wan, H., ElShahaby, F., Bazin, P.L., Prince, J.: Resolution of crossing fibers with constrained compressed sensing using diffusion tensor MRI. NeuroImage **59**, 2175–2186 (2012)
12. Li, S.Z.: Markov Random Field Modeling in Computer Vision. Springer, Berlin (1995)
13. McClymont, D., Teh, I., Whittington, H., Grau, V., Schneider, J.: Prospective acceleration of diffusion tensor imaging with compressed sensing using adaptive dictionaries. Magn. Res. Med. **76**, 248–258 (2016)
14. Merlet, S., Caruyer, E., Ghosh, A., Deriche, R.: A computational diffusion MRI and parametric dictionary learning framework for modeling the diffusion signal and its features. Med. Imag. Anal. **17**(7), 830–843 (2013)
15. Michailovich, O., Rathi, Y., Dolui, S.: Spatially regularized compressed sensing for high angular resolution diffusion imaging. IEEE Trans. Med. Imag. **30**, 1100–1115 (2011)
16. Nesterov, Y.: Smooth minimization of non-smooth functions. Math. Programm. Ser. A **103**, 127–152 (2005)
17. Ning, L., Setsompop, K., Michailovich, O., Makris, N., Shenton, M., Westin, C.F., Rathi, Y.: A joint compressed-sensing and super-resolution approach for very high-resolution diffusion imaging. NeuroImage **125**, 386–400 (2016)

18. Rathi, Y., Michailovich, O., Setsompop, K., Bouix, S., Shenton, M., Westin, C.F.: Sparse multi-shell diffusion imaging. Med. Imag. Comput. Assist. Interv. **14**, 58–65 (2011)
19. Scherrer, B., Warfield, S.: Why multiple b-values are required for multi-tensor models: evaluation with a constrained log-Euclidean model. In: IEEE ISBI, pp. 1389–1392 (2012)
20. Tuch, D., Reese, T., Wiegell, M.: High angular resolution diffusion imaging reveals intravoxel white matter fiber heterogeneity. Magn. Res. Med. **48**(4), 477–582 (2002)

Denoising Diffusion-Weighted Images Using Grouped Iterative Hard Thresholding of Multi-Channel Framelets

Jian Zhang, Geng Chen, Yong Zhang, Bin Dong, Dinggang Shen, and Pew-Thian Yap

Abstract Noise in diffusion-weighted (DW) images increases the complexity of quantitative analysis and decreases the reliability of inferences. Hence, to improve analysis, it is often desirable to remove noise and at the same time preserve relevant image features. In this paper, we propose a tight wavelet frame based approach for edge-preserving denoising of DW images. Our approach (1) employs the unitary extension principle (UEP) to generate frames that are discrete analogues to differential operators of various orders; (2) introduces a very efficient method for solving an ℓ_0 denoising problem that involves only thresholding and solving a trivial inverse problem; and (3) groups DW images acquired with neighboring gradient directions for collaborative denoising. Experiments using synthetic data with noncentral chi noise and real data with repeated scans confirm that our method yields superior performance compared with denoising using state-of-the-art methods such as non-local means.

J. Zhang
School of Information and Electrical Engineering, Hunan University of Science & Technology, Xiangtan, China

Department of Radiology and Biomedical Research Imaging Center, University of North Carolina, Chapel Hill, NC, USA
e-mail: jzhang@hnust.edu.cn

G. Chen
Data Processing Center, Northwestern Polytechnical University, Xi'an, China

Department of Radiology and Biomedical Research Imaging Center, University of North Carolina, Chapel Hill, NC, USA

Y. Zhang
Department of Psychiatry & Behavioral Sciences, Stanford University, Stanford, CA, USA

B. Dong
Beijing International Center for Mathematical Research, Peking University, Beijing, China

D. Shen • P.-T. Yap (⊠)
Department of Radiology and Biomedical Research Imaging Center, University of North Carolina, Chapel Hill, NC, USA
e-mail: ptyap@med.unc.edu

© Springer International Publishing AG 2017
A. Fuster et al. (eds.), *Computational Diffusion MRI*, Mathematics and Visualization, DOI 10.1007/978-3-319-54130-3_4

49

1 Introduction

Diffusion MRI is a powerful neuroimaging technique due to its unique ability to extract microstructural information by utilizing restricted and hindered diffusion to probe compartments that are much smaller than the voxel size. One important goal of diffusion MRI is to estimate axonal orientations, tracing of which will allow one to gauge connectivity between brain regions and will provide in vivo information on white matter pathways for neuroscience studies involving development, aging, and disorders [1–5]. In order to capture orientation information, the brain has to be scanned using a range of diffusion-sensitizing gradient directions that are ideally distributed uniformly on the unit sphere.

As shown in Fig. 1, DW images that are scanned with similar gradient directions share a lot of commonalities. However, these commonalities diminish very quickly if the difference between the gradient directions increases. As can also be seen from the figure, the images are typically very noisy and can benefit greatly from denoising. Denoising performance can be improved by borrowing information between images scanned at similar gradient directions; however, images scanned at a very different direction have to be avoided in this process to reduce artifacts.

In this paper, we take advantage of the correlation between DW images scanned with neighboring gradient directions in a group ℓ_0 minimization denoising framework that is based on tight wavelet frames. The power of tight wavelet frames lies in their ability to sparsely approximate piecewise smooth functions and the existence of fast decomposition and reconstruction algorithms associated with them. In contrast, total-variation (TV) based methods are effective in restoring images that are piecewise constant, e.g., binary or cartoon-like images. They will, however, cause staircasing effects in images that are not piecewise constant [6].

Instead of the more conventional ℓ_1 regularization, which has been shown in the theory of compressed sensing [7] to produce sparse solutions, we opted to use ℓ_0 regularization. In [8], both iterative soft and hard thresholding algorithms were adopted and the latter was found to achieve better image quality. In [9], wavelet frame based ℓ_0 regularization also shows better edge-preserving quality compared

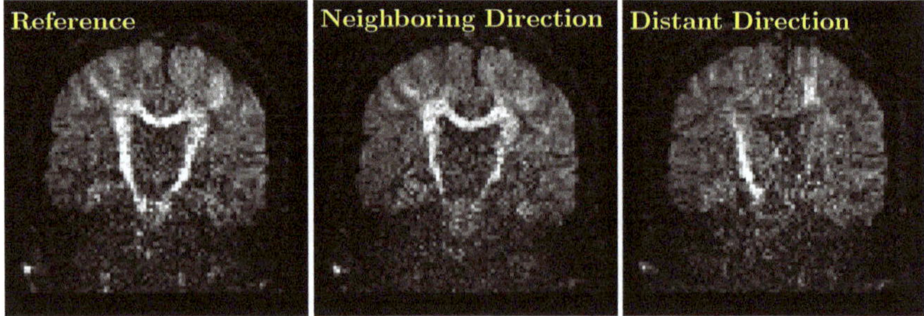

Fig. 1 Diffusion-weighted images scanned at different gradient directions. The *left and middle images* were scanned with similar gradient directions. The *right image* was scanned at a nearly perpendicular gradient direction with respect to the reference

with the conventional ℓ_1 regularization. In contrast to previous works, we propose a group version of ℓ_0 minimization to take advantage of the correlation between DW images.

Evaluations performed using synthetic data with noncentral chi noise distribution as well as real data with repeated scans indicate that the proposed method is superior to its ℓ_1 counterpart and non-local means denoising.

2 Approach

We will first provide a brief introduction to framelets, followed by details on how framelets can be incorporated into an ℓ_0 minimization framework for DWI denoising.

2.1 Tight Framelets

A system $X \subset L_2(\mathbb{R})$ is called a tight wavelet frame of $L_2(\mathbb{R})$ if

$$f = \sum_{g \in X} \langle f, g \rangle g, \quad \forall f \in L_2(\mathbb{R}), \tag{1}$$

where $\langle \cdot, \cdot \rangle$ is the inner product of $L_2(\mathbb{R})$. It is clear that an orthonormal basis is a tight frame, since the identity hold for arbitrary orthonormal bases in $L_2(\mathbb{R})$. Tight frames are generalization of orthonormal bases with greater redundancy—a property central to sparse representation and often desirable in applications such as denoising [10].

Given a set of generators $\Psi := \{\psi_1, \ldots, \psi_R\} \subset L_2(\mathbb{R}^d)$, which are desirably (anti)symmetric and compact functions, the corresponding quasi-affine system $X(\Psi)$ generated by Ψ is the collection of dilations and shifts of Ψ: $X(\Psi) = \{\psi_{l,r,k} : 1 \le r \le R; l, k \in \mathbb{Z}\}$, where $\psi_{l,n,k}$ is defined by

$$\psi_{l,r,k} := \begin{cases} 2^{\frac{l}{2}} \psi_r(2^l \cdot -k), & l \ge J, \\ 2^{\frac{l-J}{2}} \psi_r(2^l \cdot -2^{l-J}k), & l < J. \end{cases} \tag{2}$$

When $X(\Psi)$ forms an orthonormal basis of $L_2(\mathbb{R})$, $X(\Psi)$ is called an orthonormal wavelet basis. When $X(\Psi)$ forms a (tight) frame of $L_2(\mathbb{R})$, each function ψ_r, $r = 1, \ldots, R$, is called a (tight) framelet and the whole system $X(\Psi)$ is called a (tight) wavelet frame system. A tight wavelet frame is also called a Parseval frame. Note that in the literature, the affine (or wavelet) system, which corresponds to the decimated wavelet (frame) transforms, is commonly used. The quasi-affine system, introduced and analyzed in [11], corresponds to the undecimated wavelet (frame) transforms and essentially over samples the wavelet frame system starting from level $J - 1$ and downwards. In this paper, we focus on the quasi-affine system because it has been shown to work better in image restoration [12]. We set $J = 0$ and consider only $l < 0$.

The construction of Ψ is usually based on a multiresolution analysis (MRA) [12] that is generated by some refinable function ϕ with refinement mask $a_0 \in \ell_2(\mathbb{Z})$ satisfying

$$\phi = 2 \sum_{k \in \mathbb{Z}} a_0[k] \phi(2 \cdot -k). \tag{3}$$

The key is to find the masks $a_r \in \ell_2(\mathbb{Z})$ that gives

$$\psi_r = 2 \sum_{k \in \mathbb{Z}} a_r[k] \phi(2 \cdot -k), \quad r = 1, 2, \ldots, R. \tag{4}$$

The finite sequences, $a_1, \ldots, a_R$ are called wavelet frame masks, or the high pass filters of the system. The refinement mask a_0 is also known as the low pass filter. The two equations above can be combined by defining $\psi_0 := \phi$.

The unitary extension principle (UEP) [11] provides a general theory for constructing MRA-based tight wavelet frames. As long as $\{a_1, \ldots, a_R\}$ are finitely supported and their Fourier series satisfy

$$\sum_{r=0}^{R} |\widehat{a}_r(\xi)|^2 = 1 \quad \text{and} \quad \sum_{r=0}^{R} \widehat{a}_r(\xi)\overline{\widehat{a}_r(\xi + \nu)} = 0, \tag{5}$$

for all $\nu \in \{0, \pi\}$ and $\xi \in [-\pi, \pi]$, the quasi-affine system $X(\Psi)$ forms a tight frame in $L_2(\mathbb{R})$.

Consider the centered B-splines of order p, i.e.,

$$\widehat{\phi}(\xi) = e^{-ij\frac{\xi}{2}} \left(\frac{\sin(\xi/2)}{\xi/2} \right)^p, \tag{6}$$

with $j = 0$ when p is even and $j = 1$ when p is odd. The corresponding refinement mask is given as

$$\widehat{a}_0(\xi) = e^{-ij\frac{\xi}{2}} \cos^p(\xi/2), \tag{7}$$

and the p wavelet masks as

$$\widehat{a}_r(\xi) := -i^r e^{-ij\frac{\xi}{2}} \sqrt{\binom{p}{r}} \sin^r(\xi/2) \cos^{p-r}(\xi/2), \quad r = 1, 2, \ldots, p. \tag{8}$$

It is straightforward to show that the UEP conditions (5) are satisfied. Wavelet frame masks for $p = 1, 2, 4$ are shown in Table 1. It is worth noting that these masks correspond to differential operators of various orders. For example, for piecewise

Table 1 Wavelet frame masks

Piecewise constant, $p = 1$	Piecewise linear, $p = 2$	Piecewise cubic, $p = 4$
$a_0 = \frac{1}{2}[1, 1]$	$a_0 = \frac{1}{4}[1, 2, 1]$	$a_0 = \frac{1}{16}[1, 4, 6, 4, 1]$
$a_1 = \frac{1}{2}[1, -1]$	$a_1 = \frac{1}{4}[-1, 2, -1]$	$a_1 = \frac{1}{16}[1, -4, 6, -4, 1]$
	$a_2 = \frac{\sqrt{2}}{4}[1, 0, -1]$	$a_2 = \frac{1}{8}[-1, 2, 0, -2, 1]$
		$a_3 = \frac{\sqrt{6}}{16}[1, 0, -2, 0, 1]$
		$a_4 = \frac{1}{8}[-1, -2, 0, 2, 1]$

linear B-spline, the masks a_1 and a_2 correspond to the first order and second order difference operators respectively up to a scaling factor.

When a tight wavelet frame is used, the given data is considered to be sampled as a local average $u[k] = \langle f, \phi(\cdot - k) \rangle$. Noting that [12]

$$\langle f, \psi_{l-1,r,k} \rangle = \sum_{k' \in \mathbb{Z}} a_{l,r}[k'] \langle f, \psi_{l,0,k+k'} \rangle, \tag{9}$$

where the dilated sequence is defined as

$$a_{l,r}[k] = \begin{cases} a_r[2^l k], & k \in 2^{-l}\mathbb{Z}, \\ 0, & k \notin 2^{-l}\mathbb{Z}, \end{cases} \tag{10}$$

the decomposition and reconstruction down to level $-L$ [12], i.e.,

$$\mathcal{P}_0 f = \mathcal{P}_{-L} f + \sum_{r=1}^{R} \sum_{j=-L}^{-1} \sum_{k \in \mathbb{Z}} \langle f, \psi_{r,j,k} \rangle \psi_{r,j,k}, \tag{11}$$

where

$$\mathcal{P}_l f = \sum_{r=1}^{R} \sum_{j<l} \sum_{k \in \mathbb{Z}} \langle f, \psi_{r,j,k} \rangle \psi_{r,j,k}, \tag{12}$$

can be realized with convolution using the masks. We denote by W the L-level framelet decomposition, i.e.,

$$Wu = (\ldots, W_{l,r} u, \ldots)^{\top} \quad \text{for} \quad (l, r) \in \mathcal{B}_L, \tag{13}$$

with $\mathcal{B}_L := \{(1, 1), (1, 2), \ldots, (1, R), (2, 1), \ldots, (L, R)\} \cup \{(L, 0)\}$, where the level l and band r framelet decomposition is given by

$$W_{l,r} u = a_{-l,r} \otimes a_{-l+1,0} \otimes \cdots \otimes a_{0,0} \otimes u. \tag{14}$$

If we use $W^{\top}$ to denote the framelet reconstruction, we have $W^{\top} W = I$, i.e., $u = W^{\top} W u$.

Given a 1-dimensional framelet system for $L_2(\mathbb{R})$, the d-dimensional tight wavelet frame system for $L_2(\mathbb{R}^d)$ can be easily constructed by using tensor products of 1-dimensional framelets [12].

2.2 Problem Formulation

Given a vector-valued image f of an arbitrary dimension with pixel $i \in \{1, \ldots, N\}$ consisting of vector $f_i \in \mathbb{R}^M$, we are interested in restoring its denoised counterpart u by solving the following problem:

$$\min_u \left\{ \phi(u) = \|u - f\|_2^2 + \sum_{i,g,l,r} \lambda_{g,l,r} \left\| \sqrt{\sum_m w_{g,m}^2 \|(W_{l,r} u^{(m)})_i\|_2^2} \right\|_0 \right\}. \tag{15}$$

The regularization term is in fact a sum of G regularization terms, each of which grouping a set of images. The gth grouping (with associated tuning parameter $\lambda_{g,l,r}$), where $g = \{1, 2, \ldots, G\}$, is defined according to a set of weights $\{w_{g,m}\}$, where $m \in \{1, \ldots, M\}$. Channels with $w_{g,m} \neq 0$ are included in the grouping and their weighted framelet coefficients are jointly considered via ℓ_2-norm for penalization. The different groupings can possibly overlap, implying each image can be at the same time considered in different groups. This is in similar spirit as the overlapped group LASSO [13]. We set $\lambda_{g,l,r} = \lambda \left(\sum_m w_{g,m}^2\right)^{\frac{1}{2}}$ if $l, r \neq 0$ or $\lambda_{g,l,r} = 0$ if otherwise. Here λ is a constant that can be set independent of the weights.

2.3 Optimization

Problem (15) can be solved effectively using penalty decomposition (PD) [14]. Defining auxiliary variables $(v_{g,m,l,r})_i := w_{g,m}(W_{l,r} u^{(m)})_i$, this amounts to minimizing the following objective function with respect to u and $v := \{v_{g,m,l,r}\}$:

$$L_\mu(u, v) = \|u - f\|_2^2 + \sum_{i,g,l,r} \lambda_{g,l,r} \left\| \sqrt{\sum_m \|(v_{g,m,l,r})_i\|_2^2} \right\|_0$$

$$+ \frac{\mu}{2} \sum_{i,g,m,l,r} \|w_{g,m}(W_{l,r} u^{(m)})_i - (v_{g,m,l,r})_i\|_2^2. \tag{16}$$

In PD, we (1) alternate between solving for u and v using block coordinate descent (BCD). Once this converges, we (2) increase $\mu > 0$ by a multiplicative factor that is greater than 1 and repeat step (1). This is repeated until increasing μ does not result in further changes to the solution [14].

First Subproblem

We solve for v in the first problem, i.e., $\min_v L_\mu(u, v)$. This is a group ℓ_0 problem and the solution can be obtained via hard-thresholding:

$$(v_{g,m,l,r})_i = \begin{cases} w_{g,m}(W_{l,r}u^{(m)})_i, & (h_{g,l,r})_i \geq \frac{2\lambda_{g,l,r}}{\mu} \\ 0, & \text{otherwise,} \end{cases} \tag{17}$$

where

$$(h_{g,l,r})_i = \sum_{m'} \|w_{g,m'}(W_{l,r}u^{(m')})_i\|_2^2. \tag{18}$$

An ℓ_1 version of the algorithm can be obtained by using soft-thresholding instead.

Second Subproblem

By taking the partial derivative with respect to $u^{(m)}$, the solution to the second subproblem, i.e., $\min_u L_\mu(u, v)$, is for each m

$$\left(I + \frac{\mu}{2} \sum_{g,l,r} w_{g,m}^2 W_{l,r}^\top W_{l,r}\right) u^{(m)} = f^{(m)} + \frac{\mu}{2} \sum_{g,l,r} w_{g,m} W_{l,r}^\top v_{g,m,l,r}, \tag{19}$$

where we have dropped the subscript i for notation simplicity. Note that since we have $\sum_{l,r} W_{l,r}^\top W_{l,r} = I$, the the problem can be simplified to become

$$\left(1 + \frac{\mu}{2} \sum_g w_{g,m}^2\right) u^{(m)} = f^{(m)} + \frac{\mu}{2} \sum_{g,l,r} w_{g,m} W_{l,r}^\top v_{g,m,l,r}. \tag{20}$$

Solving the above equation for $u^{(m)}$ is trivial and involves only simple division.

2.4 Setting the Weights

In setting the weights $\{w_{g,m}\}$, we note that the weights should decay with the dissimilarity between gradient directions associated with a pair of diffusion-weighted images. To reflect this, we let $G = M$ and set for $g, m \in \{1, \ldots, M\}$ $w_{g,m} = e^{\kappa[(v_m^\top v_g)^2 - 1]}$ if $|v_m^\top v_g| < \cos(\theta)$ or 0 otherwise, where $\kappa \geq 0$ is a parameter that determines the rate of decay of the weight. The exponential function is in fact modified from the probability density function of the Watson distribution [15] with concentration parameter κ. Essentially, this implies that for the gth diffusion-weighted image acquired at gradient direction v_g, there is a corresponding group of images with associated weights $\{w_{g,m}\}$. The weight is maximal at $w_{g,g} = 1$ and is attenuated when $m \neq g$. To reduce computation costs, weights of images scanned at gradient directions deviating more than θ from v_g are set to 0, and the respective images are hence discarded from the group. We set $\theta = 30°$.

3　Experimental Results

In all experiments, we used the piecewise linear tight wavelet frame and set the level L to 2. The optimal λ was chosen based on grid search.

3.1　Datasets

Synthetic Data A synthetic dataset of a spiral was generated for quantitative evaluation. The parameters used for generating synthetic data simulation were consistent with the real data described next: $b = 2000 \, \text{s/mm}^2$, 48 gradient directions, $64 \times 64 \times 16$ voxels with resolution $2 \times 2 \times 2 \, \text{mm}^3$. Three levels of 32-channel noncentral Chi noise [16] was added: $\sigma = 5$, 7.5, and 10, corresponding to SNR $= 30, 20, 10$ with respect to the white matter non-diffusion-weighted signal.

Real Data The real datasets were acquired using Siemens 3T TRIO MR scanner with the same gradient directions and b-value as the synthetic dataset. The imaging protocol is as follows: 128×96 imaging matrix, voxel size of $2 \times 2 \times 2 \, \text{mm}^3$, TE=97 ms, TR=11,300 ms. Imaging acquisition was repeatedly performed on the same subject for eight times. We averaged the eight sets of DW images and removed the noncentral chi noise bias to obtain the ground truth for evaluation.

3.2　Results

The numerical results for the synthetic data, shown in Fig. 2, indicate that the proposed ℓ_0 framelet denoising method gives the best performance for all noise levels, showing improvements over ℓ_1 framelet denoising and the non-local means (NLM) algorithm [17]. The DW images, shown in Fig. 3, indicate that both ℓ_1 and ℓ_0 give sharper edges compared with NLM. Noise, however, is not totally removed for the case of ℓ_1 denoising. Only ℓ_0 denoising is able to effectively remove noise and preserve edges. Note that, for both synthetic and real data, noncentral chi bias was removed using the method described in [16]. The best tuning parameters for both ℓ_1 and ℓ_0 were selected based on grid search.

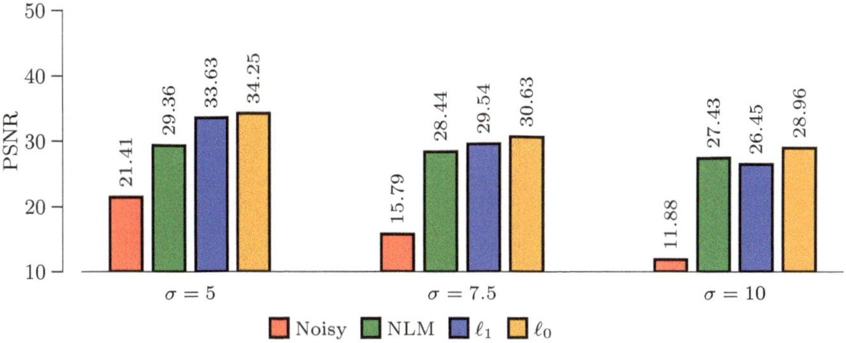

Fig. 2 Performance comparison between NLM and our method using synthetic data

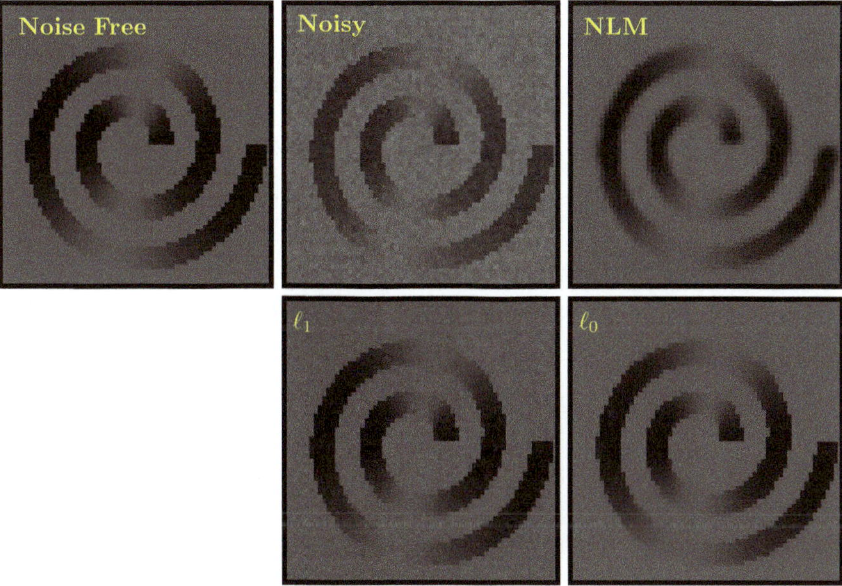

Fig. 3 Comparison of denoised DW images given by different methods ($\sigma = 5$)

For the real data, we used the average image as the ground truth for PSNR computation. The results, shown in Fig. 4, are consistent with Fig. 2, indicating that ℓ_0 gives the best performance. The visual results in Fig. 5 indicate that the results given by ℓ_0 is closest to the ground truth. In contrast, NLM over-smooths the image and edge information is hence lost.

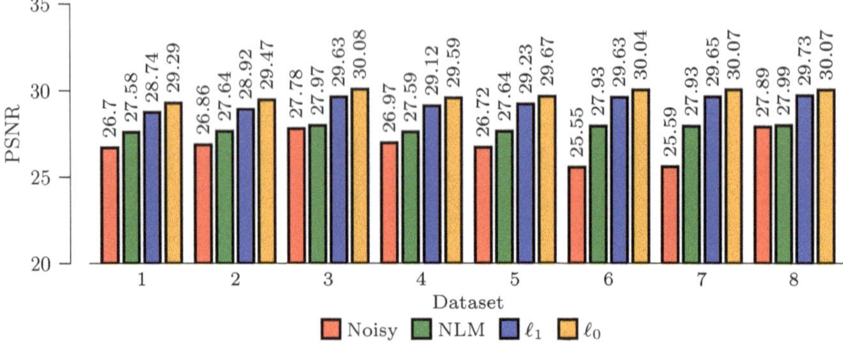

Fig. 4 Performance comparison between NLM and our method using real data

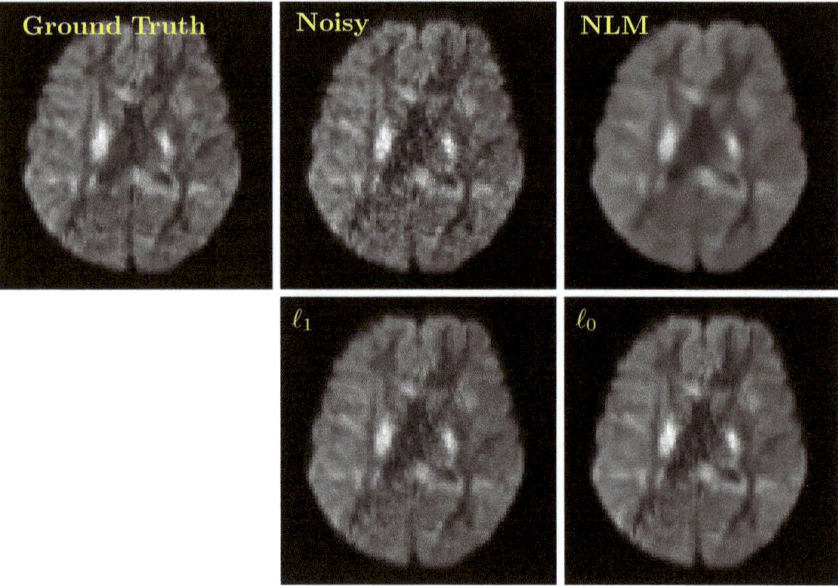

Fig. 5 Comparison of denoised DW images using the real data

4   Conclusion

In this paper, we have proposed a denoising method by using multi-channel framelet grouped iterative hard thresholding, which not only takes advantage of inter-image correlations but yields good edge-preserving property. Experiments on synthetic data with noncentral chi noise and real data with repeated scans confirm that the proposed method outperforms state-of-the-art methods such as non-local means.

Acknowledgements This work was supported in part by NIH grants (NS093842, EB006733, EB009634, AG041721, MH100217, and AA012388) and Hunan Provincial Education Department grant (15A066).

References

1. Yap, P.T., Fan, Y., Chen, Y., Gilmore, J., Lin, W., Shen, D.: Development trends of white matter connectivity in the first years of life. PLoS ONE **6**(9), e24678 (2011)
2. Wee, C.Y., Yap, P.T., Li, W., Denny, K., Brownyke, J., Potter, G., Welsh-Bohmer, K., Wang, L., Shen, D.: Enriched white-matter connectivity networks for accurate identification of MCI patients. NeuroImage **54**(3), 1812–1822 (2011)
3. Wee, C.Y., Yap, P.T., Zhang, D., Denny, K., Browndyke, J.N., Potter, G.G., Welsh-Bohmer, K.A., Wang, L., Shen, D.: Identification of MCI individuals using structural and functional connectivity networks. NeuroImage **59**(3), 2045–2056 (2012)
4. Wee, C.Y., Wang, L., Shi, F., Yap, P.T., Shen, D.: Diagnosis of autism spectrum disorders using regional and interregional morphological features. Hum. Brain Mapp. **35**(7), 3414–3430 (2014)
5. Jin, Y., Wee, C.Y., Shi, F., Thung, K.H., Yap, P.T., Shen, D.: Identification of infants at high-risk for autism spectrum disorder using multi-parameter multi-scale white matter connectivity networks. Hum. Brain Mapp. **36**(12), 4880–4896 (2015)
6. Ring, W.: Structural properties of solutions to total variation regularization problems. Mathematical Modelling and Numerical Analysis **34**, 799–810 (2000)
7. Candès, E.J., Romberg, J., Tao, T.: Robust uncertainty principles: exact signal reconstruction from highly incomplete frequency information. IEEE Trans. Inf. Theory **52**(2), 489–509 (2006)
8. Chan, R.H., Chan, T.F., Shen, L., Shen, Z.: Wavelet algorithms for high-resolution image reconstruction. SIAM J. Sci. Comput. **24**(4), 1408–1432 (2003)
9. Zhang, Y., Dong, B., Lu, Z.: ℓ_0 minimization for wavelet frame based image restoration. Math. Comput. **82**, 995–1015 (2013)
10. Mallat, S.: A Wavelet Tour of Signal Processing: The Sparse Way, 3rd edn. Academic, New York (2008)
11. Ron, A., Shen, Z.: Affine systems in $l_2(\mathbb{R}^d)$: the analysis of the analysis operator. J. Funct. Anal. **148**(2), 408–447 (1997)
12. Dong, B., Shen, Z.: MRA-based wavelet frames and applications. In: IAS Lecture Notes Series. Summer Program on "The Mathematics of Image Processing". Park City Mathematics Institute, Salt Lake City (2010)
13. Jacob, L., Obozinski, G., Vert, J.P.: Group lasso with overlap and graph lasso. In: International Conference on Machine Learning (2009)
14. Lu, Z., Zhang, Y.: Sparse approximation via penalty decomposition methods. SIAM J. Optim. **23**(4), 2448–2478 (2013)
15. Schwartzman, A., Dougherty, R.F., Taylor, J.E.: False discovery rate analysis of brain diffusion direction maps. Ann. Appl. Stat. **2**(1), 153–175 (2008)
16. Koay, C.G., Özarslan, E., Basser, P.J.: A signal transformational framework for breaking the noise floor and its applications in MRI. J. Magn. Reson. **197**(2), 108–119 (2009)
17. Coupé, P., Yger, P., Prima, S., Hellier, P., Kervrann, C., Barillot, C.: An optimized blockwise nonlocal means denoising filter for 3-D magnetic resonance images. IEEE Trans. Med. Imaging **27**(4), 425–441 (2008)

Diffusion MRI Signal Augmentation: From Single Shell to Multi Shell with Deep Learning

Simon Koppers, Christoph Haarburger, and Dorit Merhof

Abstract High Angular Resolution Diffusion Imaging makes it possible to capture information about the course and location of complex fiber structures in the human brain. Ideally, multi-shell sampling would be applied, which however increases the acquisition time. Therefore, multi-shell acquisitions are considered infeasible for practical use in a clinical setting. In this work, we present a data-driven approach that is able to augment single-shell signals to multi-shell signals based on Deep Neural Networks and Spherical Harmonics. The proposed concept is evaluated on synthetic data to investigate the impact of noise and number of gradients. Moreover, it is evaluated on human brain data from the Human Connectome Project, comprising 100 scans from different subjects. The proposed approach makes it possible to drastically reduce the signal acquisition time and performs equally well on both synthetic as well as real human brain data.

1 Introduction

Diffusion Magnetic Resonance Imaging (dMRI) is a technique that non-invasively offers insight into the course and location of neural pathways in the human brain. In order to employ dMRI in a clinical setting, Diffusion Tensor Imaging (DTI) [2] marked the first breakthrough, modeling the diffusion signal with a single Gaussian tensor. In order to fit the DTI model, images for at least six gradient directions have to be acquired. However, assuming the diffusion to be Gaussian is not generally applicable. Consequently, DTI fails to capture more complex fiber structures such as crossing, fanning and kissing fibers, which occur in 60% to 90% of the white matter voxels of the human brain [11].

In order to overcome the limitations of DTI, High Angular Resolution Diffusion Imaging (HARDI) has been proposed [15]. In case of HARDI acquisitions, images

---

Simon Koppers and Christoph Haarburger contributed equally to this work.

S. Koppers (✉) • C. Haarburger • D. Merhof
Institute of Imaging & Computer Vision, RWTH Aachen University, Aachen, Germany
e-mail: Simon.Koppers@lfb.rwth-aachen.de

A. Fuster et al. (eds.), *Computational Diffusion MRI*, Mathematics and Visualization, DOI 10.1007/978-3-319-54130-3_5

61

for more than 30 and up to several hundred gradient directions are acquired to better capture complex fiber configurations, which results in much higher acquisition times, though.

Moreover, it has been shown that fitting Multi-Tensor-Models based on dMRI signals acquired with a single diffusion weighting constant b, also known as single shell acquisitions, is an underdetermined problem [13]. Measuring the signal on several shells though additionally increases the scan time.

Despite the fact that HARDI offers a higher accuracy, DTI can still be considered as clinical standard as HARDI acquisitions are infeasible in clinical practice. Therefore, reducing the number of necessary gradient directions required for fitting HARDI models is a highly desirable asset that is addressed in this work by formulating the mapping between shells as a regression problem.

In general, classification with Deep Neural Networks (DNNs) has become very popular recently, achieving remarkable results in image classification, speech recognition and many other domains. While neural networks have been known for decades, the novel interest in this domain is due to several advances such as efficient training on GPUs, which makes it possible to use well-known training algorithms in networks with many hidden layers that are referred to as *deep*. Apart from [1, 9], where a Diffusion Kurtosis Tensor is fitted to a signal with less than the required amount of gradient directions, the application of machine learning and especially Deep Learning in Diffusion Imaging is still an open field of research.

According to [6], Spherical Harmonics (SH) adequately represent dMRI signals in a non-sparse and compact way. The signals on several shells of HARDI acquisitions are related by a non-linear transfer function [13, 15].

However, so far there are only a few approaches available for predicting another shells without any prior knowledge about this individual shell [12].

Motivated by the Universal Approximation Theorem (UAT) [4], we propose an approach based on DNNs to learn this non-linear mapping, which makes it possible to *augment* existing shells by predicting further shells from those that have actually been acquired. This novel approach is compared to the Mean Apparent Propagator (MAP) algorithm, which is considered to be one of the newest state-of-the-art algorithms [12].

In order to ensure the generalization of the non-linear mapping, we utilize data from 100 subjects of the Human Connectome Project (HCP) for training and testing. Additionally, the influence of SNR and number of gradients per shell is investigated on synthetic data.

2 Material

For evaluation purposes, the following datasets are employed:

The first dataset is based on synthetic diffusion-weighted data for 10, 20, 40 and 80 gradient directions and $b = 3000\,\mathrm{s/mm^2}$. It is simulated for different Rician noise levels (SNR $= \frac{1}{\sigma} = \{10, \infty\}$), which represent MRI scans with a high noise level and no noise, respectively. The signal is simulated based on the Multi-Tensor Model [15]. Tensor eigenvalues are set according to real DW-MRI data [3], while the number of compartments is chosen randomly between 1 and 3. Corresponding volume fractions range from 0.2 to 1 and sum up to 1. The training set consists of 40,000 voxels and the test set of 10,000 voxels for which the signal was simulated for each gradient set and noise level.

The second dataset contains data from 100 different uncorrelated healthy subjects from the Human Connectome Project (HCP). From each subject, 5000 white matter voxels were extracted randomly, resulting in 500,000 voxels in total. All three shells ($b = \{1000, 2000, 3000\}$ s/mm^2), with 90 gradient directions each, are used in this work, being either training data or target data for prediction. The dataset is split into a training set containing 450,000 voxels from 90 subjects and a test set consisting of 50,000 voxels from 10 subjects, which ensures that each subject is included in either the training or the test set. In order to create a subsampled dataset containing less, but still equidistantly distributed gradient directions, SH are fitted to the signal and subsampled by a new gradient set with 15 gradient directions. 15 gradient directions are chosen because it is the minimum number of measurements that are required to fit SH of order 4, if coefficients are calculated through matrix inversion [6].

3   Neural Network for Regression

Using DNNs for predicting the signal on an additional shell is motivated by the UAT, which states that a feed forward neural network with one hidden layer and a finite number of neurons can approximate any continuous function with arbitrary accuracy [4, 10]. However, the UAT is rather related to function *representation* with neural networks instead of learnability in practice. In order to ensure that the network parameters (i.e. weights) can be learned from training data, a sufficiently high number of training samples is required. For this reason, a large dataset consisting of 100 subjects from the HCP database is employed in the learning process.

The proposed DNN is designed to predict spherical harmonics coefficients representing a HARDI signal on one shell from HARDI signals on one or more other shells of the same voxel.

3.1   *Spherical Harmonics*

Spherical harmonics (SH) are an orthonormal basis for spherical functions that can represent dMRI signals in a compact manner. In this work, we utilize the modified SH basis as defined in [6], which restricts the SH basis to be real and symmetric. The dMRI signal $\mathbf{S}$ in matrix form can be written as a linear combination of the modified SH basis $\mathbf{B}$ and a SH coefficient vector $\mathbf{C}$, i.e. $\mathbf{S} = \mathbf{BC}$. The SH coefficients $\mathbf{C}$ are

Table 1 Topology of the neural network

#	Type	Parameters
1	Input	#neurons = #gradients
2	Fully-connected	100 neurons
3	ReLU	–
4	Fully-connected	10 neurons
5	ReLU	–
6	Fully-connected	200 neurons
7	Output	#neurons = #SH coefficients

calculated for every shell using a least-squares fit with regularization

$$\mathbf{C} = (\mathbf{B}^T \mathbf{B} + \lambda \mathbf{L})^{-1} \mathbf{B}^T \mathbf{S} \tag{1}$$

with $\lambda = 0.006$ as explained in [6].

3.2 Deep Neural Network

The DNN that predicts SH coefficients consists of an input layer which is fed with dMRI signals, three hidden layers and an output layer comprising one neuron for every SH coefficient. In contrast to the original formulation of the UAT, we incorporate several hidden layers instead of one hidden layer only, as more recent research related to deep learning suggests that deep networks represent functions more efficiently than shallow networks [5]. The activation functions between hidden layers are Rectifying Linear Units (ReLUs) with $f(x) = \max(0, x)$. With SH coefficients c_i for the corresponding shell and the predicted SH coefficients $\tilde{c}_i$ as the DNN output, we choose the loss function to be the mean squared error

$$L = \frac{1}{N} \sum_{i=1}^{N} (\tilde{c}_i - c_i)^2, \tag{2}$$

where N is the number of SH coefficients. The loss is minimized with the Adagrad optimizer [7], which is an advancement of stochastic gradient descent with an adaptive learning rate. An overview of the network's topology is provided in Table 1.

4 Results

All computations are carried out on a PC with 3.4 GHz Intel i5-4670 processor, 32 GB RAM and NVIDIA GeForce GTX 980 Ti GPU. The DNN training and prediction is implemented in TensorFlow and performed on the GPU.

In order to evaluate the proposed approach, the following experiments are performed. The impact of noise and the reduction of acquired gradient directions is assessed on synthetic data, while the prediction of other shells can only be evaluated on real human data. The DNN is compared to the MAP algorithm [12] (implemented in Dipy [8]), which represents the diffusion signal analytically utilizing a series expansion of basis functions that describe different diffusion geometries. The corresponding radial order is chosen to be $s = 2$. To confirm this setting, a radial moment order of $s \geq 4$ was evaluated and discarded due to instability issues if only few gradient directions are available.

Prediction accuracy is quantified with the Normalized Mean Square Error (NMSE), which is defined by

$$
\text{NMSE} = \frac{\left\| S_{\text{true}} - S_{\text{pred}} \right\|_2^2}{\left\| S_{\text{true}} \right\|_2^2},
\tag{3}
$$

where S_{true} represents the ground truth signal vector and S_{pred} is the predicted signal vector based on the same gradient scheme. The number of input neurons of the DNN is adjusted according to the number of gradient directions, while the SH order is chosen to be 8, which results in 45 output neurons.

4.1 Impact of Noise and Number of Gradients

The resulting impact of noise for a varying number of gradient directions is quantitatively assessed in Fig. 1. In case of high noise, the DNN achieves a slightly higher NMSE if many gradient directions are acquired. Moreover, the resulting

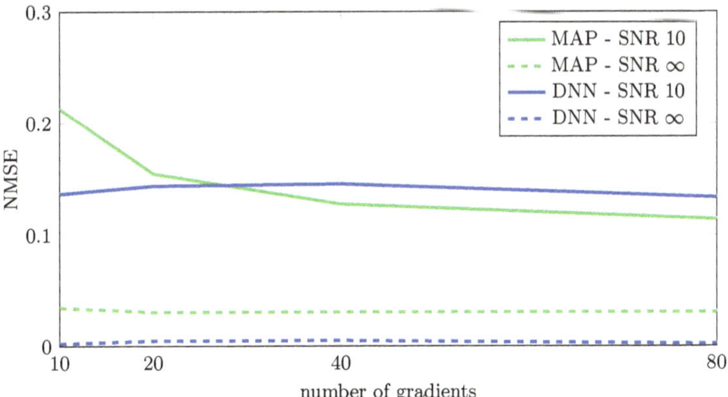

Fig. 1 Resulting NMSE of the MAP approach and the DNN for 10, 20, 40 and 80 gradient directions, SNR={10, ∞}

NMSE increases for the MAP algorithm if only few gradient directions are available, but remains rather stable in case of the DNN.

In addition, it can be seen that both algorithms achieve a low NMSE if no noise is added to the signal. Notably, the DNN achieves a lower NMSE for every gradient set.

4.2 Prediction of Another Shell

In order to evaluate the performance of predicting other shells, Tables 2 and 3 contain the resulting prediction NMSEs for every combination of input and target shells that can be generated based on the HCP dataset utilizing 15 and 90 gradient directions. DNN training is performed for each combination individually. Moreover, the resulting shell distance d between two shells is provided.

Table 2 Average NMSE for predicting the signal utilizing the DNN and the MAP approach based on 90 gradient directions on each shell

Input shell	Target shells (90 gradients)								
	Predicted 1st Shell			Predicted 2nd Shell			Predicted 3rd Shell		
	DNN	MAP	d	DNN	MAP	d	DNN	MAP	d
1st shell	1.03%	1.04%	0%	3.49%	18.06%	38.13%	5.63%	27.90%	66.21%
2nd shell	2.01%	8.08%	18.50%	2.28%	2.36%	0%	4.39%	17.81%	21.68%
3rd shell	3.58%	24.57%	33.41%	3.43%	25.99%	9.73%	3.45%	4.55%	0%
1st + 2nd shell	–	–	–	–	–	–	4.10%	14.97%	–
1st + 3rd shell	–	–	–	2.69%	16.91%	–	–	–	–
2nd + 3rd shell	1.53%	9.87%	–	–	–	–	–	–	–

In addition, d represents the NMSE between two shells without any prediction, which is comparable to a distance between two shells

Table 3 Average NMSE for predicting the signal utilizing the DNN and the MAP approach based on 15 gradient directions on each shell

Input shell	Target shells (15 gradients)								
	Predicted 1st shell			Predicted 2nd shell			Predicted 3rd shell		
	DNN	MAP	d	DNN	MAP	d	DNN	MAP	d
1st shell	1.18%	1.19%	0%	3.67%	18.32%	38.13%	5.98%	28.10%	66.21%
2nd shell	2.15%	8.13%	18.50%	2.58%	2.64%	0%	4.73%	18.09%	21.68%
3rd shell	3.89%	24.66%	33.41%	3.74%	26.11%	9.73%	3.95%	4.98%	0%
1st + 2nd shell	–	–	–	–	–	–	4.27%	20.70%	–
1st + 3rd shell	–	–	–	2.87%	15.46%	–	–	–	–
2nd + 3rd shell	1.72%	9.37%	–	–	–	–	–	–	–

In addition, d represents the NMSE between two shells without any prediction, which is comparable to a distance between two shells

In addition, it should be noted that a prediction of the third shell will always result in a higher NMSE than for the first shell, due to a smaller denominator (see Eq. (3)), which is reflected in the d.

Considering both tables, it can be seen that both algorithms result in similar NMSEs for 90 as well as for 15 gradient directions. Both algorithms achieve their lowest NMSE if the fit is performed from a input to the same target shell.

If a shell is augmented to predict another shell, the DNN generally achieves a more stable fit than the MAP algorithm. The inaccuracy grows with increasing shell distance between input and target shell. Adding a second shell to the input (i.e. predicting a third shell from two input shells) seems to stabilize the MAP algorithm and decreases the NMSE of the resulting augmented shell. Nevertheless, the DNN still achieves a much lower NMSE. In order to evaluate the results in more detail, Figure 2 exemplifies the results using the 3rd shell as target shell for 90 gradient directions. Excluding the 3rd shell as input, the MAP algorithm performs best utilizing two shells as input. In addition, its performance increases as shell

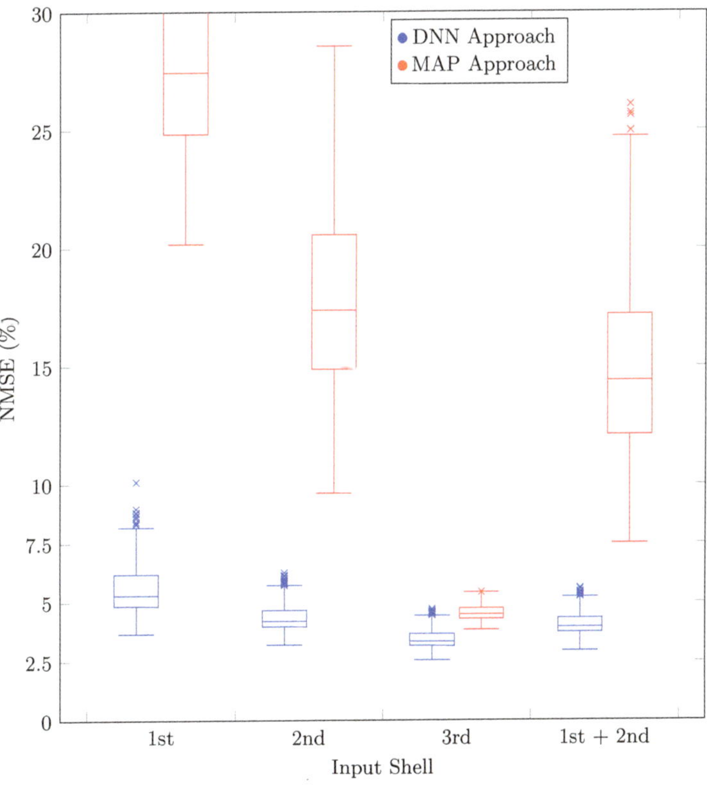

Fig. 2 Resulting NMSE of the MAP approach and the DNN utilizing only the 3rd shell as target shell presented as a boxplot for 90 gradient directions

distance between input and target shell decreases. The DNN shows similar results, but outperforms the MAP for each input scenario.

5 Discussion

For the synthetic dataset, Fig. 1 suggests that the performance of both algorithms strongly depends on the SNR, while the number of gradient directions exerts little influence. Moreover, the MAP approach outperforms DNN in terms of the NMSE for more than 30 gradient directions and a noisy signal, while its NMSE increases for less gradients. In case of noise the DNN outperforms the MAP approach for every number of gradient directions. This qualifies the DNN signal for describing a single shell, even for settings with a limited number of gradient directions and in case of high noise.

Considering the resulting real data NMSEs for the same input and target shell in Tables 2 and 3, the same effect can be seen since both algorithms achieve similarly good results, i.e. the performance is hardly influenced by the number of gradient directions. Comparing the resulting augmented data, it can be observed that the results of both algorithms diverge as the shell distance increases. In those cases, the MAP approach results in a much higher NMSE than the DNN utilizing 90 as well as 15 gradient directions. Moreover, the MAP approach completely fails in order to predict the 2nd shell using the 3rd shell as input. In this case the NMSE is higher than the NMSE of d without any prediction. Using two shells as input increases the performance of the DNN for each combination, while the MAP algorithm only improves if the 1st + 3rd shell or the 2nd + 3rd shell are used as input shell in case of 90 gradient directions. Though, the MAP approach only increases its performance in order to predict the 2nd shell given the 1st + 3rd shell as input, if only 15 gradient directions are available.

A similar behavior can be seen in Fig. 2. The variance is low if the input and target shell are identical and increases as the distance between two shells grows. As before, the MAP algorithm stabilizes if more shells are used as input since the variance, median and quantile NMSE decrease. However, only three different shells are available in the used HCP dataset.

Overall, it should be noted that only a subset of 15 gradient directions is needed for augmentation as the NMSE is only slightly higher, which reduces the scan time to $\frac{1}{6}$. For example, from data acquired with 15 gradient directions on the 2nd shell, the 1st shell can be predicted with only 2.01% NMSE while the required scan time is theoretically reduced to 50% or to 8.33% considering the original dataset with 90 gradient directions, respectively.

In terms of prediction speed, the DNN can predict one shell per voxel with $\approx 23{,}000$ voxels per second, whereas the MAP algorithm achieves a maximum rate of 150 voxels per second. Though, it should be considered that the MAP algorithm utilizes the CPU, while the DNN is based on a GPU implementation. However, the augmentation using the DNN requires less than one minute for a whole brain scan.

A limitation of this work is that the prediction is only evaluated on the scanner type that was used in the HCP. An augmentation on data from different scanners may require training with a dataset from this specific scanner. Another approach presented in [14] is to simulate individual synthetic data for a specific scan and to re-train the network utilizing the synthetic dataset. Whether or to which extent scanner-dependency is an issue will be investigated in future work.

6 Conclusion

We presented a method to augment single-shell dMRI signals to predict additional shells via a spherical harmonics representation based on a DNN. Our evaluation on both synthetic and human data shows that this augmentation is hardly influenced by the number of gradient directions, but rather depends on the noise level. The presented approach constitutes a first step towards multi-shell HARDI acquisitions in clinical scenarios.

Acknowledgements This work was supported by the International Research Training Group (IRTG 2150) of the German Research Foundation (DFG).

Data were provided by the Human Connectome Project, WU-Minn Consortium (Principal Investigators: David Van Essen and Kamil Ugurbil; 1U54 MH091657) funded by the 16 NIH Institutes and Centers that support the NIH Blueprint for Neuroscience Research; and by the McDonnell Center for Systems Neuroscience at Washington University.

References

1. Alexander, D.C., Zikic, D., Zhang, J., Zhang, H., Criminisi, A.: Image Quality Transfer via Random Forest Regression: Applications in Diffusion MRI, pp. 225–232. Springer International Publishing, Cham (2014)
2. Basser, P.J., Mattiello, J., LeBihan, D.: MR diffusion tensor spectroscopy and imaging. Biophys. J. **66**(1), 259 (1994)
3. Canales-Rodríguez, E.J., Melie-García, L., Iturria-Medina, Y.: Mathematical description of q-space in spherical coordinates: exact q-ball imaging. Magn. Reson. Med. **61**(6), 1350–1367 (2009)
4. Cybenko, G.: Approximation by superpositions of a sigmoidal function. Math. Control Signals Syst. **2**(4), 303–314 (1989)
5. Delalleau, O., Bengio, Y.: Shallow vs. deep sum-product networks. In: Shawe-Taylor, J., Zemel, R.S., Bartlett, P.L., Pereira, F., Weinberger, K.Q. (eds.) Advances in Neural Information Processing Systems, vol. 24, pp. 666–674. Curran Associates, Northampton, MA (2011)
6. Descoteaux, M., Angelino, E., Fitzgibbons, S., Deriche, R.: Apparent diffusion coefficients from high angular resolution diffusion imaging: estimation and applications. Magn. Reson. Med. **56**(2), 395–410 (2006)
7. Duchi, J., Hazan, E., Singer, Y.: Adaptive subgradient methods for online learning and stochastic optimization. J. Mach. Learn. Res. **12**, 2121–2159 (2011)
8. Garyfallidis, E., Brett, M., Amirbekian, B., Rokem, A., Van Der Walt, S., Descoteaux, M., Nimmo-Smith, I.: Dipy, a library for the analysis of diffusion mri data. Front. Neuroinform. **8**(8), 8 (2014)

9. Golkov, V., Dosovitskiy, A., Sämann, P., Sperl, J.I., Sprenger, T., Czisch, M., Menzel, M.I., Gómez, P.A., Haase, A., Brox, T., Cremers, D.: q-Space Deep Learning for Twelve-Fold Shorter and Model-Free Diffusion MRI Scans, pp. 37–44. Springer International Publishing, Cham (2015)
10. Hornik, K.: Approximation capabilities of multilayer feedforward networks. Neural Netw. **4**(2), 251–257 (1991)
11. Jeurissen, B., Leemans, A., Tournier, J.D., Jones, D.K., Sijbers, J.: Investigating the prevalence of complex fiber configurations in white matter tissue with diffusion magnetic resonance imaging. Hum. Brain. Mapp. **34**(11), 2747–2766 (2013)
12. Özarslan, E., Koay, C.G., Shepherd, T.M., Komlosh, M.E., İrfanoğlu, M.O., Pierpaoli, C., Basser, P.J.: Mean apparent propagator (MAP) MRI: a novel diffusion imaging method for mapping tissue microstructure. NeuroImage **78**, 16–32 (2013)
13. Scherrer, B., Warfield, S.K.: Why multiple b-values are required for multi-tensor models. Evaluation with a constrained log-euclidean model. In: Proceedings of IEEE International Symposium on Biomedical Imaging, pp. 1389–1392. IEEE, New York (2010)
14. Schultz, T.: Learning a Reliable Estimate of the Number of Fiber Directions in Diffusion MRI, pp. 493–500. Springer, Berlin, Heidelberg (2012)
15. Tuch, D.S., Reese, T.G., Wiegell, M.R., Makris, N., Belliveau, J.W., Wedeen, V.J.: High angular resolution diffusion imaging reveals intravoxel white matter fiber heterogeneity. Magn. Reson. Med. **48**(4), 577–582 (2002)

Multi-Spherical Diffusion MRI: Exploring Diffusion Time Using Signal Sparsity

Rutger H.J. Fick, Alexandra Petiet, Mathieu Santin, Anne-Charlotte Philippe, Stephane Lehericy, Rachid Deriche, and Demian Wassermann

Abstract Effective representation of the diffusion signal's dependence on diffusion time is a sought-after, yet still unsolved, challenge in diffusion MRI (dMRI). We propose a functional basis approach that is specifically designed to represent the dMRI signal in this four-dimensional space—varying over gradient strength, direction and diffusion time. In particular, we provide regularization tools imposing signal sparsity and signal smoothness to drastically reduce the number of measurements we need to probe the properties of this *multi-spherical* space. We illustrate a novel application of our approach, which is the estimation of time-dependent $\mathbf{q}$-space indices, on both synthetic data generated using Monte-Carlo simulations and in vivo data acquired from a C57Bl6 wild-type mouse. In both cases, we find that our regularization approach stabilizes the signal fit and index estimation as we remove samples, which may bring multi-spherical diffusion MRI within the reach of clinical application.

1 Introduction

Effective representation of the diffusion signal's dependence on diffusion time is a sought-after, yet still unsolved challenge in diffusion MRI (dMRI). Recent literature is increasingly emphasizing the need for such a representation, where accounting for the diffusion time dependence of the extra-axonal diffusion signal [1, 2] has already resulted in a more accurate estimation of the axon density and diameter [3]. To measure the *four-dimensional* dMRI signal it is necessary to go beyond a multi-shell q-space acquisition—which only varies gradient strength and direction—and also vary the diffusion time. This *multi-spherical acquisition* is hardly feasible in a clinical setting due to a large number of sample points in this four-dimensional space-time framework.

R.H.J. Fick (✉) • R. Deriche • D. Wassermann (✉)
Université Côte d'Azur, Inria, France
e-mail: rutger361988@gmail.com; demian.wassermann@inria.fr

A. Petiet • M. Santin • A.-C. Philippe • S. Lehericy
CENIR, Institut du Cerveau et de la Moelle épineère, Paris, France

© Springer International Publishing AG 2017
A. Fuster et al. (eds.), *Computational Diffusion MRI*, Mathematics and Visualization, DOI 10.1007/978-3-319-54130-3_6

To reduce the number of required samples, we propose to leverage the recently proposed representation of the multi-spherical signal in terms of an orthogonal functional basis inspired by Fick et al. [4]. Particularly, we will show that the multi-spherical dMRI signal is sparse when represented in terms of this basis. Different sparse signal reconstruction frameworks, e.g. [5, 6], have shown that signal sparsity allows for a significant reduction in the number of acquired samples. Furthermore, sparse signal reconstruction has been successfully used in different dMRI protocols, see e.g. [7–10]. However, to the best of our knowledge, we are the first to facilitate microstructural measurements by leveraging the sparsity of the spatial and temporal dMRI signal using a novel functional basis. We demonstrate that we are able to reduce the number of required samples for a multi-spherical dMRI acquisition and derive time-dependent microstructural features on both simulated data and in-vivo mouse data.

This paper is structured as follows: first, we present the theory behind our estimation method in Sect. 2. We then describe our methods of generating in-silico multi-spherical data and the parameters of our in vivo dMRI acquisition of C57Bl6 wild-type mouse in Sect. 3. In Sect. 4 we then show the results of our method, we discuss our findings and present our conclusions in Sect. 5.

2   Theory

We first provide the relation between the measured multi-spherical diffusion signal and the four-dimensional ensemble average propagator (EAP) in Sect. 2.1. We then explain the properties that we would like our multi-spherical representation to have, and provide the details on the functional basis representation and regularization which are used to impose the desired properties in Sect. 2.2.

2.1   *The Four-Dimensional Ensemble Average Propagator*

In dMRI, the EAP describes the probability density that a spin diffuses a certain distance in a given diffusion time. The EAP is estimated by obtaining diffusion-weighted images (DWIs). A DWI is obtained by applying two sensitizing diffusion gradients of pulse length δ to the tissue, separated by separation time Δ. The resulting signal is 'weighted' by the average particle movements along the applied gradient direction. When these gradients are considered infinitely short ($\delta \rightarrow 0$), which can only be approximated in practice, the relation between the measured signal $S(\mathbf{q}, \tau)$ and the EAP $P(\mathbf{r}; \tau)$ is given by a Fourier transform [11] as

$$E(\mathbf{q}, \tau) = \int_{\mathbb{R}^3} P(\mathbf{R}; \tau)e^{-2\pi i\mathbf{q}\cdot\mathbf{r}}d\mathbf{R} \quad \text{with} \quad \mathbf{q} = \frac{\gamma\delta\mathbf{G}}{2\pi} \quad \text{and} \quad \tau = \Delta - \delta/3, \quad (1)$$

where $E(\mathbf{q}, \tau) = S(\mathbf{q}, \tau)/S_0$ is the normalized signal attenuation measured at diffusion encoding position $\mathbf{q}$, and S_0 is the baseline image acquired without diffusion sensitization ($q = 0$). We denote $q = |\mathbf{q}|$, $\mathbf{q} = q\mathbf{u}$ and $\mathbf{R} = R\mathbf{r}$, where $\mathbf{u}$ and $\mathbf{r}$ are 3D unit vectors and $q, R \in \mathbb{R}^+$. The wave vector $\mathbf{q}$ on the right side of Eq. (1) is related to pulse length δ, nuclear gyromagnetic ratio γ and the applied diffusion gradient vector $\mathbf{G}$.

The four-dimensional EAP has boundary conditions with respect to $\{\mathbf{q}, \tau\}$:

- $\{\mathbf{q}, \tau = 0\}$: When $\tau = 0$ the spins have no time to diffuse and the EAP is a spike function at the origin, i.e., $P(\mathbf{R}; \tau = 0) = \delta(R)$. Following Eq. (1), the signal attenuation will not attenuate for any value of $\mathbf{q}$, i.e., $E(\mathbf{q}, \tau = 0) = 1$.
- $\{\mathbf{q}, \lim_{\tau \to \infty}\}$: When $\lim_{\tau \to \infty} E(\mathbf{q}, \tau)$ the signal attenuation is in the long diffusion time limit and only signal contributions from restricted compartments remain [12]. In this case, given infinite gradient strength and some assumptions on tissue composition [13, 14], q-space indices such as the Return-To-Axis Probability (RTAP) are related to the mean apparent axon diameter.
- $\{\mathbf{q} = 0, \tau\}$: When $\mathbf{q} = 0$ there is no diffusion sensitization so $E(\mathbf{q} = 0, \tau) = 1$. With Fourier relationship in Eq. (1), this point also corresponds to the zeroth harmonic of the EAP, which as a probability density integrates to one.
- $\{\lim_{\mathbf{q} \to \infty}, \tau\}$: $\lim_{\mathbf{q} \to \infty} E(\mathbf{q}, \tau) = 0$, as even an infinitesimally small spin movement will attenuate the signal completely.

2.2 Multi-Spherical Signal Representation

In dMRI, functional basis approaches have been used to efficiently represent the diffusion signal with little assumptions on its shape. Following this methodology, we represent the measured multi-spherical signal $E(\mathbf{q}, \tau)$ in terms of a continuous functional basis $\hat{E}(\mathbf{q}, \tau; \mathbf{c})$, where the signal is now represented in terms of coefficients $\mathbf{c} \in \mathbb{R}^{N_c}$. An effective representation $\hat{E}(\mathbf{q}, \tau; \mathbf{c})$ should be able to

1. closely approximate the measured multi-spherical dMRI signal,
2. smoothly interpolate between and outside the measured $\{\mathbf{q}, \tau\}$ points,
3. have a sparse representation in $\mathbf{c}$,
4. be able to reconstruct the EAP from the fitted signal.

Requirements 1–3 are described in Eq. (2), while the fourth will follow by choosing a functional basis that is also a *Fourier* basis.

$$\underset{\mathbf{c}}{\mathrm{argmin}} \overbrace{\iint \left[E(\mathbf{q}, \tau) - \hat{E}(\mathbf{q}, \tau; \mathbf{c})\right]^2 d\mathbf{q}d\tau}^{(1)\ \text{Data Fidelity}} + \overbrace{\iint \left[\nabla^2 \hat{E}(\mathbf{q}, \tau; \mathbf{c})\right]^2 d\mathbf{q}d\tau}^{(2)\ \text{Smoothness}} + \overbrace{||\mathbf{c}||_1}^{(3)\ \text{Sparsity}}$$

$$\text{subject to } E(0, \tau; \mathbf{c}) = 1,\ E(\mathbf{q}, 0; \mathbf{c}) = 1,\ \hat{P}(\mathbf{R}, \tau; \mathbf{c}) = \mathrm{IFT}\left(\hat{E}(\mathbf{q}, \tau; \mathbf{c})\right) \qquad (2)$$

Note that the integrals over three-dimensional $\mathbf{q}$ have limits $[-\infty, \infty]$ and those over τ have limits $[0, \infty]$. As stated in Sect. 2.1, the boundary constraints are important to respect the Fourier relationship between the fitted signal attenuation and the EAP.

Functional Basis Signal Representation

We represent the multi-spherical signal using an orthogonal basis that allows for the implementation of all our previously stated requirements. As we assume an infinitely short gradient pulse ($\delta \rightarrow 0$), we follow Callaghan et al.'s description of time-dependent diffusion in pores and assume separability in the dependence of the dMRI signal to $\mathbf{q}$ and τ [12]. Following this hypothesis, we can independently choose any representation for these two spaces. We represent the combined space $\hat{E}(\mathbf{q}, \tau; \mathbf{c})$ using the cross-product between the spatial basis $\Phi(\mathbf{q})$ and temporal basis $T(\tau)$ as

$$\hat{E}(\mathbf{q}, \tau; \mathbf{c}) = \sum_i^{N_{\mathbf{q}}} \sum_k^{N_\tau} \mathbf{c}_{ik}\, \Phi_i(\mathbf{q})\, T_k(\tau), \tag{3}$$

where $N_{\mathbf{q}}$ and N_τ are the maximum expansion order of each basis and $\mathbf{c}_{ik}$ weights the contribution of the ikth basis function to $\hat{E}(\mathbf{q}, \tau; \mathbf{c})$.

A plethora of functional bases to represent $\mathbf{q}$ have been proposed, e.g. [8, 9, 13, 15]. Of these bases, we use the Mean Apparent Propagator (MAP) basis [13] as it neatly fulfills all four previously stated requirements; (1) being an orthogonal basis, it can accurately represent any signal over $\mathbf{q}$ using few coefficients; (2) it allows to impose smoothness using analytic Laplacian regularization [14]; (3) the isotropic MAP implementation was successfully used to obtain sparse signal representation [8] and (4) MAP is a Fourier basis. It is worth noting that this basis is different than Fick et al.'s basis, who used the isotropic implementation (3D-SHORE) to represent $\mathbf{q}$ [4].

MAP's signal basis is a product of three orthogonal Simple Harmonic Oscillator-based Reconstruction and Estimation (SHORE) functions $\phi_n(u)$ [16]:

$$\Phi_{N(i)}(\mathbf{q}, \mathbf{A}) = \phi_{n_1}(q_x, u_x)\phi_{n_2}(q_y, u_y)\phi_{n_3}(q_z, u_z)$$

$$\text{with } \phi_n(q, u) = \frac{i^{-n}}{\sqrt{2^n n!}}e^{-2\pi^2 q^2 u^2} H_n(2\pi u q) \tag{4}$$

with its Fourier transform, the EAP basis as

$$\Psi_{N(i)}(\mathbf{R}, \mathbf{A}) = \psi_{n_1}(R_x, u_x)\psi_{n_2}(R_y, u_y)\psi_{n_3}(R_z, u_z)$$

$$\text{with } \psi_n(R, u) = \frac{1}{\sqrt{2^{n+1}\pi n! u}}e^{-R^2/(2u^2)} H_n(R/u) \tag{5}$$

where H is a physicist's Hermite polynomial of order n and u is a data-dependent scale factor. As in MAP [13], before fitting, the data is rotated such that the DTI eigenvectors are aligned with the coordinate axis and we can use the data-dependent scaling matrix $\mathbf{A} = \mathrm{Diag}(u_x^2, u_y^2, u_z^2)$ to scale the MAP basis functions according to the anisotropy of the data. The zeroth order is a purely Gaussian function while higher orders use the Hermite to correct this approximation to the true shape of the data. For a given radial order N_{rad} the number of coefficients is $N_{\mathbf{q}} = (N_{\mathrm{rad}} + 2)(N_{\mathrm{rad}} + 4)(2N_{\mathrm{rad}} + 3)/24$.

Our functional basis to describe τ was introduced in Fick et al. [4]. As a limiting case the diffusion signal dependence on τ is exponential for pure Gaussian diffusion and constant for diffusion in restricted geometries. To represent τ we, therefore, choose a product of the negative exponential and a Laguerre polynomial L, which together form an orthogonal basis over τ

$$T_p(\tau, u_t) = \exp(-u_t\tau/2)L_o(u_t\tau) \tag{6}$$

with basis order p and temporal scaling factor u_t. The zeroth order is a pure exponential function and higher orders use the Laguerre polynomials to correct this approximation to the true shape of the signal.

For the rest of this work we will linearize the ordering of our multi-spherical basis such that we use one basis index i with notation

$$\hat{E}(\mathbf{q}, \tau; \mathbf{c}) = \sum_i^{N_c} \mathbf{c}_i \, \Xi_i(\mathbf{q}, \tau, \mathbf{A}, u_t) = \sum_i^{N_c} \mathbf{c}_i \, \Phi_{N(i)}(\mathbf{q}, \mathbf{A}) \, T_{p(i)}(\tau, u_t) \tag{7}$$

where the total number of fitted coefficients is $N_c = (N_\tau + 1)(N_{\mathbf{q}} + 2)(N_{\mathbf{q}} + 4)(2N_{\mathbf{q}} + 3)/24$. Using this notation, the fitted signal $\hat{E}(\mathbf{q}, \tau; \mathbf{c})$ in the *Data Fidelity* term in Eq. (2), with measured signal $\mathbf{y} \in \mathbb{R}^{N_y}$ and N_y the number of samples, can be represented as $\hat{\mathbf{y}} = \Phi\mathbf{c}$ with $\Phi \in \mathrm{R}^{N_y \times N_c}$ with values $\Phi_{ij} = \Xi_j(\mathbf{q}_i, \tau_i, \mathbf{A}, u_t)$.

The multi-spherical EAP can be reconstructed using MAP's Fourier properties [13]. The Fourier transform only concerns the $\mathbf{q}$-space, so the EAP is found simply by switching $\Phi(\mathbf{q}, \mathbf{A})$ in Eq. (7) by its Fourier transform in Eq. (5).

Analytic Laplacian Regularization

We impose smoothness in the multi-spherical signal reconstruction by using the squared norm of the Laplacian of the reconstructed signal as a regularizer. We define the *Smoothness* term in Eq. (2) as Laplacian functional $U(\mathbf{c})$ as

$$U(\mathbf{c}) = \iint \left[\nabla^2\hat{E}(\mathbf{q}, \tau; \mathbf{c})\right]^2 d\mathbf{q}d\tau \tag{8}$$

where, due to our choice of basis, the Laplacian of the reconstructed signal can be estimated as $\nabla^2 E_\mathbf{c}(\mathbf{q}, \tau) = \sum_i c_i \nabla^2 \Xi_i(\mathbf{q}, \tau, \mathbf{A}, u_t)$. Equation (8) can be further rewritten in quadratic form as $U(\mathbf{c}) = \mathbf{c}^T \mathbf{U} \mathbf{c}$ with

$$\mathbf{U}_{ik} = \iint \nabla^2 \Xi_i(\mathbf{q}, \tau, \mathbf{A}, u_t) \cdot \nabla^2 \Xi_k(\mathbf{q}, \tau, \mathbf{A}, u_t) d\mathbf{q}\, d\tau \tag{9}$$

where the subscript ik indicates the ikth position in the regularization matrix. We use the orthogonality of the basis functions (standard inner product on $[0, \infty]$) to compute the values of the regularization matrix to a closed form depending only on the basis orders and scale factors. We provide $\mathbf{U}$ in Appendix.

Coefficient Estimation from Multi-Spherical Data

We represent the multi-spherical signal $E(\mathbf{q}, \tau)$ in terms of a sparse coefficient vector $\mathbf{c}$ as $\mathbf{y} = \Phi \mathbf{c} + \epsilon$ with Φ the observation matrix, $\mathbf{y}$ the signal values and ϵ the acquisition noise. We frame the numerical implementation of our approach in the same way as we did continuously in Eq. (2):

$$\operatorname{argmin}_\mathbf{c} \overbrace{||\mathbf{y} - \Phi \mathbf{c}||_2}^{\text{(1) Data Fidelity}} + \overbrace{\beta ||\mathbf{c}^T \mathbf{U} \mathbf{c}||_2}^{\text{(2) Smoothness}} + \overbrace{\alpha ||\mathbf{c}||_1}^{\text{(3) Sparsity}} \tag{10}$$

$$\text{subject to } \Phi^{\text{constraints}} \mathbf{c} = \mathbf{1}$$

where we described the *Data Fidelity* and *Smoothness* term in Sect. 2.2, and the *Sparsity* term and constraints are imposed by framing our problem as a convex optimization using the open-source package CVXPY [17]. We find optimal values for regularization weights α and β using cross-validation and implemented the surrounding code infrastructure inside the DiPy framework [18].

2.3   *Estimation of τ-Dependent q-Space Indices*

Once coefficients $\mathbf{c}$ are known, our basis allows us to freely explore, for any diffusion time, all previously proposed scalar metrics for the three-dimensional EAP [13, 14], also known as $\mathbf{q}$-space indices. We can do this because our basis reduces to the MAP basis when the temporal basis is evaluated for a particular diffusion time. In this work we illustrate this using the τ-dependent Return-To-Origin Probability (RTOP) and Mean Squared Displacement (MSD):

$$MSD(\tau) \triangleq \int_{\mathbb{R}^3} \hat{P}(\mathbf{R}, \tau; \mathbf{c}) \mathbf{R}^2 d\mathbf{R} \quad \text{and} \quad RTOP(\tau) \triangleq \hat{P}(0, \tau; \mathbf{c}) \tag{11}$$

3 Data Set Specification

Acquisition Scheme We will use the same acquisition scheme for both our synthetic and in vivo mouse experiments. An illustration of this scheme is given in Fig. 1. We acquire 32 different "shells" with 21 uniformly spread DWIs and one b0 each using pulse duration $\delta = 5$ ms. Over these shells, we measure four equispaced "τ-shells" $\Delta = \{8.7, 12.2, 15.8, 19.4\}$ ms and eight approximately equispaced "gradient shells" between $\{50 - 520\}$ mT/m. The minimum b-value is $b_{\min} = 48$ s/mm^2 and maximum b-value is $b_{\max} = 8590$ s/mm^2.

In Silico Data Sets with Camino We use Camino [19] to reproduce diffusion signals originating from tissues containing realistic axon diameter distributions and packings. As we illustrate in Table 1, we use five gamma distributions from Aboitiz et al. [20] and six from Lamantia et al. [21]. Similarly as in Alexander et al. [22], we simulate the overall diffusion signal from these 11 distributions from the same distributions with doubled axonal diameters and two different packing densities, resulting in a total of 44 distributions.

Mouse Acquisition Data A spin echo sequence was acquired from a C57Bl6 wild-type mouse on an 11.7 T Bruker scanner. The data consists of $96 \times 160 \times 12$ voxels of size $110 \times 110 \times 500$ μm. We manually created a brain mask and corrected the data from eddy currents and motion artifacts using FSL's eddy_correct [23]. We then

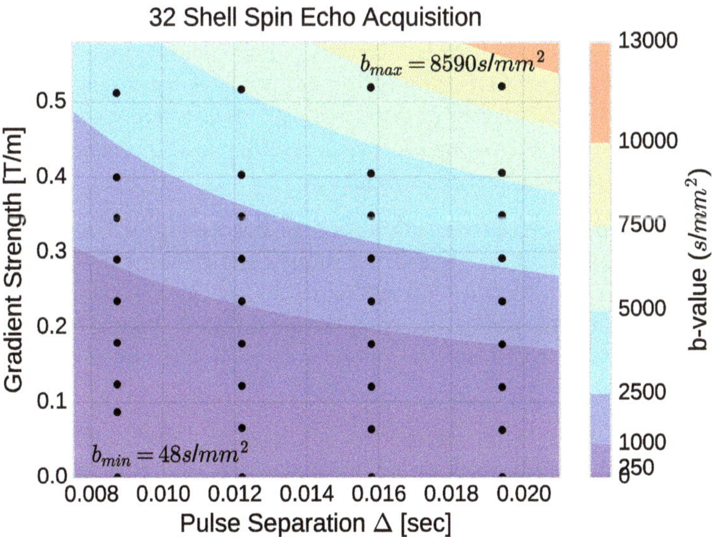

Fig. 1 Acquisition scheme for multi-spherical acquisition. Every *dot* represents a shell with 21 DWIs and one b0 image. The contours represent b-value isolines, whose values are given in the *colorbar*

Table 1 Simulated Gamma
distributions, sorted by mean
axonal diameter $\langle D \rangle$

Origin	Shape (α)	Scale (β)	$\langle D \rangle$ (μm)
Aboitiz	3.2734	2.4563e−07	1.60
Aboitiz	2.8771	2.4932e−07	1.43
Aboitiz	4.8184	1.3008e−07	1.25
Aboitiz	3.5027	1.6331e−07	1.14
Aboitiz	5.3316	1.0242e−07	1.09
Lamantia	5.2051	1.0227e−07	1.06
Lamantia	5.2357	9.3946e−08	0.98
Lamantia	10.1960	3.6983e−08	0.75
Lamantia	8.5358	3.7369e−08	0.64
Lamantia	5.9242	5.3249e−08	0.63
Lamantia	16.2750	1.4282e−08	0.46

drew a region of interest consisting of 72 voxels in the middle slice in the corpus
callosum, see Fig. 4, where we know the tissue is reasonably coherent.

4 Experiments and Results

Radial and Temporal Order Fitting In this noiseless experiment, we find the
optimal choice of radial and temporal order to accurately fit the diffusion signal with
the lowest number of coefficients. We fit our multi-spherical basis to the Camino
data using different radial and temporal orders and calculate the mean squared error
(MSE) of the fitted signal to the original signal. We show the result in Fig. 2a. We
find that the mean absolute error of the signal over all distributions falls below 1%
at a radial order of 6 and temporal order of 2, resulting in 150 coefficients. We will
use this combination in our next experiments.

Comparison with DTI Approximation In Fig. 2b we compare the MSE of fitting
DTI, the basis of Fick et al. [4] and our multi-spherical approach to subsets of
the noiseless data with increasing maximum b-values. As the maximum b-value
increases, data with higher gradients strengths and diffusion times are included (see
Fig. 1). Our approach fits diffusion restriction over $\mathbf{q}$ and τ best of the three methods
regardless of b-value.

Multi-Spherical Signal Reconstruction and q-Space Index Estimation To
reduce the number of measurements, we regularize the basis fitting with a
combination of imposing smoothness in the fitted signal and sparsity in the basis
coefficients. To study its effectiveness, we first add Rician noise to the Camino data
such that the signal-to-noise (SNR)-ratio is 20. We then randomly subsample, fit and
then recover the data from our model and estimate the MSE with the noiseless data.
The experiment for every chosen number of samples is repeated 50 times for all 44
voxels with each a different noise instance. The result can be seen in Fig. 3a, where

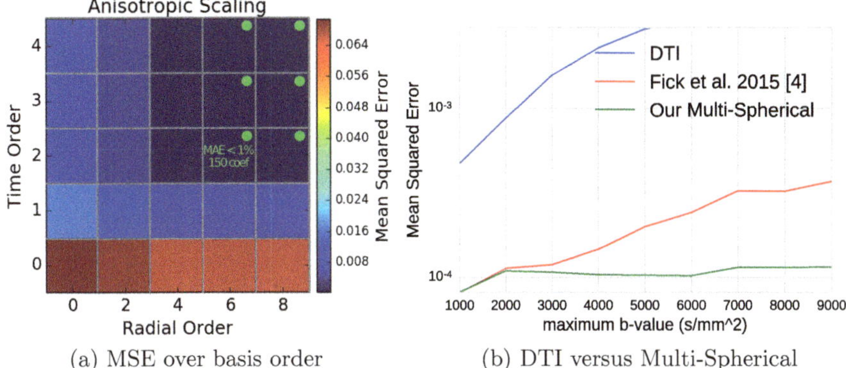

(a) MSE over basis order   (b) DTI versus Multi-Spherical

Fig. 2 (**a**) Noise free fitting of Camino data set using different radial and time orders using our multi-spherical basis. The *color* intensity shows the mean squared error and the *green dots* indicate orders for which the mean absolute error of the reconstruction is smaller than 1% of the b0 value. (**b**) Comparison of the fitting error between DTI, the approach of Fick et al. [4] and our multi-spherical approach over maximum b-value

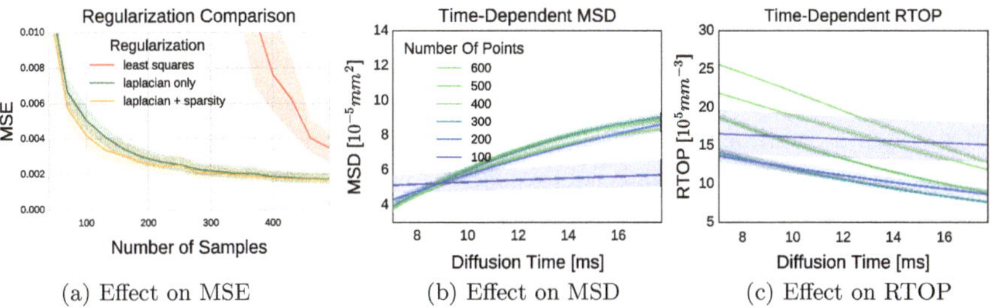

(a) Effect on MSE   (b) Effect on MSD   (c) Effect on RTOP

Fig. 3 Effect of random subsampling at SNR=20 on (**a**) mean squared error (MSE) for different regularization techniques, (**b**) the time-dependent Return-To-Origin Probability (RTOP) and (**c**) Mean Squared Displacement (MSD). (**a**) Our combined sparsity and Laplacian regularization (*yellow*) has lower MSE than only Laplacian (*green*) and least squares (*red*). (**b**) and (**c**) show the MSD and RTOP using 600 samples (*green*) to 100 samples (*blue*)

our combined approach (yellow) has the lowest MSE, followed by using only the Laplacian (green) and the worst is least squares (red). We also show the effects of using between 600 samples (green) and 100 samples (blue) on the estimation of the Mean Squared Displacement (MSD) and the **q**-space index Return-To-Origin probability (RTOP) in Fig. 3b, c. We see that MSD increases as time increases, while its profile does not change much until the profile flattens for 100 samples. In contrast, we see that RTOP decreases over time and as the number of samples reduces, the overall RTOP values decrease. Again for 100 samples, the profile flattens out.

Application to In-Vivo Mouse Acquisition Finally, we apply our method to in vivo acquired data from a C57Bl6 wild-type mouse. The results are shown in Fig. 4. First, we estimate MSD and RTOP for the whole data and show their values for

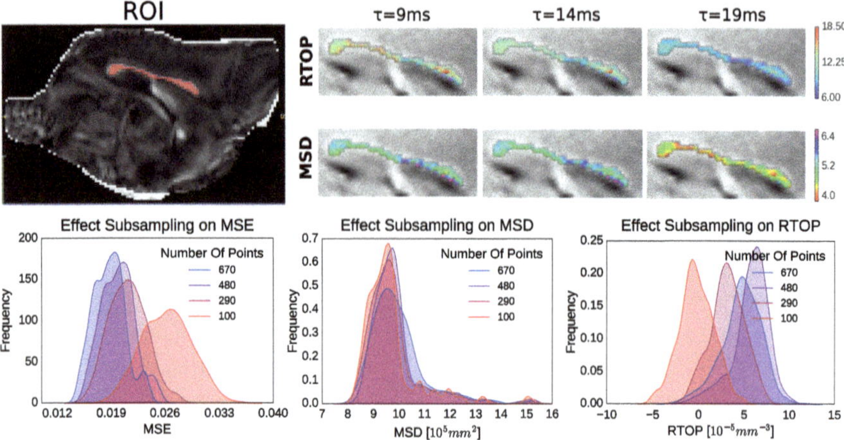

Fig. 4 (*top-left*) Region of interest in mouse corpus callosum. (*top-right*) Maps of RTOP and MSD for different diffusion times. (*bottom*) Histograms of the MSE (*left*), MSD (middle) and RTOP (*right*) for different numbers of fitted points. The RTOP and MSD were calculated for $\tau = 14$ ms

different diffusion times on the top left. RTOP decreases as time increases, which corresponds with the in-silico experiments. In MSD we first find an overall increase, after which a small decrease is seen. The latter phenomenon does not correspond with what we previously found. We then again randomly subsample the data for all voxels in the ROI and estimate the MSE, together with the MSD and RTOP for a chosen diffusion time of $\tau = 14$ ms. The trends for all markers correspond with the synthetic data: MSE increases, RTOP decreases, and MSD stays the same as the number of samples decreases.

5 Discussion and Conclusion

In this work, we proposed a novel functional basis to efficiently represent the multi-spherical diffusion signal over both three-dimensional **q**-space and diffusion time. We regularized this basis by imposing both smoothness in the fitted signal using Laplacian regularization and sparsity in the fitted coefficients. Compared to the work by Fick et al. [4], the main methodological differences are the **q**-space representation, where we use the MAP basis instead of 3D-SHORE, and the sparsity term. As Fig. 2b shows, using MAP allows us to fit the multi-spherical signal better than [4] using the same number of coefficients. We remark that DTI fits the multi-spherical signal worst as it cannot describe diffusion restriction over **q** or τ. This limitation becomes more apparent at higher b-values, which is exactly where the diffusion signal is most characterizing of the underlying tissue.

This work is also the first to estimate and study the progress of three-dimensional **q**-space indices over diffusion time. Our basis is especially well-suited for this exploration. For any evaluated diffusion time the basis reduces to MAP, which allows us to calculate all of its previously proposed indices [13, 14]. For now, we focused on the well-known Mean Squared Displacement (MSD) and Return-to-Origin Probability (RTOP). We found that the recovered trends in synthetic data correspond with what we expect from theory (Fig. 3b, c). As diffusion time increases, spins get more time to diffusive, so MSD increases and RTOP decreases. Decreasing the number of samples did not influence MSD trends so much, but RTOP trends did lower, possibly related to removal of samples along the "restricted" direction in the signal. Overall, a lower bound of reliable index estimation seems to be around 200 samples using random subsampling, as both profiles flatten out at this point.

Applying our method to real multi-spherical data from a mouse produces mostly coherent results with the simulated data. Again we find that RTOP drops as diffusion time increases, and lowering the number of samples decreases the RTOP and leaves MSD mostly unaffected. As fewer samples were used, we found more negative (infeasible) RTOP values. To avoid this, our framework could still be improved by adding a positivity constraint like in Özarslan et al. [13].

Regardless, our multi-spherical basis is the first of its kind in being specifically designed to represent the four-dimensional EAP and analyzing its properties. Our proposed regularization allows us to significantly reduce the number of measured samples, which may eventually bring multi-spherical diffusion MRI within the reach of clinical application.

Acknowledgements This work was partly supported by ANR "MOSIFAH" under ANR-13-MONU-0009-01, the ERC under the European Union's Horizon 2020 research and innovation program (ERC Advanced Grant agreement No 694665:CoBCoM), MAXIMS grant funded by ICM's The Big Brain Theory Program and ANR-10-IAIHU-06.

Appendix: Analytic Laplacian Regularization

We provide the analytic form of the Laplacian regularization matrix in Eq. (9). As our basis is separable in $\mathbf{q}$ and τ, the Laplacian of our basis function Ξ_i is

$$\nabla^2 \Xi_i(\mathbf{q}, \tau, u_s, u_t) = \left(\nabla_{\mathbf{q}}^2 \Phi_i(\mathbf{q}, u_s)\right) T_i(\tau, u_t) + \Phi_i(\mathbf{q}, u_s) \left(\nabla_{\tau}^2 T_i(\tau, u_t)\right) \qquad (12)$$

with $\nabla_{\mathbf{q}}^2$ and ∇_{τ}^2 the Laplacian to either $\mathbf{q}$ or τ. We then rewrite Eq. (9) as

$$\mathbf{U}_{ik} = \int_{\mathbb{R}} (\nabla_{\mathbf{q}}^2 \Phi_i)(\nabla_{\mathbf{q}}^2 \Phi_k) d\mathbf{q} \int_{\mathbb{R}} T_i T_k d\tau + \int_{\mathbb{R}} \Phi_i \Phi_k d\mathbf{q} \int_{\mathbb{R}} (\nabla_{\tau}^2 T_i)(\nabla_{\tau}^2 T_k) d\tau$$

$$+ \int_{\mathbb{R}} (\nabla_{\mathbf{q}}^2 \Phi_i) \Phi_k d\mathbf{q} \left(\int_{\mathbb{R}} T_i(\nabla_{\tau}^2 T_k) d\tau + \int_{\mathbb{R}} (\nabla_{\tau}^2 T_i) T_k d\tau \right) \qquad (13)$$

Equation (13) can be calculated to a closed form using the orthogonality of physicists' Hermite polynomials with respect to weighting function e^{-x^2} on $[-\infty, \infty]$.

Let us first consider the integrals with respect to $\mathbf{q}$, which all parts of the Laplacian regularization functional of the MAP basis [14]. Writing the second order derivative as a double apostrophe $''$, the Laplacian of the spatial basis is given in terms of the 1D-SHORE functions as $\nabla_{\mathbf{q}}^2 \Phi_i = \phi_{n_x}'' \phi_{n_y} \phi_{n_z} + \phi_{n_x} \phi_{n_y}'' \phi_{n_z} + \phi_{n_x} \phi_{n_y} \phi_{n_z}''$. The integral of the product of two Laplacians therefore becomes a sum of nine terms, but can be described using the following three equations:

$$U_n^m(u) = \int_{\mathbb{R}} \phi_n'' \phi_m'' d\mathbf{q} = u^3 2(-1)^n \pi^{7/2} \left(\delta_n^m 3(2n^2 + 2n + 1) + \delta_n^{m+4} \sqrt{n!/m!} \right.$$

$$\left. + \delta_{n+2}^m (6 + 4n) \sqrt{m!/n!} + \delta_{n+4}^m \sqrt{m!/n!} + \delta_n^{m+2}(6 + 4m) \sqrt{n!/m!} \right)$$

$$V_n^m(u) = \int_{\mathbb{R}} \phi_n'' \phi_m d\mathbf{q} = u(-1)^{n+1} \pi^{3/2} \left(\delta_n^m (1 + 2n) \quad + \delta_n^{m+2} \sqrt{n(n-1)} + \delta_{n+2}^m \sqrt{m(m-1)} \right)$$

$$(14)$$

$$W_n^m(u) = \int_{\mathbb{R}} \phi_n \phi_m d\mathbf{q} = u^{-1} \delta_n^m (-1)^n / (2\pi^{1/2})$$

Using the functions in Eq. (14) we define the $\mathbf{q}$-dependent parts of Eq. (13):

$$\int_{\mathbb{R}} (\nabla_{\mathbf{q}}^2 \Phi_i)(\nabla_{\mathbf{q}}^2 \Phi_k) d\mathbf{q} = \frac{u_x^3}{u_y u_z} U_{x_i}^{x_k} W_{y_i}^{y_k} W_{z_i}^{z_k} + 2\frac{u_x u_y}{u_z} V_{x_i}^{x_k} V_{y_i}^{y_k} W_{z_i}^{z_k} + \frac{u_y^3}{u_z u_x} U_{y_i}^{y_k} W_{z_i}^{z_k} W_{x_i}^{x_k}$$

$$+ 2\frac{u_y u_z}{u_x} V_{y_i}^{y_k} V_{z_i}^{z_k} W_{x_i}^{x_k} + \frac{u_z^3}{u_x u_y} U_{z_i}^{z_k} W_{x_i}^{x_k} W_{y_i}^{y_k} + 2\frac{u_x u_z}{u_y} V_{x_i}^{x_k} V_{z_i}^{z_k} W_{y_i}^{y_k}$$

$$\int_{\mathbb{R}} (\nabla_{\mathbf{q}}^2 \Phi_i)(\Phi_k) d\mathbf{q} = \frac{u_x}{u_y u_z} V_{x_i}^{x_k} W_{y_i}^{y_k} W_{z_i}^{z_k} + \frac{u_y}{u_x u_z} V_{x_i}^{x_k} W_{y_i}^{y_k} W_{z_i}^{z_k} + \frac{u_z}{u_x u_y} V_{x_i}^{x_k} W_{y_i}^{y_k} W_{z_i}^{z_k}$$

$$\int_{\mathbb{R}} \Phi_i \Phi_k d\mathbf{q} = \frac{1}{u_x u_y u_z} W_{x_i}^{x_k} W_{y_i}^{y_k} W_{z_i}^{z_k}$$

For terms with τ, we denote the operator $M_{x_1}^{x_2} = \min(x_1, x_2)$ for the minimal value of x_1, x_2 and H_x the Heaviside step function with $H_x = 1$ iff $x \geq 0$.

$$\int_{\mathbb{R}} (\nabla_\tau^2 T_i)(\nabla_\tau^2 T_k) d\tau = \left(\frac{1}{4}|o(i) - o(k)| + \frac{1}{16}\delta_{o(i)}^{o(k)} + M_{o(i)}^{o(k)} \right.$$

$$+ \sum_{p=1}^{M_{o(i)}^{o(k)}+1} (o(i) - p)(o(k) - p)H_{M_{o(i)}^{o(k)}-p} + H_{o(i)-1}H_{o(k)-1}\left(o(i) + o(k) - 2 \right.$$

$$+ \sum_{p=0}^{M_{o(i)-1}^{o(k)-2}} p + \sum_{p=0}^{M_{o(i)-2}^{o(k)-1}} p + M_{o(i)-1}^{o(k)-1} (|o(i) - o(k)| - 1) H_{(|o(i)-o(k)|-1)} \left. \right) \left. \right)$$

$$\left(\int_{\mathbb{R}} T_i(\nabla_\tau^2 T_k) d\tau + \int_{\mathbb{R}} (\nabla_\tau^2 T_i) T_k d\tau \right) = u_t \left(\frac{1}{2}\delta_{o(i)}^{o(k)} + (1 - \delta_{o(i)}^{o(k)}) \cdot |o(i) - o(k)| \right)$$

$$\int_{\mathbb{R}} T_i T_k d\tau = 1/u_t \delta_{o(k)}^{o(i)}$$

References

1. Novikov, D.S., et al.: Revealing mesoscopic structural universality with diffusion. Proc. Natl. Acad. Sci. **111**(14), 5088–5093 (2014)
2. Burcaw, L.M., et al.: Mesoscopic structure of neuronal tracts from time-dependent diffusion. NeuroImage **114**, 18–37 (2015)
3. De Santis, S., et al.: Including diffusion time dependence in the extra-axonal space improves in vivo estimates of axonal diameter and density in human white matter. NeuroImage **130**, 91–103 (2016)
4. Fick, R., et al.: A unifying framework for spatial and temporal diffusion in diffusion MRI. In: Information Processing in Medical Imaging. Springer International Publishing, Cham (2015)
5. Candès, E.J., Wakin, M.B.: An introduction to compressive sampling. IEEE Signal Process. Mag. **25**(2), 21–30 (2008)
6. Candès, E.J., et al.: Robust uncertainty principles: exact signal reconstruction from highly incomplete frequency information. IEEE Trans. Inf. Theory **52**(2), 489–509 (2006)
7. Paquette, M., et al.: Comparison of sampling strategies and sparsifying transforms to improve compressed sensing diffusion spectrum imaging. Magn. Reson. Med. **73**(1), 401–416 (2015)
8. Merlet, S.L., Deriche, R.: Continuous diffusion signal, EAP and ODF estimation via compressive sensing in diffusion MRI. Med. Image Anal. **17**(5), 556–572 (2013)
9. Rathi, Y., et al.: Multi-shell diffusion signal recovery from sparse measurements. Med. Image Anal. **18**(7), 1143–1156 (2014)
10. Bilgic, B., et al.: Accelerated diffusion spectrum imaging with compressed sensing using adaptive dictionaries. Magn. Reson. Med. **68**(6), 1747–1754 (2012)
11. Stejskal, E.O.: Use of spin echoes in a pulsed magneticfield gradient to study anisotropic, restricted diffusion and flow. J. Chem. Phys. **43**(10), 3597–3603 (1965)
12. Callaghan, P.T.: Pulsed-gradient spin-echo NMR for planar, cylindrical, and spherical pores under conditions of wall relaxation. J. Magn. Reson. Ser. A **113**(1), 53–59 (1995)
13. Özarslan, E., et al.: Mean apparent propagator (MAP) MRI: a novel diffusion imaging method for mapping tissue microstructure. NeuroImage **78**, 16–32 (2013)
14. Fick, R.H.J., et al.: MAPL: tissue microstructure estimation using Laplacian-regularized MAP-MRI and its application to HCP data. NeuroImage **134**, 365–385 (2016)
15. Hosseinbor, A.P., et al.: Bessel fourier orientation reconstruction (BFOR): an analytical diffusion propagator reconstruction for hybrid diffusion imaging and computation of q-space indices. NeuroImage **64**, 650–670 (2013)
16. Özarslan, E., et al.: Nuclear magnetic resonance characterization of general compartment size distributions. New J. Phys. **13**(1), 015010 (2011)
17. Diamond, S., Boyd, S.: CVXPY: a python-embedded modeling language for convex optimization. J. Mach. Learn. Res. **17**(83), 1–5 (2016)
18. Garyfallidis, E., et al.: Dipy, a library for the analysis of diffusion MRI data. Front. Neuroinform. **8**, 8 (2014)
19. Cook, P.A., et al.: Camino: open-source diffusion-MRI reconstruction and processing. In: 14th ISMRM, Seattle, WA, p. 2759 (2006)
20. Aboitiz, F., et al.: Fiber composition of the human corpus callosum. Brain Res. **598**(1), 143–153 (1992)
21. Lamantia, A.S., Rakic, P.: Cytological and quantitative characteristics of four cerebral commissures in the rhesus monkey. J. Comp. Neurol. **291**(4), 520–537 (1990)
22. Alexander, D.C., et al.: Orientationally invariant indices of axon diameter and density from diffusion MRI. NeuroImage **52**(4), 1374–1389 (2010)
23. Andersson, J.L.R., Sotiropoulos, S.N.: An integrated approach to correction for off-resonance effects and subject movement in diffusion MR imaging. NeuroImage **125**, 1063–1078 (2016)

Sensitivity of OGSE ActiveAx to Microstructural Dimensions on a Clinical Scanner

Lebina S. Kakkar, David Atkinson, Rachel W. Chan, Bernard Siow, Andrada Ianus, and Ivana Drobnjak

Abstract Axon diameter can play a key role in the function and performance of nerve pathways of the central and peripheral nervous system. Previously, a number of techniques to measure axon diameter using diffusion MR I have been proposed, majority of which uses single diffusion encoding (SDE) spin-echo sequence. However, recent theoretical research suggests that low-frequency oscillating gradient spin echo (OGSE) offers benefits over SDE for imaging diameters when fibres are of unknown orientation. Furthermore, it suggests that resolution limit for clinical scanners (gradient strength of 60–80 mT/m) is $\approx 6\,\mu$m. Here we investigate the sensitivity of OGSE to fibre diameters experimentally on a clinical scanner, using microcapillaries of unknown orientation. We use the orientationally invariant OGSE ActiveAx method to image microcapillaries with diameters of 5, 10 or 20 μm. As predicted by theory, we find that 5 μm diameters are undistinguishable from zero. Furthermore, we find accurate and precise estimates for 10 and 20 μm. Finally, we find that low frequency oscillating gradient waveforms are optimal for accurate diameter estimation.

1 Introduction

Non-invasive estimation of axon diameter plays an important role in biomedical imaging. For instance, the conduction velocity of signal transmission throughout the nerve pathways in the central nervous system (CNS) [1] is directly influenced by axon diameter. Thus, estimating this tissue feature can provide essential information on the performance and function of white matter pathways [2]. Moreover, changes

L.S. Kakkar (✉) • A. Ianus • I. Drobnjak
Centre for Medical Image Computing, University College London, London, UK
e-mail: lebina.shrestha.11@ucl.ac.uk

D. Atkinson • R.W. Chan
Centre for Medical Imaging, Wolfson House, 4 Stephenson Way, London, UK

B. Siow
Centre for Advanced Biomedical Imaging, University College London, London, UK

© Springer International Publishing AG 2017

A. Fuster et al. (eds.), *Computational Diffusion MRI*, Mathematics and Visualization, DOI 10.1007/978-3-319-54130-3_7

in axon diameter estimates can be used to study the effect of ageing [3], as well as of various CNS diseases, such as amyotrophic lateral sclerosis [4], autism [5], and schizophrenia [6], where axonal degeneration can lead to abnormal axon diameters.

A number of methods for estimating axon diameter using diffusion weighted magnetic resonance imaging (DW-MRI) have been proposed. These include q-space imaging (QSI) [7], double pulsed field gradient (dPFG) [8, 9], AxCaliber [10] and ActiveAx [11]. The majority of these techniques are based on single diffusion encoding (SDE) sequences. However, various authors suggest that oscillating gradient spin echo (OGSE) offers benefits over SDE for imaging fibre diameter [12–15].

A common argument is that high-frequency OGSE sequences provide shorter effective diffusion time than SDE and hence are able to probe smaller length scales. This is clearly an advantage for measuring the free diffusivity in small fibres because it minimises the effects of restriction [16, 17]. However, it is not clear whether it is advantageous for measuring fibre diameter where contrast at the long diffusion time limit may be more informative.

Recently, a thorough numerical approach has been used to compare directly the sensitivity to axon diameter of SDE and OGSE sequences in a wide space of clinically plausible sequence parameters [12]. The research showed that for the simple case of diffusion gradient direction perfectly perpendicular to straight parallel fibres, SDE with the longest gradient duration always gives maximum sensitivity for small diameters. However, in real-world scenarios where fibres have unknown and/or dispersed orientation, OGSE provides higher sensitivity. This happens because the oscillating waveforms can achieve high sensitivity to fibre diameters at a modest b-value, which in turn enables OGSE sequences to retain their sensitivity by avoiding excessive signal attenuation from unrestricted displacements along the fibre direction. These results were confirmed analytically in a recent study by Nillson et al. [18]. Both groups also found diameter resolution limits for a range of different gradient strengths and SNRs. Their results show that on typical clinical scanners the limit is around $6\,\mu$m, i.e. axon diameters below that limit are undistinguishable from zero.

This study aims to explore experimentally, on a clinical scanner, the sensitivity of OGSE sequences to fibre diameter in a phantom consisting of cylindrical micro-capillaries with unknown orientation. We use water-filled micro-capillaries array plates as a model for axons, and fit a single restricted component. We use a rotationally invariant HARDI acquisition with 32 directions as we assume micro-capillaries of unknown orientation. The micro-capillary diameters used here are 5, 10 or $20\,\mu$m, which is within the limits of axon diameters in the body (0.2–$20\,\mu$m) [2]. We use a trapezoidal OGSE with a range of frequencies for imaging and OGSE ActiveAx [14, 19] for the estimation of microstructure parameters.

2 Methods

2.1 Diffusion MR Model

We use a single restricted compartment of unknown orientation as a model for our phantoms. All microcapillaries (representing axons) are parallel and non-abutting cylinders, with equal radii and impermeable walls. The parameters of the model are (1) intrinsic diffusivity, D_i, (2) microcapillary diameter, a and (3) microcapillary direction, $\mathbf{n}$.

The restricted diffusion signal, S_r, can be written as the product of components arising from displacements parallel, $S_{r\parallel}$, and perpendicular, $S_{r\perp}$, to the long axis of the microcapillary as described in [20]. The model for $S_{r\perp}$ is calculated using the Gaussian phase distribution approximation (GPD) [21] for a diffusion gradient perpendicular to the microcapillary with strength $|\mathbf{G}|\sin\theta$, where θ is the angle between $\mathbf{n}$ and $\mathbf{G}$. $S_{r\parallel}$ describes free diffusion with D_i for a diffusion gradient parallel to the microcapillary with strength $|\mathbf{G}|\cos\theta$, and is calculated using $S_{r\parallel} = \exp(-b\cos^2\theta D_i)$, where the b-value for trapezoidal OGSE is from [22].

The total signal accounting for both components ($S_{r\parallel}$ and $S_{r\perp}$) is:

$$S = S_0 S_r = S_0 S_{r\parallel} S_{r\perp}. \tag{1}$$

where S_0 is the MR signal without diffusion weighting.

2.2 Phantom Experiments

Sample Preparation

The microcapillaries array plates (as shown in Fig. 1a) are thin square plates (each of dimensions $20\,\text{mm} \times 20\,\text{mm} \times 1\,\text{mm}$) made up of borosilicate glass (Incom, inc). The microcapillaries array plates will simply be referred to as 'plates' from here onwards. Each plate consists of many microcapillaries. This study uses three pairs of plates with nominal microcapillary diameters of 5, 10 or $20\,\mu\text{m}$, and an open area fraction between 60 and 65 % (Fig. 1b–d). The ground truth diameters of the microcapillaries are provided by the manufacturer and these are the only available sizes which broadly mimic the possible in vivo axon diameters that are encountered in the central nervous system [2].

The three pairs of plates are slotted into a phantom holder containing distilled water such that the microcapillaries are aligned parallel to the main magnetic field in order to reduce susceptibility artefacts. They are soaked in the distilled water for 1 week to ensure that the microcapillaries are filled and to remove air bubbles at the plate surface.

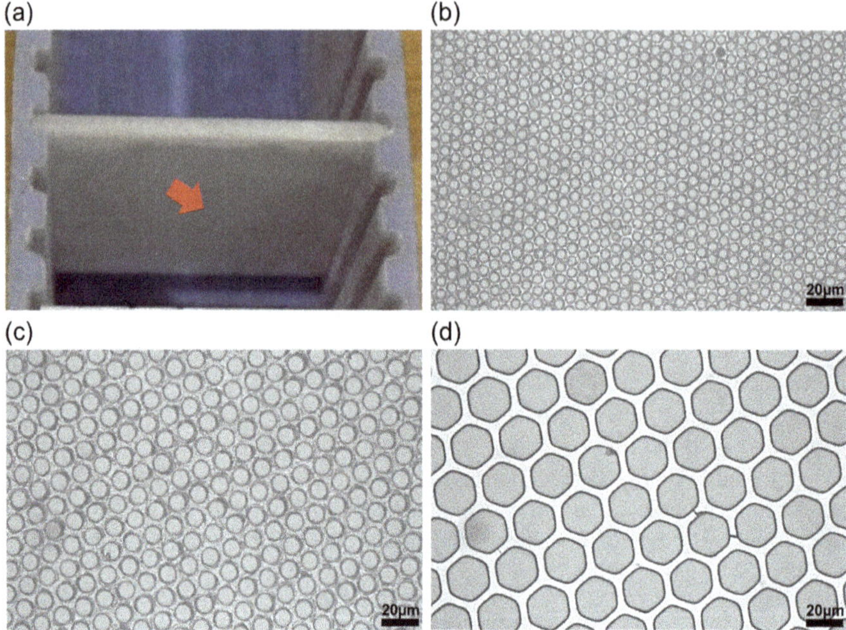

Fig. 1 (**a**) Photograph of an example microcapillaries array plate with microcapillary diameters of 5 μm (plate 1). Each plate is vertically slotted into a phantom holder containing distilled water. Magnified light microscopy images of (**b**) 5 μm (plate 1), (**c**) 10 μm (plate 1) and (**d**) 20 μm (plate 1), at the approximate point indicated by the *red arrow*, to show the cross-section of the microcapillaries array plate

Image Acquisition

Trapezoidal OGSE diffusion sequences, as shown in Fig. 2, are implemented on a Philips Achieva 3.0T TX MRI system (University College London Hospital, London, UK). We choose trapezoidal OGSE waveforms with a fixed maximum gradient strength as it has been shown previously that these are the most sensitive to microcapillary diameters [19, 23]. The main user controlled parameters are echo time (TE), pulse duration (δ), diffusion time (Δ) and number of half period oscillations, referred to as 'lobes' (N). Gradient strength, **G**, and slew rate for the trapezoid waveforms are fixed at 62 mT/m and 68.9 mT/m/ms, respectively, to adhere to manufacturer set threshold for peripheral nervous stimulation (PNS). The b-value for the OGSE sequences with trapezoidal gradient are calculated as in [22].

The plates are scanned during the same session using Philips SENSE Flex Surface coils. A room temperature of 20 °C is maintained throughout the experiment. The diffusion protocol consists of nine HARDI shells with b-values 120–20,000 s/mm^2, each with 32 gradient directions and one b=0 s/mm^2. The shells have a fixed pulse duration ($\delta = 39$ ms, $\Delta = 63$ ms) but the number of lobes varies from N = 1 to N = 9 (i.e. frequencies between 12.8–115 Hz), and consequently the

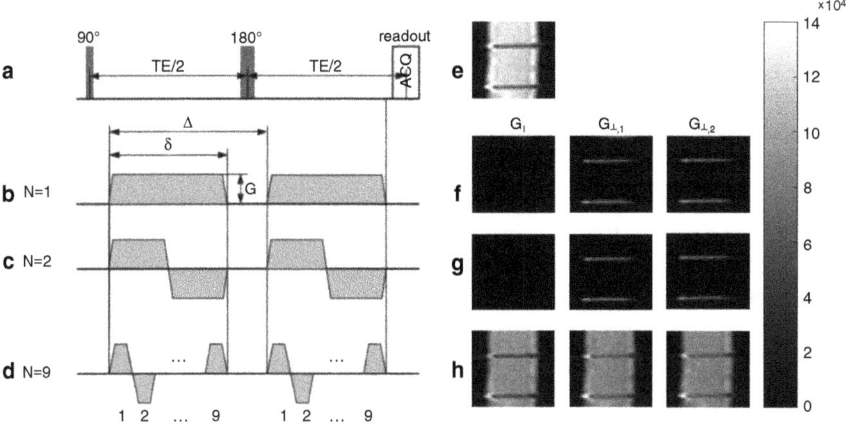

Fig. 2 Schematic representation of the OGSE diffusion imaging protocols (*left*) and corresponding plate example images (*right*). The protocol included (**a**) the single shot echo planar imaging (SS-EPI) sequence containing the excitation, refocusing pulse and readout timings; and the OGSE sequences with (**b**) N = 1, (**c**) N = 2 and (**d**) N = 9. The parameters depicted here are: echo time (TE), pulse duration (δ), diffusion time (Δ), gradient strength (**G**) and number of lobes (N). The example plate images show the 5 μm pair (immersed vertically in water) scanned perpendicular to the plane of the plate. (**e**) is the non-diffusion weighted image. (**f**), (**g**) and (**h**) display diffusion weighted images for OGSE sequence shown in (**b**), (**c**) and (**d**) respectively. The diffusion weighted images are in the parallel and two nearly perpendicular directions relative to the long axis of the microcapillaries. These are only three example directions of the 32 gradient directions that were used in this study. High signal attenuation is seen in the parallel gradient direction indicating free diffusion of water along the long axis of the microcapillaries. Signal appears bright in the perpendicular directions which comes from the restricted diffusion of water across the long axis of the microcapillaries

b-values varied (see Fig. 2). An additional, standard SDE diffusion sequence (N = 1, δ = 10 ms, Δ = 92 ms) with a b-value of 1860 s/mm^2 is also included for comparison.

All diffusion protocols use single-shot-echo-planar imaging (SS-EPI). Each acquired image has one slice of thickness 10 mm, which is orthogonal to the plane of the plate (see Fig. 2). The imaging matrix is 76 × 19 with a resolution of 0.4 × 1.6 mm, which is used to ensure at least one row of the voxels does not contain partial volume effects. In order to obtain sufficient diffusion weighting for all N, we extend the diffusion gradient duration by using a long echo time (in terms of clinical scanning) TE = 120 ms for all shells. Other sequence parameters are: Half Fourier = 0.8, TR = 3 s, repetitions = 1 and acquisition time per protocol = 1.75 min.

2.3 Data Analysis

Data Processing

The acquired images are registered using FMRIB Software Library (FSL, FMRIB, Oxford) rigid-body registration [24] to account for any potential vibrations from the oscillating gradient waveforms. The SNR is calculated from the mean and standard deviation across 9 b = 0 images per voxel. The region of interest (ROI) is chosen from the b = 0 images by manually excluding edges of the plate to avoid voxels affected by partial volume effect. The ROIs of all plates has a mean SNR > 45. Additionally, as the direction of the microcapillaries, $\mathbf{n}$, is assumed to be unknown, $\mathbf{n}$ is estimated using OGSE diffusion tensor imaging and then is inputted into our model fitting procedure described below.

ActiveAx Model Fitting

A voxel-wise two stage model fitting procedure, as defined in [11], is used to estimate diameter and diffusivity of the plate samples. The procedure consists of an initial grid search followed by a non-linear fitting of the model described in (1) to the measured signal. The gradient descent optimisation is constrained with user-defined limits for all parameters (lower and upper bound limits: $a = 0.002$ and $30.0\,\mu$m, and $D_i = 0.002$ and $6.0\,\mu$m^2/ms, respectively) to speed up the fitting. The microcapillary diameters and diffusivities are estimated for each voxel in the ROI, then the mean and standard deviation of the parameters for each plate are calculated across the chosen ROI.

3 Results

First we test whether the microcapillary diameter and the intrinsic diffusivity can be estimated based on the entire trapezoidal OGSE imaging protocol in Fig. 2. We then test which of the OGSE sequences out of those in Fig. 2 provide the most accurate parameter estimates by analysing each shell separately, and we compare the results with the parameters obtained from the standard SDE with long diffusion time.

Figure 3a, b display the parameter maps (diameter and diffusivity, respectively) for the ROIs of our plates. Both pairs of 10 and 20 μm plates have accurate and precise (indicated by the homogeneous maps) estimates. The parameter maps for the 5 μm plates are partially inhomogeneous and they significantly underestimate the diameter. Figure 3c, d reflect the accuracy and precision of the parameters, displayed in Fig. 3a, b, as the mean and standard deviation of the estimated a and D_i calculated across the ROI. The figure also shows very similar parameter estimates within each pair of plates suggesting that the results are reproducible. For the first set of 5, 10 and 20 μm plates, the estimates of mean±standard deviation for

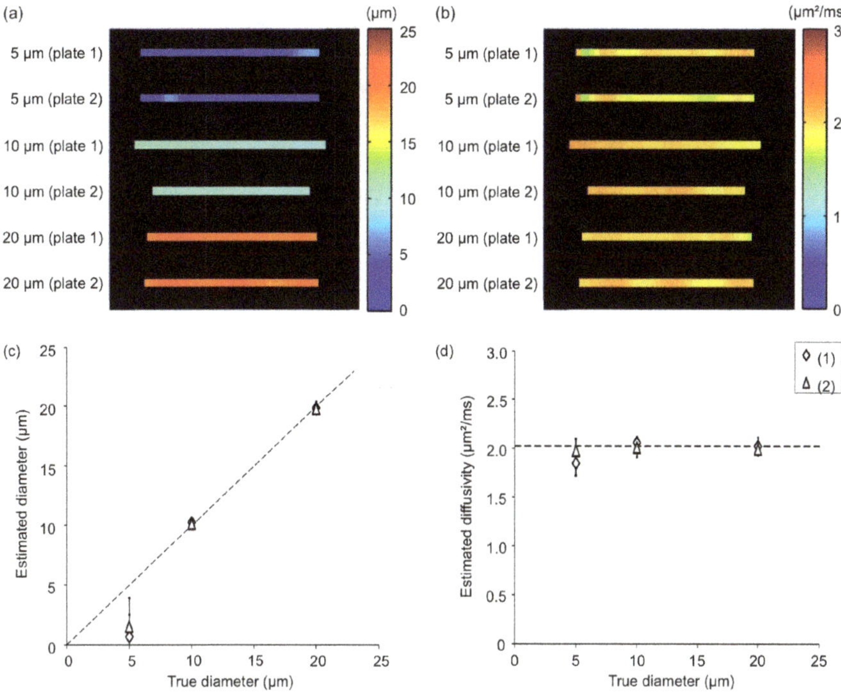

Fig. 3 The (**a**) diameter, a, and (**b**) diffusivity, D_i, maps, respectively, across the ROIs of the 5 μm (plates 1 & 2), 10 μm (plates 1 & 2) and 20 μm (plates 1 & 2) plates. All images have been cropped and magnified by the same amount for visual clarity. The graphs show the mean and standard deviation of the (**c**) diameters of the microcapillaries (μm) and (**d**) intrinsic diffusivities (μm²/ms), which are calculated over the ROIs. The diamond and triangle data points represent the first and second set of plates, respectively. The *dashed line* represent the line of equality for (**c**), and for (**d**) it represents the theoretical water diffusivity calculated using [25] for water at 20 °C

$[a, D_i]$ are $[1.5 \pm 2.4\,\mu\text{m},\ 2.0 \pm 0.1\,\mu\text{m}^2/\text{ms}]$, $[10.1 \pm 0.5\,\mu\text{m},\ 2.0 \pm 0.1\,\mu\text{m}^2/\text{ms}]$ and $[19.8 \pm 0.4\,\mu\text{m},\ 2.0 \pm 0.1\,\mu\text{m}^2/\text{ms}]$, respectively. For the second set of 5, 10 and 20 μm plates, the values of $[a, D_i]$ are: $[0.7 \pm 1.9\,\mu\text{m},\ 1.9 \pm 0.1\,\mu\text{m}^2/\text{ms}]$, $[10.3 \pm 0.2\,\mu\text{m}, 2.1 \pm 0.1\,\mu\text{m}^2/\text{ms}]$ and $[19.8 \pm 0.6\,\mu\text{m},\ 2.0 \pm 0.1\,\mu\text{m}^2/\text{ms}]$, respectively. We observe the highest accuracy and precision for 10 μm plate pairs, and the worst for 5 μm plate pairs.

Figure 4 shows the quality of fit by comparing measurements with predictions from the fitted model (dashed line) and the ground truth (solid line) in the central voxel of each plate ROI. The ground truth curve was generated using the manufacturer provided diameters and a diffusivity constant (2.0 μm²/ms) calculated for the free water compartment at 20 °C [25]. The representative voxels chosen here are typical for the ROIs. A good agreement can be observed between the measurements and the fitted curve and the ground truth curve for 10 μm and 20 μm plates. However, slight differences between the fitted curve and the ground truth

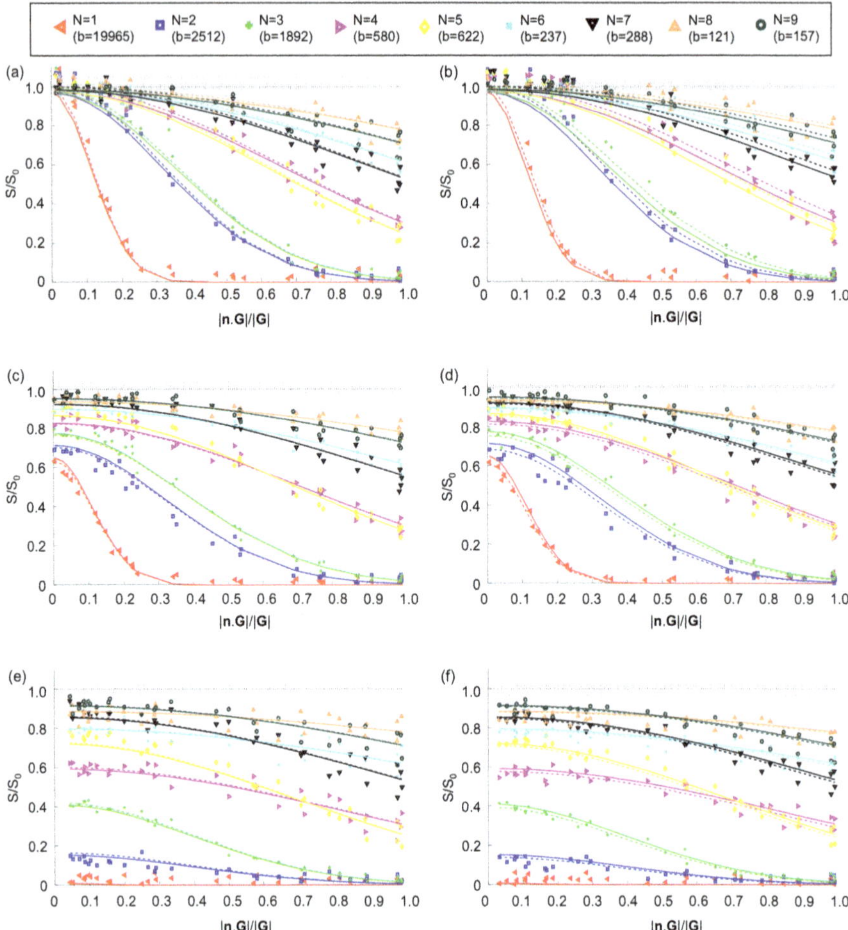

Fig. 4 Plots of normalised signal from central voxel of each ROI in Fig. 3a against absolute dot product between the gradient directions and the estimated direction of the microcapillaries; signals from perpendicular gradient direction are towards 0 on the x-axis, and from parallel directions towards 1. The measurements are represented by markers, while the *solid* (–) and *dashed* (- -) lines show the predicted signal from the ground truth and estimated parameters, respectively. The colours indicate the different N of the imaging protocol. The black dotted lines show the b=0 measurements. All measurements are normalised by the averaged b0 signal per voxel. The parameter estimates for the representative voxels here are: $[a,D_i] = [0.0\,\mu\text{m}, 2.0\,\mu\text{m}^2/\text{ms}], [10.2\,\mu\text{m}, 2.0\,\mu\text{m}^2/\text{ms}]$ and $[20.1\,\mu\text{m}, 2.0\,\mu\text{m}^2/\text{ms}]$ for the first pair of 5, 10 and 20 μm plates, respectively. For the second pair, the respective $[a,D_i]$ are $[0.0\,\mu\text{m}, 1.8\,\mu\text{m}^2/\text{ms}]$, $[10.4\,\mu\text{m}, 2.1\,\mu\text{m}^2/\text{ms}]$ and $[20.5\,\mu\text{m}, 2.1\,\mu\text{m}^2/\text{ms}]$. (**a**) 5 μm, plate 1; (**b**) 5 μm, plate 2; (**c**) 10 μm, plate 1; (**d**) 10 μm, plate 2; (**e**) 20 μm, plate 1 (**f**) 20 μm, plate 2

curve can be observed in the second plates of 10 and 20 μm. This can be due to the overestimated diffusion constant caused potentially by partial volume effects. For this central voxel, in the case of 5 μm plates (Fig. 4a, b), some differences can be seen between the measurements, the fitted curve and the ground truth curve. In this case, due to the low signal attenuation for gradients almost perpendicular to the fibre, measurement noise results in normalized signal values $S/S_0 > 1$ which are not well captured by the model. Moreover, the differences between signals predicted using the known parameters $[a,D_i] = [5.0\,\mu m, 2.0\,\mu m^2/ms]$ and model estimates $[a, D_i] = [0.0\,\mu m, 2.0\,\mu m^2/ms]$ for the first 5 μm plate are small, despite the model estimates of diameter being so different. The difference is slightly larger in the second 5 μm plate ($[a,D_i] = [0.0\,\mu m, 1.8\,\mu m^2/ms]$) but this is most likely due to an underestimation in the diffusion constant. These results suggest the change in measured signal is negligible for microcapillaries with diameters at or below 5 μm, i.e the measured signal is not very sensitive to diameters at or below 5 μm.

Figure 5 shows the mean and standard deviation of the estimated diameter and diffusivity obtained by separately analysing each individual shell with N lobes (from Fig. 2). Here, results from a standard SDE sequence ($N = 1$, $\delta = 10$ ms) are also included for comparison. 10 and 20 μm plate diameter estimates are close to the ground truth values for the majority of N, whereas 5 μm estimates are largely underestimated for all N. Focusing on 10 and 20 μm plates, $N \in \{2,3,4\}$ perform very well, while for $N \geq 5$, the estimates are progressively less accurate and precise as N increases. This is due to insufficient diffusion weighting as N increases. At

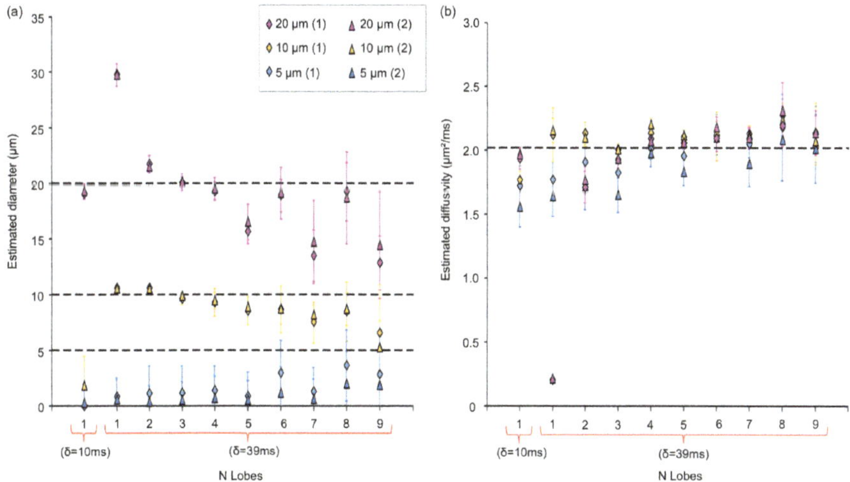

Fig. 5 Mean diameter (**a**) and diffusivity (**b**) estimates calculated for each N from Fig. 2 (labelled as 1–9 (39 ms), where $\delta = 39$ ms) and also from the standard SDE sequence (labelled as 1 (10 ms), where $\delta = 10$ ms), for all plates. The same central row of voxels, as in Fig. 3, is used to calculate the mean and the standard deviation. The *dashed lines* represents the real nominal diameters in (**a**), and the calculated diffusivity from [25] in (**b**). $N = 3$ produces the best diameter and diffusivity for both pairs of 10 μm and 20 μm plates

low N ($N = 1$ ($\delta = 39$ ms)), the fitting fails to correctly estimate the parameters for $20\,\mu$m plates because of the strong diffusion attenuation, forcing the model to fit to the noise floor. As a sanity check we compare the results to ($N = 1, \delta = 10$ ms) and find that diameter and diffusivity of microcapillaries with diameter of $20\,\mu$m are estimated accurately for this SDE sequence, however, $10\,\mu$m plates are poorly estimated. Hence, for this particular TE and diffusion gradient duration, we find that $N > 1$ gives better results overall.

$N = 3$ gives the best estimates for both 10 and $20\,\mu$m plates. $N = 3$ outputs $[a, D_i]$ of $[9.7 \pm 0.5\,\mu\text{m}, 2.0 \pm 0.0\,\mu\text{m}^2/\text{ms}]$ and $[20.1 \pm 0.5\,\mu\text{m}, 1.9 \pm 0.1\,\mu\text{m}^2/\text{ms}]$ for the first pairs of 10 and $20\,\mu$m plates, respectively. We also see consistency in our estimates because the estimates ($[a, D_i]$) for the second pair are $[9.9 \pm 0.3\,\mu\text{m}, 2.1 \pm 0.0\,\mu\text{m}^2/\text{ms}]$ and $[20.1 \pm 0.8\,\mu\text{m}, 1.9 \pm 0.1\,\mu\text{m}^2/\text{ms}]$. The diameter estimates from $N = 3$ are close to the ground truth and are also within the confidence limits of the estimates from the combined OGSE protocol shown in Fig. 3. The diffusivity estimates have slightly higher accuracy and slightly lower precision for both pairs of 10 and $20\,\mu$m plates in comparison to the combined OGSE protocol. The diffusivity estimates are also very close to the estimates from the combined OGSE protocol. These results suggest that, for the case of idealised systems, one OGSE shell can perform similarly compared to a combination of OGSE shells.

4 Discussion

In this article we explore the sensitivity of OGSE to microstructural dimensions of microcapillaries of unknown orientation on a clinical scanner. We find that 10 and $20\,\mu$m micro-capillary diameters can be accurately and precisely estimated whereas $5\,\mu$m estimates are neither accurate nor precise. We also find that low frequency OGSE sequences give the best results and are optimal for parameter estimation. In particular, $N = 3$ OGSE sequence can be used on its own to give estimates that are very similar to those of the combined OGSE frequencies ($N = 1$ to $N = 9$).

Our observations support the theoretical findings in [12, 18] regarding the clinical scanner diameter resolution limit which, based on their calculations, for gradient strength of $\mathbf{G} = 62$ mT/m, is approximately $6\,\mu$m for SNR ≈ 50. We get excellent estimates for 10 and $20\,\mu$m plates and can assume that the same would be true for the diameters of microcapillaries within this range ($a \in [10, 20]\,\mu$m). On the other hand, $5\,\mu$m diameters cannot be estimated as they fall bellow the resolution limit. In our study, we used idealised phantom plates (homogeneously and densely packed with microcapillaries), which were imaged with a HARDI type acquisition, pushed to the clinically feasible limits. We used a 'long' TE $= 120$ ms (in terms of standard clinical settings) in order to allow for larger diffusion weighting which is necessary to improve the sensitivity to the smaller diameter microcapillaries ($5\,\mu$m). We also maximised SNR (≥ 45) on the clinical scanner by imaging the phantom ensemble with a surface coil and using water as the substrate (long T2 relaxation time ≈ 1500 ms). Yet for a gradient strength of 62 mT/m, the diffusion weighted signal for the 5 μm microcapillaries could not be differentiated from a diffusion signal for 0μm microcapillaries. This highlights that diameters of 5 μm cannot be estimated on clinical scanners even under idealised conditions. On the other hand, when we place the same 5 μm plates in a pre-clinical scanner with 800 mT/m gradients we estimate 5 μm perfectly (data not shown), suggesting that the sole reason for the results is the insufficient gradient strength.

Our analysis of individual OGSE sequences shows that there is an optimal range of OGSE lobes, for estimation of diameters of microcapillaries and intrinsic diffusivity. The optimal OGSE shells are with low number of lobes, ($N \in \{2, 3, 4\}$) and their parameter estimates are accurate and precise, especially for $N = 3$. Our experimental findings are consistent with the recent ActiveAx simulation study [12] and spectroscopy study [17], which show that OGSE with lower N are optimal for the measurement of fibre diameters. The result highlights the importance of optimisation for microstructure indices estimation.

In this work we analysed the sensitivity of OGSE sequences to fibre diameter in micro-capillaries. Based on theoretical studies which compare OGSE and SDE sequences [12, 18], we do not expect SDE based techniques to provide better diameter estimates, with the same gradient constraints. Although we have not directly compared the sensitivity of other more complex sequences (e.g. NOGSE [26]), similar conclusions hold, as the sensitivity and resolution limit is driven by the maximum gradient strength and pulse duration [18].

The phantom we use in this study is much simpler than in vivo nerve tissue. However, the purpose of this work is to test the innate sensitivity of OGSE sequences to fibre diameters on a clinical scanner, which requires ideal diffusion substrates. We expect that results for in vivo nerve tissue to be similar or worse. For instance, resolution limit would be lower, i.e. since 5 μm diameter can not be estimated in an ideal phantom with extremely long T2 of pure water and simple parallel cylindrical capillaries, then its potential to be estimated in vivo is further reduced. As for the optimal frequency of the OGSE , the exact value would be different, however it is predictable that it would be low frequency. The benefits of using physical phantoms with known geometry and microstructural characteristics are numerous. They are not degradable over time and are easy to use in validating microstructure imaging protocols [27], even over multiple clinical trial sites. There are other ongoing development of more complex phantoms such as biomimetic phantoms [28] being developed for validating diffusion MR imaging. However, the simplicity of the plates used in this study is also ideal for validation and calibration purposes. In future, we plan to develop an integrated phantom with a more finely graded range of microcapillary diameters to explore the resolution limit with more accuracy.

Overall, our results suggest that imaging axon diameters in vivo in the brain using standard clinical scanners with gradient strength of 60–80 mT/m would be very challenging. This work, combined with the theoretical work by Drobnjak et al. [12] and Nillson et al. [18], provides further evidence for validity of models of brain nerve tissue where axons are represented as sticks and not as cylinders [29]. On the other hand, our work also demonstrates that axon diameter mapping is still a possibility in the peripheral nervous system, where axons are larger (1–8 μm [30]).

Axon diameter imaging of the peripheral nerves using clinical scanners can potentially play a crucial role in the understanding of nerve tissue regeneration—a mechanism unique to peripheral nerves and with correlation to axon diameters [31].

Acknowledgements We thank EPSRC for funding the research studentship of Lebina Shrestha Kakkar. EPSRC grants EP/I018700/1 and EP/H046410/1 also contributed to this work. The study was undertaken at UCH and UCL, both of whom are part-funded by the Department of Health NIHR Biomedical Research Centres funding scheme.

References

1. Ritchie, J.M.: On the relation between fibre diameter and conduction velocity in myelinated nerve fibres. Proc. R. Soc. Lond. Ser. B **217**(1206), 29–35 (1982)
2. Hildebrand, C., Remahl, S., Persson, H., Bjartmar, C.: Myelinated nerve fibres in the CNS. Prog. Neurobiol. **40**, 319–384 (1993)
3. Marner, L., Nyengaard, J.R., Tang, Y.Y., Pakkenberg, B.: Marked loss of myelinated nerve fibers in the human brain with age. J. Comput. Neurosci. **462**(2), 144–152 (2003)
4. Cluskey, S., Ramsden, D.B.: Mechanisms of neurodegeneration in amyotrophic lateral sclerosis. Mol. Pathol. **54**(6), 386 (2001)
5. Piven, J., Bailey, J., Ranson, B.J., Arndt, S.: An MRI study of the corpus callosum in autism. Am. J. Psychiatr. **154**(8), 1051 (1997)
6. Rice, D., Barone, S. Jr.: Critical periods of vulnerability for the developing nervous system: evidence from humans and animal models. Environ. Health Perspect. **108**(Suppl 3), 511 (2000)
7. Ong, H.H., Wehrli, F.W.: Quantifying axon diameter and intra-cellular volume fraction in excised mouse spinal cord with q-space imaging. Neuroimage **51**, 1360–1366 (2010)
8. Shemesh, N., Özarslan, E., Komlosh, M.E., Basser, P.J., Cohen, Y.: From single-pulsed field gradient to double-pulsed field gradient MR: gleaning new microstructural information and developing new forms of contrast in MRI. NMR Biomed. **23**, 757–780 (2010)
9. Komlosh, M.E., Özarslan, E., Lizak, M.J., Horkayne-Szakaly, I., Freidlin, R.Z., Horkay, F., Basser, P.J.: Mapping average axon diameters in porcine spinal cord white matter and rat corpus callosum using d-PFG MRI. Neuroimage **78**, 210–216 (2013)
10. Assaf, Y., Blumenfeld-Katzir, T., Yovel, Y., Basser, P.J.: AxCaliber: a method for measuring axon diameter distribution from diffusion MRI. Magn. Reson. Med. **59**(6), 1347–1354 (2008)
11. Alexander, D.C., Hubbard, P.L., Hall, M.G., Moore, E.A., Ptito, M., Parker, G.J., Dyrby, T.B.: Orientationally invariant indices of axon diameter and density from diffusion MRI. NeuroImage **52**, 1374–1389 (2010)
12. Drobnjak, I., Zhang, H., Ianus, A., Kaden, E., Alexander, D.C.: PGSE, OGSE, and sensitivity to axon diameter in diffusion MRI: insight from a simulation study. Magn. Reson. Med. **75**(2), 688–700 (2016)
13. Li, H., Jiang, X., Xie, J., Gore, J.C., Xu, J.: Impact of transcytolemmal water exchange on estimates of tissue microstructural properties derived from diffusion MRI. Magn. Reson. Med. (2016)
14. Siow, B., Drobnjak, I., Chatterjee, A., Lythgoe, M.F., Alexander, D.C.: Estimation of pore size in a microstructure phantom using the optimised gradient waveform diffusion weighted NMR sequence. J. Magn. Reson. **214**, 51–60 (2012)
15. Parsons, E.C., Does, M.D., Gore, J.C.: Temporal diffusion spectroscopy: theory and implementation in restricted systems using oscillating gradients. J. Magn. Reson. **55**, 75–84 (2006)
16. Callaghan, P.T.: Translational Dynamics and Magnetic Resonance: Principles of Pulsed Gradient Spin Echo NMR, 1st edn. Oxford University Press, Oxford (2011)

17. Li, H., Gore, J.C., Xu, J.: Fast and robust measurement of microstructural dimensions using temporal diffusion spectroscopy. J. Magn. Reson. **242**, 4–9 (2014)
18. Nilsson, M., Lasic, S., Topgaard, D., Westin, C.F.: Estimating the axon diameter from intra-axonal water diffusion with arbitrary gradient waveforms: resolution limit in parallel and dispersed fibers. In: ISMRM Annual Meeting, vol. 24, p. 663 (2016). ISMRM Abstract
19. Drobnjak, I., Siow, B., Alexander, D.C.: Optimizing gradient waveforms for microstructure sensitivity in diffusion-weighted MR. J. Magn. Reson. **206**, 41–51 (2010)
20. Assaf, Y., Freidlin, R.Z., Rohde, G.K., Basser, P.J.: New modeling and experimental framework to characterize hindered and restricted water diffusion in brain white matter. Magn. Reson. Med. **52**(5), 965–978 (2004)
21. Murday, J.S., Cotts, R.M.: Self-diffusion coefficient of liquid lithium. J. Chem. Phys. **48**(11), 4938–4945 (1968)
22. Ianus, A., Siow, B., Drobnjak, I., Zhang, H., Alexander, D.C.: Gaussian phase distribution approximations for oscillating gradient spin echo diffusion MRI. J. Magn. Reson. **227**, 25–34 (2013)
23. Drobnjak, I., Cruz, G., Alexander, D.C.: Optimising oscillating waveform-shape for pore size sensitivity in diffusion-weighted MR. Microporous Mesoporous Mater. **178**, 11–14 (2013)
24. Jenkinson, M., Bannister, P., Brady, J.M., Smith, S.M.: Improved optimisation for the robust and accurate linear registration and motion correction of brain images. NeuroImage **17**(2), 825–841 (2002)
25. Holz, M., Heila, S.R., Saccob, A.: Temperature-dependent self-diffusion coefficients of water and six selected molecular liquids for calibration in accurate 1H NMR PFG measurements. Phys. Chem. Chem. Phys. **2**, 4740–4742 (2000)
26. Shemesh, N., Alvarez, G.A., Frydman, L.: Size distribution imaging by non-uniform oscillating-gradient spin echo (NOGSE) MRI. PLoS One **10**(7), e0133201 (2015)
27. Komlosh, M.E., Özarslan, E., Lizak, M.J., Horkay, F., Schram, V., Shemesh, N., Cohen, Y., Basser, P.J.: Pore diameter mapping using double pulsed-field gradient MRI and its validation using a novel glass capillary array phantom. J. Magn. Reson. **208**, 128–135 (2011)
28. Hubbard, P.L., Zhou, F.L., Eichhorn, S.J., Parker, G.J.M.: Biomimetic phantom for the validation of diffusion magnetic resonance imaging. Magn. Reson. Med. **73**, 299–305 (2015)
29. Behrens, T.E.J., Woolrich, M.W., Jenkinson, M., Johansen-Berg, H., Nunes, R.G., Clare, S., Matthews, P.M., Brady, J.M., Smith, S.M.: Characterization and propagation of uncertainty in diffusion-weighted MR imaging. Magn. Reson. Med. **50**, 1077–1088 (2003)
30. Schroder, J.M., Bohl, J., Brodda, K.: Changes of the ratio between myelin thickness and axon diameter in the human developing sural nerve. J. Neurosurg. Sci. **76**(5), 114–120 (1988)
31. Sanders, F.K.: The thickness of the myelin sheaths of normal and regenerating peripheral nerve fibres. Proc. R. Soc. Lond. Ser. B **135**(880), 323–357 (1948)

Groupwise Structural Parcellation of the Cortex: A Sound Approach Based on Logistic Models

Guillermo Gallardo, Rutger Fick, William Wells III, Rachid Deriche, and Demian Wassermann

Abstract Current theories hold that brain function is highly related with long-range physical connections through axonal bundles, namely *extrinsic connectivity*. However, obtaining a groupwise cortical parcellation based on extrinsic connectivity remains challenging. Current parcellation methods are computationally expensive; need tuning of several parameters or rely on ad-hoc constraints. Furthermore, none of these methods present a model for the cortical extrinsic connectivity. To tackle these problems, we propose a parsimonious model for the extrinsic connectivity and an efficient parcellation technique based on clustering of tractograms. Our technique allows the creation of single subject and groupwise parcellations of the whole cortex. The parcellations obtained with our technique are in agreement with anatomical and functional parcellations in the literature. In particular, the motor and sensory cortex are subdivided in agreement with the human homunculus of Penfield. We illustrate this by comparing our resulting parcels with an anatomical atlas and the motor strip mapping included in the Human Connectome Project data.

1 Introduction

The human brain is arranged in areas based on criteria such as cytoarchitecture or axonal connectivity. Current hypotheses attribute specialized functions to several of these areas. Hence, parcellating the cortex into such areas and characterizing their interaction is key to understanding brain function. Diffusion MRI (dMRI) enables the in vivo exploration of long-rage physical connections through axonal bundles, namely *extrinsic connectivity* . Current theories hold that extrinsic connectivity is strongly related to brain function, e.g. this has been shown in macaques [15]. Hence, parcellating the cortex based on its extrinsic connectivity can help to understand the internal organization of the brain. However, obtaining a whole-cortex

G. Gallardo (✉) • R. Fick • R. Deriche • D. Wassermann
Université Côte d'Azur, Inria, France
e-mail: guillermo.gallardo-diez@inria.fr

W. Wells III
Harvard Medical School, Boston, MA, USA

© Springer International Publishing AG 2017
A. Fuster et al. (eds.), *Computational Diffusion MRI*, Mathematics and Visualization, DOI 10.1007/978-3-319-54130-3_8

groupwise parcellation based on extrinsic connectivity remains challenging [9]. Current extrinsic connectivity parcellation methods are computationally expensive; need tuning of several parameters or rely on ad-hoc constraints. For example, Clarkson et al. [4] propose to iteratively refine an anatomical parcellation using information from dMRI. This technique's main drawback is the strong dependence on the initial anatomical parcellation. Lefranc et al. [10] calculate the average connectivity profile of regions using a watershed-driven dimension reduction, but they work parcellating predefined gyri. Parisot et al. [14] estimate a consistent parcellation across subjects using a spectral clustering approach, without averaging subject's connectivity profiles. Nevertheless, the method needs tuning of several parameters, including the expected number of parcels specified a priori. Moreno-Dominguez et al. [12] present a parcelling method based on hierarchical clustering parcellation, in which it's not necessary to set an a priori number of clusters. However, they use the cosine distance to compare tractograms and the centroid of tractograms to represent their union. This can lead to an erroneous parcellation since the centroid criterion doesn't minimize the cosine distance between points. These examples show that an efficient groupwise parcelling technique alongside a sound model for the extrinsic connectivity is still needed.

In this work we present a parsimonious model for the cortical connectivity and an efficient parcelling technique based on it, both summarized in Fig. 1. Our model assumes that the cortex is divided in patches of homogeneous extrinsic connectivity.

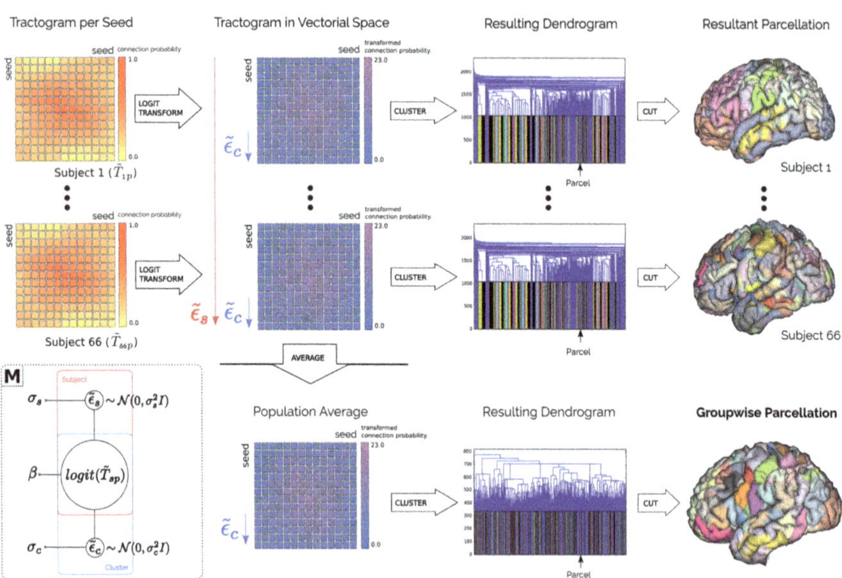

Fig. 1 *Lower left corner*: graphical model of the linear relationship between a tractogram ($\widetilde{T}_{sp}$); the intra-cluster ($\widetilde{\epsilon}_c$) and across-subject ($\widetilde{\epsilon}_s$) variability. We transform the tractograms into a vectorial space while explicitly accounting for the variability, allowing us to propose a clustering technique in accordance

That is, nearby neurons in the cortex share approximately the same long-ranged physical connections, we call this the *local coherence criterion*. Our assumption is based on histological results in the macaque brain [19]. As in clustered data models in statistics [16] we allow intra-patch variability and across-subject variability in the patches.

Nowadays, the most common tool to estimate the extrinsic connectivity of a point on the cortex in vivo is dMRI-based tractography [9] . To frame tractography within our cortical connectivity model, we use Logistic Random Effects Models [19]. This allows us to explicitly denote the relationship between tractography and the variability present in our model. Taking advantage of this, we propose an efficient clustering technique to create single subject and groupwise parcellations of the whole-cortex. Inspired by the method of Moreno-Dominguez et al.[12], our technique creates a dendrogram: a structure that comprises different levels of granularity for the same parcellation. We also create the dendrogram while imposing the local coherence criterion using only one parameter: the minimum size of each parcel. Then, by choosing cutting criteria, we can explore different parcellation granularities without recomputing the dendrogram.

We validate our technique by taking advantage of the information available in the Human Connectome Project (HCP). Using our technique, we create single-subject and groupwise parcellations for 66 subjects. Then, we compare our purely structural parcellations against an anatomical atlas [5] and responses to functional stimuli [2]. We show that our parcels subdivide some well-known anatomical structures in accordance with functional responses on the cortex.

2   Methods

2.1   Data and Preprocessing

In this work we used 66 male subjects aged 31–35 from the group S500 of the Human Connectome Project (HCP), all preprocessed with the HCP minimum pipeline [7]. The main advantages of using this public data base are: each subject possess a dense mesh representing their cortical surface, we use it to create seed-points for tractography; all the mesh's vertices are coregistered across subjects, property that we use to create the groupwise parcellation; each subject possess the Desikan Atlas [5] parcellation already computed over their cortical mesh; for each cortical mesh there are also different z-score maps representing the response to different stimuli obtained with functional MRI (fMRI) [2]. Finally, the group S500 contains z-score maps representing the average functional response to stimuli for 100 unrelated subjects (U100). These studies are used to validate our technique's results.

2.2 Cortical Connectivity Model and Tractography

Our model assumes that the cortex is divided in clusters of homogeneous extrinsic connectivity. That is, nearby neurons in the cortex share approximately the same long-ranged physical connections, we call this the *local coherence criterion*. Our assumption is based on histological results in the macaque brain [19]. As in clustered data models in statistics [16] we allow intra-cluster and across-subject variability. We formalize this concept as:

$$K = \bigcup_{i=1}^{k} K_i, \forall_{1 \leq i,j \leq k}, i \neq j \to K_i \cap K_j = \emptyset \wedge \mathrm{conn}(K_i) \neq \mathrm{conn}(K_j) \qquad (1)$$

where the set of points on the cortex K is the disjoint union of each cluster K_i and $\mathrm{conn}(\cdot)$ is the extrinsic connectivity fingerprint of a cluster. We will make the notion of variability explicit in Eq. (3). In this work, the connectivity fingerprint of a seed-point in the brain is a binary vector denoting to which other seed-points it is connected through axonal bundles. This is, the physical connections of a point $p \in K_i$ in the brain are represented by its connectivity fingerprint $\mathrm{conn}(p) = \mathrm{conn}(K_i)$.

Nowadays, the most common tool for estimating the extrinsic connectivity fingerprint of a point in vivo is probabilistic tractography [9]. Given a seed-point in the brain, probabilistic tractography creates a *tractogram*: an image where each voxel is valued with its probability of being connected to the seed through axonal bundles. One way of calculating these probabilities is with a Monte Carlo procedure, simulating the random walk of water particles through the white matter [3]. Each one of these paths is known as a streamline. If we think these streamlines as Bernoulli trials, were we get a value for the connection from our seed with other points (1 if they connected by the streamline, 0 if not) [3], then we can model the tractogram of the subject s in the seed-point p as:

$$T_{sp} = [P(\tilde{C}_{spi} = 1)]_{1 \leq i \leq n} = [\theta_{spi}]_{1 \leq i \leq n}, \ \tilde{C}_{spi} \sim \mathrm{Bernoulli}(\theta_{spi}) \ , \qquad (2)$$

where $\tilde{C}_{spi}$ is a Bernoulli random variable[1] representing "the point p of the subject s is connected to the voxel i". Each Bernoulli's parameter (θ_{spi}) represents the probability of being connected, and is estimated as the proportion of success in the Bernoulli trials of each seed.

To formulate the tractogram in accordance to our hypothesis of cortical connectivity, we model a tractogram as a vector of random variables. In our model, each element in a tractogram comes from a random variable depending of the point's cluster alongside its intra-cluster and across-subject variability:

$$p \in K_c \to \tilde{T}_{sp} = [P(\tilde{C}_{spi} = 1 \,|\, \mathrm{conn}(K_c), \, \tilde{\epsilon}_{ci}, \, \tilde{\epsilon}_{si})]_{1 \leq i \leq n} \ , \qquad (3)$$

---

[1]For the sake of clarity we denote all random variables with a tilde, e.g. $\tilde{C}$.

in this case, the point p belongs to the cluster c; $\tilde{\epsilon}_{ci}$ represents the intra-cluster variability and $\tilde{\epsilon}_{si}$ represents the across-subject variability for the connectivity to voxel i in the cluster c.

Since each $\tilde{C}_{spi}$ follows a Bernoulli distribution [Eq. (2)] it's difficult to find an explicit formulation for $P(\tilde{C}_{spi} = 1 \mid \mathrm{conn}(K_c), \tilde{\epsilon}_{ci}, \tilde{\epsilon}_{si})$ accounting for the variabilities. For this, we use the generalized linear model (GLM) theory. In this theory, the data is assumed to follow a linear form after being transformed with an appropriate link function [11]. Using the following notation abuse:

$$\mathrm{logit}(\tilde{T}_{sp}) \triangleq [\mathrm{logit}(P(\tilde{C}_{spi} = 1 \mid \mathrm{conn}(K_c), \tilde{\epsilon}_{ci}, \tilde{\epsilon}_{si})]_{1 \leq i \leq n}, \tag{4}$$

we derive from GLM a logistic random-effects model [16] for each point p:

$$\mathrm{logit}(\tilde{T}_{sp}) = \beta_c + \tilde{\epsilon}_c + \tilde{\epsilon}_s \in \mathbb{R}^n, \quad \tilde{\epsilon}_c \sim \mathcal{N}(\mathbf{0}, \sigma_c^2 Id), \ \tilde{\epsilon}_s \sim \mathcal{N}(\mathbf{0}, \sigma_s^2 Id), \tag{5}$$

where ϵ_c and ϵ_s represent the intra-cluster and across-subject variability respectively. According to GLM theory $\beta_c \in \mathbb{R}^n$ is the extrinsic connectivity fingerprint of cluster K_c transformed:

$$\mathrm{logit}^{-1}(\beta_c) = E(\tilde{T}_{sp}) = \mathrm{conn}(K_c) \ . \tag{6}$$

The choice of logit as link function is based on the work of Pohl et al. [17]. There, they show that the logit function's codomain is a Euclidean space, which allows us to transform and manipulate the tractograms in a well-known space.

2.3 Single Subject and Groupwise Parcelling Methodologies

In the previous section we hypothesised that the cortex is divided in clusters with homogeneous extrinsic connectivity, alongside intra-cluster and across-subject variability. In using the previous hypothesis, it is important to remark that we don't have a priori knowledge of the cluster's location or their variability. But, thanks to the proposed logistic random effects model, we formulated the problem of finding these clusters as a well-known clustering problem. This is because, after transforming the tractograms with the logit function as in Eq. (4) they will be in a Euclidean space [17]. Even more, Eq. (5) states that the transformed tractograms come from a mixture of Gaussian distributions. This is known as a Gaussian mixture model.

To solve the Gaussian mixture model and find the clusters, we use a modified Agglomerative Hierarchical Clustering (AHC) algorithm. This was inspired by the method of Moreno-Dominguez et al. [12]. To enforce the local coherence criterion we also modify the algorithm to accept one parameter: the minimum size of the resulting clusters. Clusters smaller than this size are merged with neighbors, i.e. physically close clusters in the cortex. As we are working in a Euclidean space, we use the Euclidean distance and the centroid as similarity and linkage functions, improving performance. Our technique's time complexity is $O(n^2 log(n))$, with n the number of tractograms to cluster [13]. AHC creates a dendrogram: a structure that comprises different levels of granularity for the same parcellation. This allows us to explore different parcellation granularities by choosing cutting criteria, without the need of recomputing each time.

The main advantage of the model we proposed in the previous section is that it allows us to create a groupwise parcellation using linear operations. Assuming direct seed correspondence across subjects, as in the HCP data set, our model lets us remove the subject variability of each seed's tractogram by calculating the expected value across subjects:

$$E_s(g(\tilde{T}_{sp})) = E_s(\beta_c + \tilde{\epsilon}_c + \tilde{\epsilon}_s), = \beta_c + \tilde{\epsilon}_c + E_s(\tilde{\epsilon}_s) = \beta_c + \tilde{\epsilon}_c. \qquad (7)$$

where the last equality is due to $E_s(\tilde{\epsilon}_s) = 0$ [Eq. (5)]. This allows us to create population-representative tractograms for each seed free of across-subject variability, which then can be clustered to create a groupwise parcellation.

3 Experiments and Results

3.1 *Reliability of the Clustering Algorithm for the Model*

In the previous sections we presented a model for the cortical extrinsic connectivity and a clustering technique to parcellate the brain. Our technique allows us to create single subject and groupwise parcellations, encoded with different levels of granularity in a dendrogram. However, is not immediate that the chosen clustering algorithm (AHC) solves a Gaussian mixture model [Eq. 5] since it was not designed for this particular case [13]. That is, it's not immediate that the algorithm finds the clusters if they are stated as in the model [Eq. 5]. Now we show that the modified version of the algorithm (Sect. 2.3) to enforce the local coherence criterion (Sect. 2.2), solves the model for reasonable levels of variability. Moreover, it retrieves the right clusters using one of the simplest criterion to cut the dendrogram: the horizontal cut, i.e. cutting the dendrogram just by choosing the cut's height.

To test the technique, we started by creating synthetic data from the model [Eq. (5)]. We randomly took ten subjects from our chosen set alongside their extant Desikan parcellations. Then, we created synthetic connectivity fingerprints representing the connections between their Desikan areas. Next, for each vertex in their cortical surface we: replicated those fingerprints; transformed them with the logit function and added cluster-specific variability and across-subject variability as in our model. Finally, we grouped the vertex based on their connectivity using our clustering technique.

If our parcelling technique is able to solve the model, then the Desikan Areas should be encoded in the resulting dendrogram. To show that the Desikan areas were encoded in the resulting dendrogram, we calculated the best obtainable overlap between each Desikan area and the clusters in the dendrogram using the Dice coefficient. To evince the accuracy of the horizontal cut criterion, we compared every obtainable parcellation through cutting our dendrogram in the average subject case against the Desikan atlas using the corrected Rand index [8]. A Rand index of 1 means that the two parcellations were equal.

Figure 2-left shows the best dice coefficients obtained for every Desikan region under different levels of variability. The Signal-to-Noise-Ratio (SNR) in the figure represents the amount of variability added respect to the original variability of the synthetic connectivity fingerprint. The result in Fig. 2-left shows that parcels were retrieved and well-encoded inside the dendrogram for reasonable levels of variability, specially in the average case (dark blue line) were we get ride of the across-subject variability by averaging. Figure 2-right shows the best obtainable rand index using horizontal cut on the dendrogram under different levels of variability. The high Rand indices obtained show that we can solve our model by simply using the horizontal cut criterion.

3.2 Parcelling Subjects From the Human Connectome Project

We next applied our parcellation technique to the HCP data. First, we performed Constrained Spherical Deconvolution (CSD) based tractography [20] from a dense set of points in the cortex. Then, we used our technique to parcellate the cortex by clustering the tractograms. Specifically, since each subject has a surface representing their gray-matter/white-matter interface, we used their vertices as seeds to create tractograms. To avoid superficial cortico-cortical fibers [18], we shrank each of the 66 surfaces 3 mm into the white matter. For each subject, we fitted a CSD model [20] to their diffusion data using Dipy (version 0.11) [6] and created 15,000 streamlines per seed-voxel using the implementation of probabilistic tractography in Dipy. Later, we created a tractogram as in [Eq. (2)] by calculating the fraction of particles that visited each white-matter voxel. Then, we transformed each tractogram with the logit function [17] as in Eq. (4). We clustered the tractograms of each subject using the modified AHC algorithm while imposing a minimum cluster size of $3 \, \text{mm}^2$ in the finest granularity.

To create the groupwise parcellation, we took advantage of the vertex correspondence across subjects in the HCP data set. Since we are in a vectorial space we calculated the average tractogram of each seed. Then, we created the groupwise parcellation by clustering the average tractograms with our proposed technique (Sect. 2.3). The resulting dendrogram for the groupwise case, alongside some of the obtainable parcellations, are in Fig. 3.

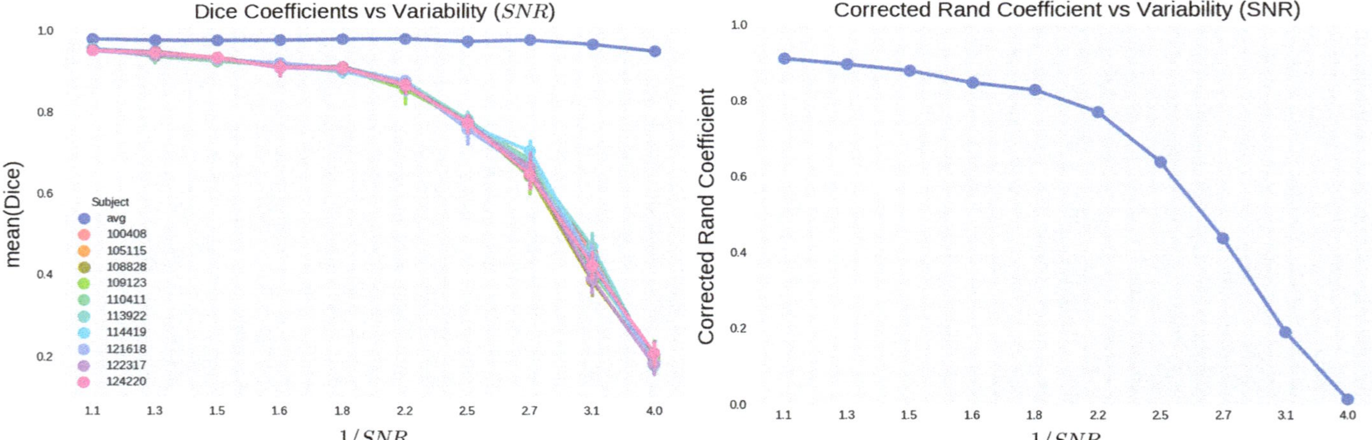

Fig. 2 Clustering performance for different levels of variability. *SNR* comprises both intra-cluster and across-subject variability, at smaller *SNR* more variability is present. *Left*, best overlap between synthetic regions and clusters in the dendrogram. *Right*, best corrected rand coefficient for horizontal cutting. The coefficients close to 1, specially in the average case (*dark blue line*), show the compatibility between our parcellation technique and the proposed model

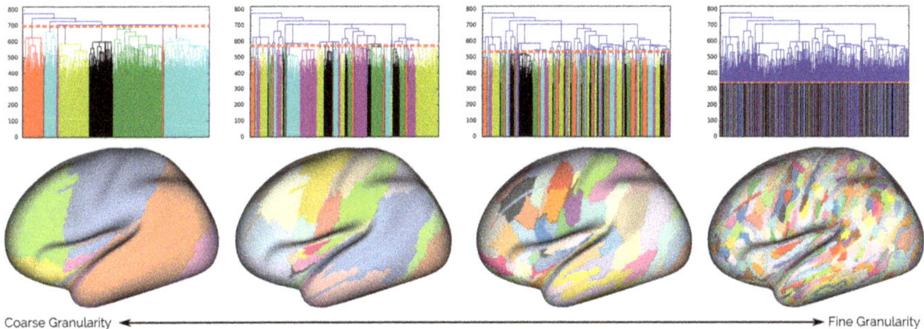

Fig. 3 Groupwise dendrogram created by our technique. We can retrieve different granularities of the same parcellation by choosing cutting height, shown as a *red dotted line*. Motor and Sensory cortex appear at coarse levels of granularity

3.3 *Functional and Anatomical Comparison*

Here we present a proof of concept that our resulting dendrograms encode parcellations with both anatomical and functional meaning by comparing our results against an anatomical atlas and a functional study. To make the comparisons we extracted a parcellation from each subject's dendrogram using the horizontal cut criterion since it showed good accuracy in Sect. 3.1. We manually searched for parcellations with a minimum of 36 parcels and a maximum of 150. This was made to get parcellations with coarse granularity while having at least the amount of parcels in the anatomical atlas of Desikan [5].

Anatomical Comparison

To assess if some anatomical structures were present in the dendrogram and if our resulting parcels were subdividing them, we compared the extracted parcellation with the Desikan atlas [5]. It's important to remark that each subject in the HCP already has this atlas computed. We projected the Desikan regions over our parcels and then calculated: how many of our parcels were inside each projection and how many of them had more than 90% of its area inside the projection. Comparisons with eight regions of the Desikan atlas for the single-subject and the groupwise case are in Figs. 4-left and 5 respectively. Table 1 shows the fraction of parcels inside of each projections that were well contained. Our division of the inferior frontal cortex differs from the Desikan's [5] (regions 1 and 2 in Fig. 5). However, it's similar to that of Anwander et al. [1]. In particular, our orange and cyan parcels inside regions 1 and 2 correspond with their blue and green parcels in Fig. 4, panels I, II, IV and V [1]. The Insula; Motor and Sensory cortex (regions 3, 4 and 5 in Fig. 5) were well subdivided for both single subject and groupwise parcellations.

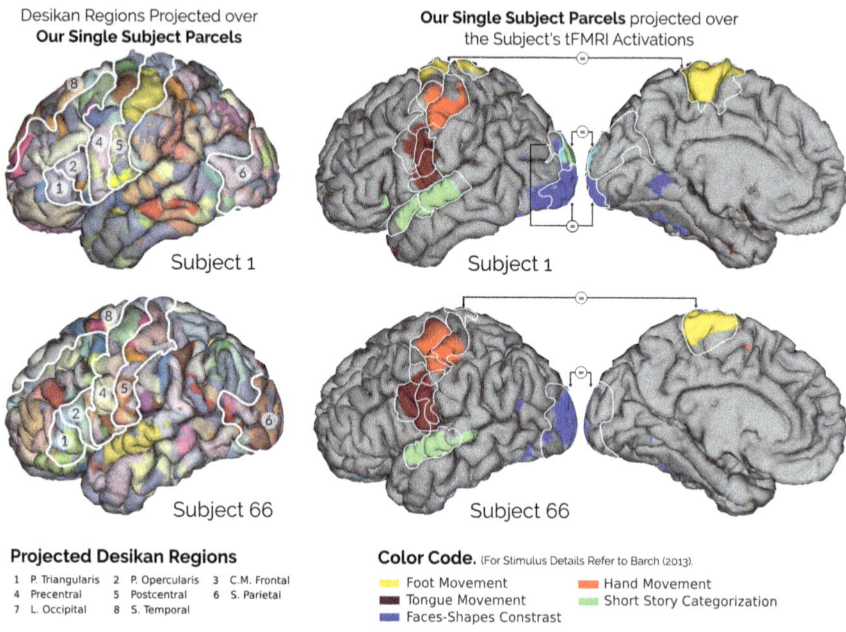

Fig. 4 Single subject parcellations created with our technique, alongside both anatomical (*left*) and functional (*right*) comparisons from Sect. 3.3. Motor and Sensory Cortex (regions 4 and 5) appear to be found and their subdivision is consistent with the motor strip mapping in HCP

Functional Comparison

We studied if our parcels were related to brain function. To do so we calculated their overlap with thresholded maps representing responses to functional stimuli [2]. These maps are also available for each subject in the HCP. Figure 4-right shows the functional comparison for two single subject parcellations. Figure 6 shows a projection from our groupwise parcels over averaged tFMRI activations. Each color encodes the response to a different stimulus thresholded with a z-score > 5. The comparison for the average-subject case was done against the average functional responses in the Unrelated100 population from the HCP. Table 2 shows the highest dice coefficient achieved by one of our regions for each task. Here it is important to remark than, in general, each stimulus will generate a functional response in both motor and sensory cortex. Our hypothesis is that this happens because, for example, while a subject is moving the hand he's also feeling it. Therefore, an overlapping of 0.5 suggests that at least one of our parcels in the motor or sensory cortex is having a good overlapping with the functional response, as confirmed visually. Table 2 shows high dice coefficients for each subject, but shows even higher coefficients for the average subject. We hypothesize that averaging tractograms in the Euclidean space is removing the across-subject variability.

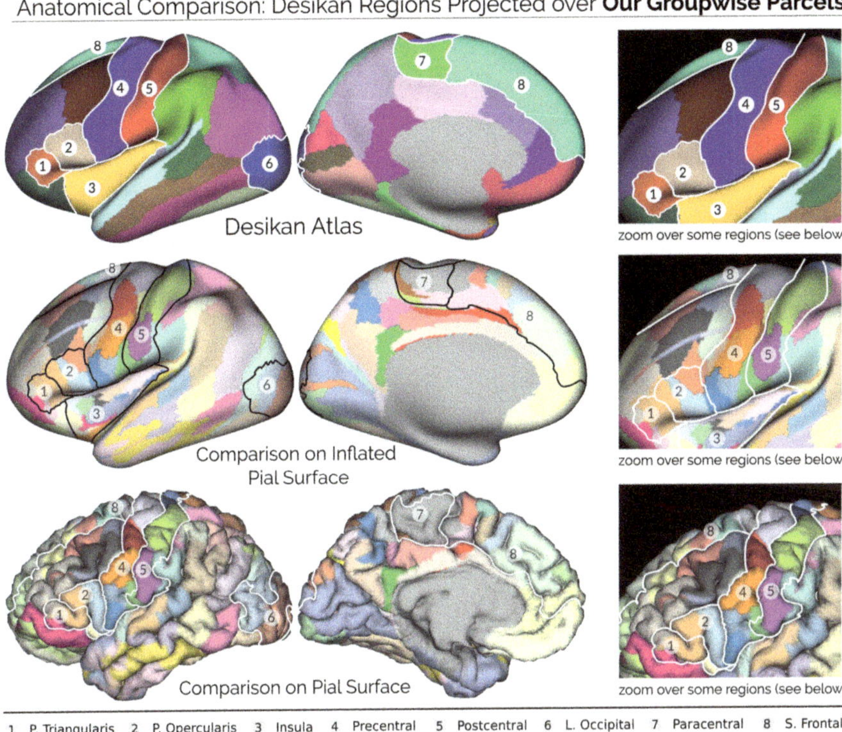

Fig. 5 Relation between our pure extrinsic parcellation and the anatomical atlas of Desikan [5]. Some regions from Desikan projected over a parcellation with less than 150 parcels. Motor and Sensitive cortex appears to be found

Table 1 Area proportion contained for parcels inside Desikan projections

	Area proportion contained (see Fig. 4-left)								
	1	2	3	4	5	6	7	8	Variability
Single subj.	0.4	0.6	0.8	0.8	0.8	0.7	0.2	0.6	$\pm 0.1, min : 0.07, max : 0.16$
Average subj.	0.0	0.3	0.9	0.8	0.8	0.3	0.2	0.6	N/A

4 Discussion and Conclusion

In this work we presented a parsimonious model for the long-range structural connectivity. Our model assumes that the cortex is divided in patches of homogeneous extrinsic connectivity, with intra-patch and across-subject variability. Then, using Logistic Random Effects Models we formulate tractography in accordance to our model. This allowed us to transformed the tractograms into a Euclidean space. Working within this sound framework enabled us to easily manipulate and compare tractograms. Taking advantage of this we presented an efficient technique

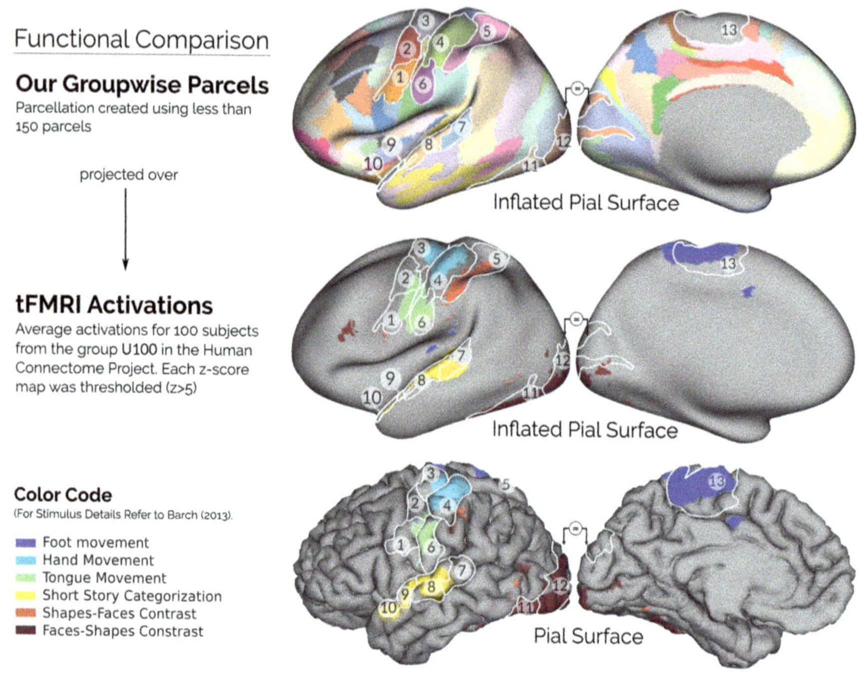

Fig. 6 Relation between our pure extrinsic parcellation and a functional study [2]. Some of our groupwise parcels projected over responses to task-related functional activations. Our division of the Motor and Sensitive cortex appears to be consistent with the motor strip mapping

Table 2 Best dice coefficient obtained for each functional task

	Best dice coefficient for task (see Fig. 4-right)				
	Foot	Hand	Tongue	Story	Shape/face
Single subj.	0.54 ± 0.10	0.46 ± 0.09	0.50 ± 0.1	0.43 ± 0.09	0.56 ± 0.19
Average subj.	0.62	0.60	0.58	0.65	0.54

Our parcels are mostly contained inside one anatomical region and overlap well with the activations

to parcellate the whole cortex in single subject and groupwise cases. The groupwise case assumes seed correspondence across-subject, we expect our model to account errors in seeds coregistration as across-subject variability. Our technique creates a dendrogram using only one comprehensive parameter: the minimum size of each cluster. Then, different parcellation granularities can be obtained just by choosing at which height to cut the dendrogram. Also, as a preliminary validation of our results we showed that our pure structural parcellation had good agreement with anatomical and functional parcellations.

Acknowledgements This work has received funding from the European Research Council (ERC) under the European Union's Horizon 2020 research and innovation program (ERC Advanced Grant agreement No 694665 : CoBCoM).

References

1. Anwander, A., Tittgemeyer, M., von Cramon, D., Friederici, A., Knosche, T.: Connectivity-based parcellation of Broca's area. Cereb. Cortex **17**(4), 816–825 (2006)
2. Barch, D.M., Burgess, G.C., Harms, M.P., Petersen, S.E., Schlaggar, B.L., Corbetta, M., Glasser, M.F., Curtiss, S., Dixit, S., Feldt, C., Nolan, D., Bryant, E., Hartley, T., Footer, O., Bjork, J.M., Poldrack, R., Smith, S., Johansen-Berg, H., Snyder, A.Z., Van Essen, D.C.: Function in the human connectome: task-fMRI and individual differences in behavior. Neuroimage **80**, 169–189 (2013)
3. Behrens, T., Woolrich, M., Jenkinson, M., Johansen-Berg, H., Nunes, R., Clare, S., Matthews, P., Brady, J., Smith, S.: Characterization and propagation of uncertainty in diffusion-weighted MR imaging. Magn. Reson. Med. **50**(5), 1077–1088 (2003)
4. Clarkson, M.J., Malone, I.B., Modat, M., Leung, K.K., Ryan, N., Alexander, D.C., Fox, N.C., Ourselin, S.: A Framework for Using Diffusion Weighted Imaging to Improve Cortical Parcellation. Lecture Notes in Computer Science, vol. 6362. Springer, Berlin, Heidelberg (2010)
5. Desikan, R.S., Ségonne, F., Fischl, B., Quinn, B.T., Dickerson, B.C., Blacker, D., Buckner, R.L., Dale, A.M., Maguire, R.P., Hyman, B.T., Albert, M.S., Killiany, R.J.: An automated labeling system for subdividing the human cerebral cortex on MRI scans into gyral based regions of interest. Neuroimage **31**(3), 968–980 (2006)
6. Garyfallidis, E., Brett, M., Amirbekian, B., Rokem, A., van der Walt, S., Descoteaux, M., Nimmo-Smith, I.: Dipy, a library for the analysis of diffusion MRI data. Front. Neuroinform. **8**, 8 (2014). http://journal.frontiersin.org/article/10.3389/fninf.2014.00008/full
7. Glasser, M.F., Sotiropoulos, S.N., Wilson, J.A., Coalson, T.S., Fischl, B., Andersson, J.L., Xu, J., Jbabdi, S., Webster, M., Polimeni, J.R., Van Essen, D.C., Jenkinson, M.: The minimal preprocessing pipelines for the Human Connectome Project. Neuroimage **80**, 105–124 (2013)
8. Hubert, L., Arabie, P.: Comparing partitions. J. Classif. **2**(1), 193–218 (1985)
9. Jbabdi, S., Behrens, T.E.: Long-range connectomics. Ann. N.Y. Acad. Sci. **1305**(1), 83–93 (2013)
10. Lefranc, S., Roca, P., Perrot, M., Poupon, C., Le Bihan, D., Mangin, J.F., Rivière, D.: Group-wise connectivity-based parcellation of the whole human cortical surface using watershed-driven dimension reduction. Med. Image Anal. **30**, 11–29 (2016)
11. McCullagh, P., Nelder, J.A.: Generalized Linear Models, 2nd edn. Chapman & Hall/CRC, London (1989)
12. Moreno-Dominguez, D., Anwander, A., Knösche, T.R.: A hierarchical method for whole-brain connectivity-based parcellation. Hum. Brain Mapp. **35**(10), 5000–5025 (2014)
13. Murtagh, F., Contreras, P.: Methods of Hierarchical Clustering. Empir. Econ. **38**(1), 23–45 (2011)
14. Parisot, S., Arslan, S., Passerat-Palmbach, J., Wells, W.M., Rueckert, D.: Tractography-driven groupwise multi-scale parcellation of the cortex. Inf. Process. Med. Imaging **24**, 600–612 (2015)
15. Passingham, R.E., Stephan, K.E., Kötter, R.: The anatomical basis of functional localization in the cortex. Nat. Rev. Neurosci. **3**(8), 606–616 (2002)
16. Pendergast, J.F., Gange, S.J., Newton, M.A., Lindstrom, M.J., Palta, M., Fisher, M.R.: A survey of methods for analyzing clustered binary response data. Int. Stat. Rev./Rev. Int. Stat. **64**(1), 89 (1996)
17. Pohl, K.M., Fisher, J., Bouix, S., Shenton, M., McCarley, R.W., Grimson, W.E.L., Kikinis, R., Wells, W.M.: Using the logarithm of odds to define a vector space on probabilistic atlases. Med. Image Anal. **11**(5), 465–477 (2007)

18. Reveley, C., Seth, A.K., Pierpaoli, C., Silva, A.C., Yu, D., Saunders, R.C., Leopold, D.A., Ye, F.Q.: Superficial white matter fiber systems impede detection of long-range cortical connections in diffusion MR tractography. Proc. Natl. Acad. Sci. **112**(21), E2820–E2828 (2015)
19. Schmahmann, J.D., Pandya, D.N.: Fiber Pathways of the Brain, vol. 1. Oxford University Press, Oxford (2006)
20. Tournier, J.D., Calamante, F., Gadian, D.G., Connelly, A.: Direct estimation of the fiber orientation density function from diffusion-weighted MRI data using spherical deconvolution. Neuroimage **23**(3), 1176–1185 (2004)

Robust Construction of Diffusion MRI Atlases with Correction for Inter-Subject Fiber Dispersion

Zhanlong Yang, Geng Chen, Dinggang Shen, and Pew-Thian Yap

Abstract Construction of brain atlases is generally carried out using a two-step procedure involving registering a population of images to a common space and then fusing the aligned images to form an atlas. In practice, image registration is not perfect and simple averaging of the images will blur structures and cause artifacts. In diffusion MRI, this is further complicated by the possibility of within-voxel fiber misalignment due to natural inter-subject orientation dispersion. In this paper, we propose a method to improve the construction of diffusion atlases in light of inter-subject fiber dispersion. Our method involves a novel q-space (i.e., wavevector space) patch matching mechanism that is incorporated in a mean shift algorithm to seek the most probable signal at each point in q-space. Our method relies on the fact that the mean shift algorithm is a *mode seeking* algorithm that converges to the mode of a distribution and is hence robustness to outliers. Our method is therefore in effect seeking the most probable signal profile at each voxel given a distribution of profiles. Experimental results confirm that our method yields cleaner fiber orientation distribution functions with less artifacts caused by dispersion.

Z. Yang and G. Chen contributed equally to this work.

Z. Yang
College of Marine, Northwestern Polytechnical University, Xi'an, China

Department of Radiology and BRIC, UNC Chapel Hill, Chapel Hill, NC, USA

G. Chen
Data Processing Center, Northwestern Polytechnical University, Xi'an, China

Department of Radiology and BRIC, UNC Chapel Hill, Chapel Hill, NC, USA

D. Shen • P.-T. Yap (⊠)
Department of Radiology and BRIC, UNC Chapel Hill, Chapel Hill, NC, USA
e-mail: ptyap@med.unc.edu

© Springer International Publishing AG 2017

A. Fuster et al. (eds.), *Computational Diffusion MRI*, Mathematics and Visualization, DOI 10.1007/978-3-319-54130-3_9

1 Introduction

Brain atlases [1, 2] capture the common features of image populations and play crucial roles in the processing and analysis of brain images. They are widely used for guiding brain tissue segmentation, normalization of images to a common space, and brain labeling with regions of interest. Unlike atlases of T_1-weighted images, diffusion MRI atlases afford additional white matter microstructural information that can be harnessed for tissue characterization and axonal tracing. To ensure that the microstructural information captured at each voxel location is properly encoded in the atlas, dedicated techniques are needed.

Atlas construction generally involves fusing a population of images that are registered to a common space. However, in practice, perfect registration is difficult, if not impossible. Averaging misaligned images to construct an atlas blurs structures and introduces artifacts. In diffusion MRI [3], the problem is even more challenging, since the alignment of gross anatomical structures does not necessarily guarantee the alignment of the microstructural information captured in each voxel. In this situation, it is unclear for example how signals characterizing fiber bundles of varying orientations, which can occur naturally across subjects, should be fused to form the atlas. Moreover, the commonly used simple averaging method is sensitive to outliers. For instance, if the distribution of signal profiles of single-directional fiber bundles is contaminated with a small number of signal profiles of crossing fibers, simple averaging will result in a crossing profile, albeit with a small secondary peak. This outcome apparently is not representative of the majority.

In this paper, we propose a novel q-space patch-matching mechanism that is incorporated in a mean shift algorithm to seek the most probable signal at each point in q-space. Mean shift is a versatile non-parametric iterative algorithm that can be used for mode seeking [4]. Instead of the mean, our method employs the mean shift algorithm to determine the mode of a distribution of signal profiles. The mean shift algorithm uses a kernel to measure the distance between signals. To increase robustness to noise, we measure the distance between signals using patches defined in the q-space. Patch matching is key to the success of many state-of-the-art denoising algorithms, such as non-local means [5]. We perform patch matching in q-space with the help of azimuthal equidistant projection [6] and rotation invariant features [7]. Experimental results confirm that our method yields diffusion atlases with cleaner fiber orientation distribution functions and less artifacts caused by inter-subject fiber dispersion.

2 Approach

Our method employs neighborhood matching in q-space for effective atlas construction. For each point in the x-q space, $(\mathbf{x}_i, \mathbf{q}_k)$, where $\mathbf{x}_i \in \mathbb{R}^3$ is a voxel location and $\mathbf{q}_k \in \mathbb{R}^3$ is a wavevector, we define a spherical patch, $\mathcal{P}_{i,k}$, centered at

$\mathbf{q}_k$ with fixed $q_k = |\mathbf{q}_k|$ and subject to a neighborhood angle α_p. The diffusion measurements on this spherical patch are mapped to a disc using azimuthal equidistant projection (AEP) before computing the rotation invariant features via polar complex exponential transform (PCET) (Sect. 2.1) [7] for patch matching (Sect. 2.2). The similarity weights resulting from patch matching will be used in the mean shift algorithm (Sect. 2.3) to determine the most probable signal at each point in q-space.

2.1 Patch Features

Azimuthal equidistant projection (AEP) [6] maps the coordinates on a sphere to a plane where the distances and azimuths of points on the sphere are preserved with respect to a reference point [6]. This provides a good basis for subsequent computation of invariant features for matching. The reference point (ϕ_0, λ_0), with ϕ being the latitude and λ being the longitude, corresponds in our case to the center of the spherical patch and will be projected to the center of a disc. Viewing the reference point as the 'North pole', all points along a given azimuth, θ, will project along a straight line from the center of the disc. In the projection plane, this line subtends an angle θ with the vertical. The distance from the center to another projected point is given as ρ. The projection can be described as $\mathbf{q} \to (q, \rho, \theta)$. Based on [6], distance ρ associated with a point (ϕ, λ) on the sphere is computed as the great circle distance between the point and the reference (ϕ_0, λ_0) and is given by

$$\cos \rho = \sin \phi_0 \sin \phi + \cos \phi_0 \cos \phi \cos(\lambda - \lambda_0). \tag{1}$$

The angle θ is computed as the azimuth of the point in relation to the reference:

$$\tan \theta = \frac{\cos \phi \sin(\lambda - \lambda_0)}{\cos \phi_0 \sin \phi - \sin \phi_0 \cos \phi \cos(\lambda - \lambda_0)}. \tag{2}$$

Note that, since the diffusion signals are antipodal symmetric, we map antipodally all the points on the sphere to the same hemisphere as the reference point prior to performing AEP. After projection, the q-space spherical patch $\mathcal{P}$ is mapped to a 2D circular patch $\widehat{\mathcal{P}}$.

After AEP, we proceed with the computation of rotation invariant features. We choose to use the polar complex exponential transform (PCET) [7] for its computation efficiency. PCET with order n, $|n| = 0, 1, 2, \ldots, \infty$, and repetition l, $|l| = 0, 1, 2, \ldots, \infty$, of AEP-projected signal profile $S(\mathbf{x}, q, \rho, \theta)$ is defined as

$$M_{n,l}(\widehat{\mathcal{P}}) = \frac{1}{\pi} \int_{(\mathbf{x},q,\rho,\theta)\in\widehat{\mathcal{P}}} [H_{n,l}(\rho, \theta)]^* S(\mathbf{x}, q, \rho, \theta) \rho \, d\rho \, d\theta, \tag{3}$$

where $[\cdot]^*$ denotes the complex conjugate and $H_{n,l}(\rho, \theta)$ is the basis function defined as

$$H_{n,l}(\rho, \theta) = e^{i2\pi n\rho^2} e^{il\theta}. \tag{4}$$

For each patch $\widehat{\mathcal{P}}$ consisting of signal vector $\mathbf{S}(\widehat{\mathcal{P}})$, the associated PCET features $\{|M_{n,l}(\widehat{\mathcal{P}})|\}$ computed up to maximum order m (i.e., $0 \leq l, n \leq m$) are concatenated into a feature vector $\mathbf{M}(\widehat{\mathcal{P}})$.

2.2 Patch Matching

The similarity of a reference patch $\widehat{\mathcal{P}}_{i,k}$ with another patch $\widehat{\mathcal{P}}_{j,l}(d)$ associated with the d-th subject is characterized by weight

$$w_{i,k;j,l}(d) = \frac{1}{Z_{i,k}} \exp\left\{ -\frac{\|\mathbf{M}(\widehat{\mathcal{P}}_{i,k}) - \mathbf{M}(\widehat{\mathcal{P}}_{j,l}(d))\|_2^2}{h_{\mathbf{M}}^2(i,k)} \right\} \exp\left\{ -\frac{\|\mathbf{x}_i - \mathbf{x}_j\|_2^2}{h_{\mathbf{x}}^2} \right\}, \tag{5}$$

where $Z_{i,k}$ is a normalization constant to ensure that the weights sum to one. Here $h_{\mathbf{M}}(i,k)$ is a parameter that controls the attenuation of the exponential function. As in [8], we set $h_{\mathbf{M}}(i,k) = \sqrt{2\beta\hat{\sigma}_{i,k}^2|\mathbf{M}(\widehat{\mathcal{P}}_{i,k})|}$, where β is a constant [8] and $\hat{\sigma}_{i,k}^2$ is the estimated noise standard deviation, which can be computed globally as shown in [9] or spatial-adaptively as shown in [8]. The former is used in this paper. Parameter $h_{\mathbf{x}} = \sqrt{2}\sigma_{\mathbf{x}}$ controls the attenuation of the second exponential function, where $\sigma_{\mathbf{x}}$ is a scale parameter. $|\mathbf{M}(\widehat{\mathcal{P}}_{i,k})|$ denotes the length of the vector $\mathbf{M}(\widehat{\mathcal{P}}_{i,k})$.

Given D subjects, a "mean" signal can be computed based on the weights resulting from patch matching:

$$\bar{S}(\mathbf{x}_i, \mathbf{q}_k) = \sqrt{\sum_{d=1}^{D} \sum_{(\mathbf{x}_j,\mathbf{q}_l)\in\mathcal{V}_{i,k}} w_{i,k;j,l}(d)S^2(\mathbf{x}_j, \mathbf{q}_l; d) - 2\sigma^2}, \tag{6}$$

where $S(\mathbf{x}_i, \mathbf{q}_k; d)$ is the measured signal associated with the d-th subject at location $\mathbf{x}_i \in \mathbb{R}^3$ with wavevector $\mathbf{q}_k \in \mathbb{R}^3$. $\mathcal{V}_{i,k}$ is a local x-q space neighborhood associated with $(\mathbf{x}_i, \mathbf{q}_k)$, defined by a radius r_s in x-space and an angle α_s in q-space. Note the bias associated with the Rician noise distribution is removed in this process [9]. σ is the Gaussian noise standard deviation that can be estimated from the image background [9]. Without patch matching, a "simple averaging" version of (6) is given as

$$\bar{S}(\mathbf{x}_i, \mathbf{q}_k) = \sqrt{\frac{1}{D} \sum_{d=1}^{D} S^2(\mathbf{x}_i, \mathbf{q}_k; d) - 2\sigma^2}. \tag{7}$$

2.3 Mean Shift

Given a set of diffusion signal profiles $\{S(\mathbf{x}_j, \mathbf{q}_l; d) : (\mathbf{x}_j, \mathbf{q}_l) \in \mathcal{V}_{i,k}, d = 1, \ldots, D\}$, we want to determine the modal profile $\tilde{S}(\mathbf{x}_i, \mathbf{q}_k)$. This is achieved using a mean shift algorithm [4] that is modified to take advantage of the patch matching mechanism described above. Mean shift is a non-parametric algorithm for locating the maxima of a density function and is hence a mode-seeking algorithm. It is an iterative algorithm where the mean is progressively updated by using the mean computed in the previous iteration as the reference for computing sample similarity.

We first note that the weights computed using (5) is dependent on the signal vector $\mathbf{S}(\widehat{\mathcal{P}})$ of a patch $\widehat{\mathcal{P}}$. To explicitly express this dependency, we write $w_{i,k;j,l}(d) := w\left(\bar{\mathbf{S}}(\widehat{\mathcal{P}}_{i,k}), \mathbf{S}(\widehat{\mathcal{P}}_{j,l}(d))\right)$. Note that we have made here the mean signal vector $\bar{\mathbf{S}}(\widehat{\mathcal{P}}_{i,k})$ the reference for weight computation. Our implementation of the mean shift algorithm involves the following steps. For iteration $t = 1, 2, \ldots, T$,

1. Update weights $w_{i,k;j,l}^{(t)}(d) = w\left(\bar{\mathbf{S}}^{(t-1)}(\widehat{\mathcal{P}}_{i,k}), \mathbf{S}(\widehat{\mathcal{P}}_{j,l}(d))\right)$ based on (5).
2. Update the mean at each location $(\mathbf{x}_i, \mathbf{q}_i)$ using (6) with weights $\{w_{i,k;j,l}^{(t)}(d)\}$ and $\{S(\mathbf{x}_j, \mathbf{q}_l; d)\}$ for $(\mathbf{x}_j, \mathbf{q}_l) \in \mathcal{V}_{i,k}$.
3. Repeat steps above with $t \leftarrow t + 1$.

3 Experimental Results

Quantitative and qualitative experiments using synthetic and real data were performed to evaluate the proposed method. In all experiments, we set $r_s = 2$ voxels, $\beta = 0.1$, $\alpha_p = 30°$, $\alpha_s = 30°$, and $m = 4$. We use peak signal-to-noise ratio (PSNR) as the metric for performance evaluation.

3.1 Synthetic Data

A synthetic dataset consisting of one- and two-directional fiber bundles was generated for the quantitative evaluation of the proposed method. The dataset was simulated with $b = 1000\,\text{s/mm}^2$ and 81 non-collinear gradient directions. In order to simulate the dispersion of fiber orientations across subjects, we generate a set of diffusion signal profiles of fiber bundles oriented according to the Watson probability distribution function [10], which in modified form is given as

$$f(\theta|\kappa) \propto \exp\left[-\kappa(1 - \cos^2(\theta))\right], \tag{8}$$

where θ is the angle of deviation from the ground truth direction and the concentration parameter κ is defined as $\kappa = 2(1 - \cos^2(\theta_T))^{-1}$. Parameter θ_T determines the degree of dispersion of the orientations of the fiber bundles. We set $\theta_T = 15°, 30°, 45°$. The fiber orientation distribution functions (ODFs) [11] of some diffusion profiles are shown in Fig. 1. The "atlas" is computed using this distribution of diffusion signal profiles and the outcome is compared with the ground truth without deviation. Four levels of Rician noise (3%, 5%, 7% and 9%) were added to the dataset. Rician noise was simulated by adding Gaussian noise [i.e. $\mathcal{N}(0, v(p/100))$] to the complex domain of the signal with noise variance determined by noise-level percentage p and maximum signal value v (150 in our case).

As shown in Figs. 2 and 3, for the various noise levels, our method improves the PSNRs over simple averaging for both cases of one- and two-directional fiber bundles. The PSNR improvement is over 2 dB and sometimes even up to 3 dB. The fiber ODFs of some representative results, shown in Fig. 4, indicate that simple averaging causes artifacts and that the proposed method yields results that are very close to the ground truth.

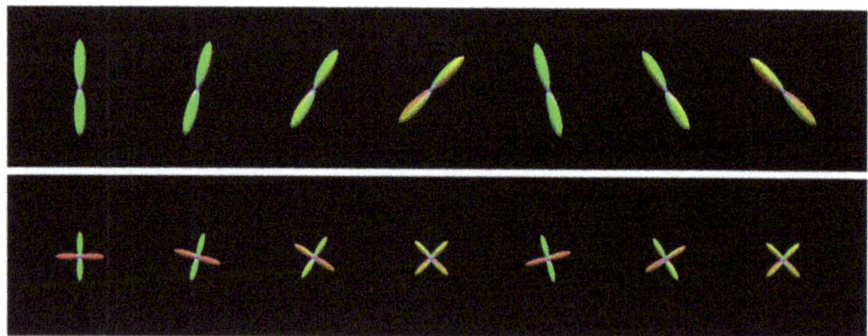

Fig. 1 Examples from the synthetic dataset simulating (*top*) one- and (*bottom*) two-direction fiber bundles

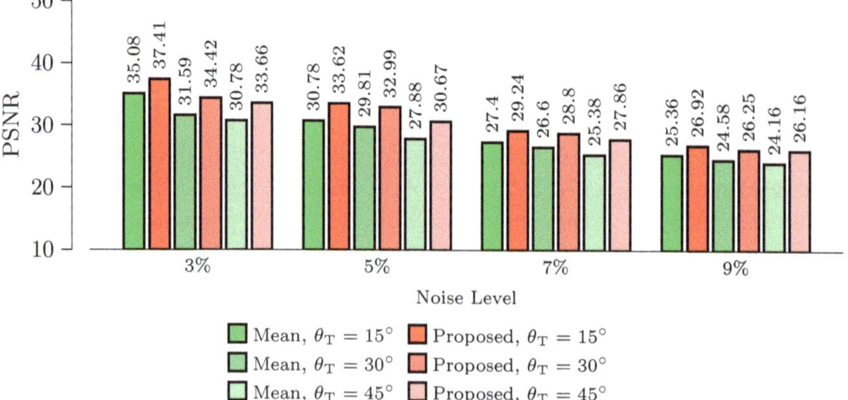

Fig. 2 PSNR comparison of results given by the mean, computed via simple averaging, and the proposed method for the case of one-direction fiber bundles

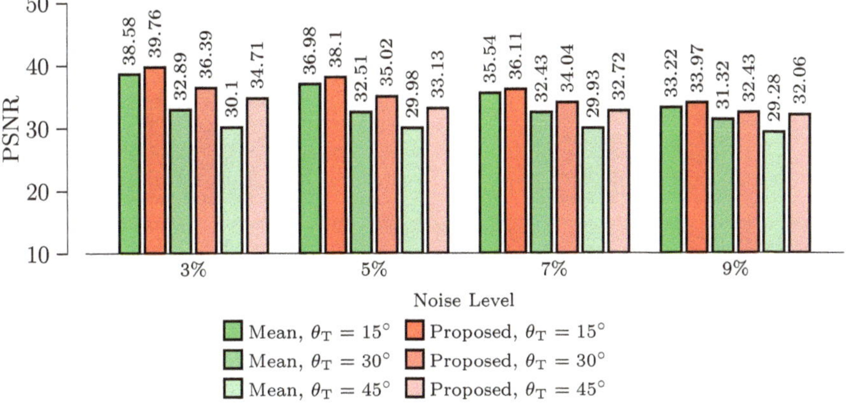

Fig. 3 PSNR comparison of results given by the mean, computed via simple averaging, and the proposed method for the case of two-direction fiber bundles

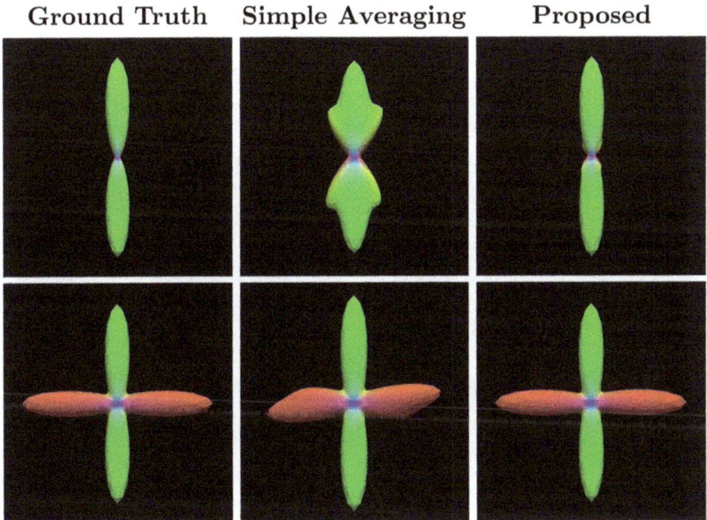

Fig. 4 Comparison of fiber ODFs. (*Left*) Ground-truth ODFs. (*Middle*) ODFs given by simple averaging. (*Right*) ODFs given by the proposed method. The results were generated using synthetic dataset with 9% noise and $\theta_T = 45°$ and 5% noise and $\theta_T = 15°$ respectively for the one- and two-direction cases

3.2 Real Data

All images were acquired using a Siemens 3T TRIO MR scanner following a standard imaging protocol: 30 diffusion directions uniformly distributed on a hemisphere, $b = 1000\,\mathrm{s/mm^2}$, one image with no diffusion weighting, 128×128 imaging matrix, voxel size of $2 \times 2 \times 2\,\mathrm{mm^3}$, TE=81 ms, TR=7618 ms.

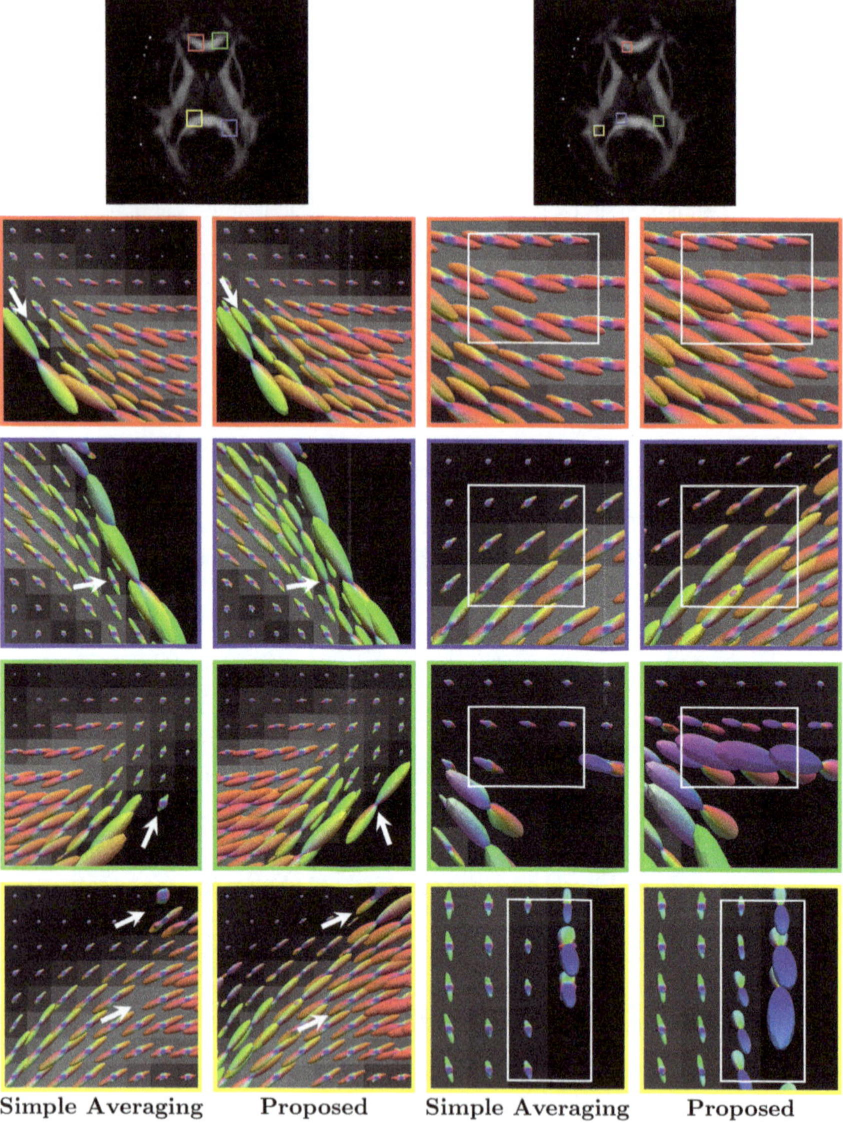

Fig. 5 Comparisons of white matter fiber ODFs given by the simple averaging method (columns 1 and 3) and our method (columns 2 and 4). The fractional anisotropy images at the *top* are shown for reference. Visible differences between the methods are marked by *arrows* and *boxes*

As shown in Fig. 5, our method obtains ODFs that are more consistent and exhibit stronger directionality. Visible differences are marked using arrows and boxes. For simple averaging, the ODF glyphs are generally shorter, indicating weaker directionality. In contrast, our method gives sharper and longer ODF glyphs, indicating its superiority.

4 Conclusion

In this paper, we propose a novel patch-based mean-shift algorithm for constructing diffusion MRI atlases. Our method is less sensitive to outliers and is able to deal with inter-subject fiber dispersion. Preliminary experimental results indicate that our method yields improvements over the commonly used simple averaging method and generates diffusion atlases with cleaner fiber orientations and less artifacts caused by inter-subject orientation dispersion.

Acknowledgements This work was supported in part by NIH grants (NS093842, EB006733, EB009634, AG041721, MH100217, and AA012388) and the National Natural Science Foundation of China (No. 61540047).

References

1. Evans, A.C., Janke, A.L., Collins, D.L., Baillet, S.: Brain templates and atlases. Neuroimage **62**(2), 911–922 (2012)
2. Deshpande, R., Chang, L., Oishi, K.: Construction and application of human neonatal DTI atlases. Front. Neuroanat. **9**, 138 (2015)
3. Johansen-Berg, H., Behrens, T.E.J.: Diffusion MRI: From Quantitative Measurement to In Vivo Neuroanatomy, 2nd edn. Academic, San Diego (2014). ISBN 9780123964601, http://dx.doi.org/10.1016/B978-0-12-396460-1.01001-5
4. Comaniciu, D., Meer, P.: Mean shift: a robust approach toward feature space analysis. IEEE Trans. Patt. Anal. Mach. Intell. **24**(5), 603–619 (2002)
5. Buades, A., Coll, B., Morel, J.M.: A review of image denoising algorithms, with a new one. Multisc. Model. Simul. **4**(2), 490–530 (2005)
6. Wessel, P., Smith, W.H.: The Generic Mapping Tools (1995). http://gmt.soest.hawaii.edu
7. Yap, P.T., Jiang, X., Kot, A.C.: Two-dimensional polar harmonic transforms for invariant image representation. IEEE Trans. Patt. Anal. Mach. Intell. **32**(7), 1259–1270 (2010)
8. Coupé, P., Yger, P., Prima, S., Hellier, P., Kervrann, C., Barillot, C.: An optimized blockwise nonlocal means denoising filter for 3-D magnetic resonance images. IEEE Trans. Med. Imag. **27**(4), 425–441 (2008)
9. Manjón, J.V., Carbonell-Caballero, J., Lull, J.J., García-Martí, G., Martí-Bonmatí, L., Robles, M.: MRI denoising using non-local means. Med. Image Anal. **12**(4), 514–523 (2008)
10. Schwartzman, A., Dougherty, R.F., Taylor, J.E.: False discovery rate analysis of brain diffusion direction maps. Ann. Appl. Stat. **2**(1), 153–175 (2008)
11. Yap, P.T., Zhang, Y., Shen, D.: Multi-tissue decomposition of diffusion MRI signals via ℓ_0 sparse-group estimation. IEEE Trans. Image Process. **25**(9), 4340–4353 (2016)

Parcellation of Human Amygdala Subfields Using Orientation Distribution Function and Spectral K-means Clustering

Qiuting Wen, Brian D. Stirling, Long Sha, Li Shen, Paul J. Whalen, and Yu-Chien Wu

Abstract Amygdala plays an important role in fear and emotional learning, which are critical for human survival. Despite the functional relevance and unique circuitry of each human amygdaloid subnuclei, there has yet to be an efficient imaging method for identifying these regions in vivo. A data-driven approach without prior knowledge provides advantages of efficient and objective assessments. The present study uses high angular and high spatial resolution diffusion magnetic resonance imaging to generate orientation distribution function, which bears distinctive microstructural features. The features were extracted using spherical harmonic

Q. Wen • L. Shen
Department of Radiology and Imaging Sciences, Center for Neuroimaging, Indiana University School of Medicine, Goodman Hall, 355 West 16th Street, Suite 4100, Indianapolis, IN, 46202, USA
e-mail: wenq@iupui.edu

B.D. Stirling
Division of Biokinesiology and Physical Therapy, University of Southern California, Los Angeles, CA, 90089, USA

Department of Psychological and Brain Sciences and Dartmouth Brain Imaging Center, Dartmouth College, 6207, Moore Hall, Hanover, NH, 03755, USA
e-mail: bstirlin@usc.edu

L. Sha
Neuroscience Institute, New York University, New York, NY, 10016, USA

Department of Psychological and Brain Sciences and Dartmouth Brain Imaging Center, Dartmouth College, 6207, Moore Hall, Hanover, NH, 03755, USA

P.J. Whalen
Department of Psychological and Brain Sciences and Dartmouth Brain Imaging Center, Dartmouth College, 6207, Moore Hall, Hanover, NH, 03755, USA

Y.-C. Wu (✉)
Division of Biokinesiology and Physical Therapy, University of Southern California, Los Angeles, CA, 90089, USA

Department of Psychological and Brain Sciences and Dartmouth Brain Imaging Center, Dartmouth College, 6207, Moore Hall, Hanover, NH, 03755, USA
e-mail: yucwu@iupui.edu

© Springer International Publishing AG 2017

A. Fuster et al. (eds.), *Computational Diffusion MRI*, Mathematics and Visualization, DOI 10.1007/978-3-319-54130-3_10

decomposition to assess microstructural similarity within amygdala subfields that are identified via similarity matrices using spectral k-mean clustering. The approach was tested on 32 healthy volunteers and three distinct amygdala subfields were identified including medial, posterior-superior lateral, and anterior-inferior lateral.

1 Introduction

The amygdala, a subcortical structure in the human brain, is associated with fear and emotional learning [1]; with such, it regulates social behavior and perception, and memory consolidation in other brain regions [2]. These functionalities of the amygdala, especially fear learning and conditioning, are critical for survival. Functionally distinct subfields compose the whole amygdala, coarsely separated into the lateral, basolateral, and centromedial nuclei [3]. The lateral and basolateral nuclei receive afferent fibers that deliver highly processed sensory information from cortices while the centromedial nuclei project efferent fibers to hypothalamus and limbic nuclei. Conventionally, our knowledge of the amygdala and its subfields has been derived from studies of compromised human brain using direct electrical stimulation [4]. Thus, having an accessible approach for imaging the amygdala is valuable for advancing amygdala research in vivo.

In vivo studies of function and structure of the human amygdala have been made possible through neuroimaging, notably functional magnetic resonance imaging (fMRI) and diffusion magnetic resonance imaging (dMRI). The whole amygdala appears as a compact small region of grey matter in conventional magnetic resonance T1-weighted (T1W) imaging. Finer granularity of amygdala subfields may be parceled using ultra-high resolution T1W imaging [5], dMRI probability tractography [6, 7], or combining tasked fMRI and diffusion tensor imaging (DTI) streamline tractography [8]. These studies, however, require priori knowledge. The ultra-high resolution T1W imaging segmentation requires manually tracing with prior knowledge of amygdala histology; studies involving dMRI tractography call for pre-defined amygdala-cortical projections.

Alternatively, a data-driven approach without prior knowledge provides advantages of efficient and objective assessments. Spectral clustering algorithm has been applied to DTI principle directions (i.e., major eigenvector of the diffusion tensor), and yielded two directionally coherent subfields separated by a boundary called septa [9]. However, in the DTI framework, the water diffusion is approximated by an ellipsoid with a major eigenvector representing an overall direction of underlying microstructural organization [10]. Thus, local complexity and important features of microstructures may be lost in the simplified tensor model [11, 12]. To overcome DTI limitations, orientation distribution function (ODF) was proposed [13–18]. Compared to DTI major eigenvector, which has only three vector components, ODF describes a three-dimensional diffusion probability function defined on the surface of a unit sphere. ODF elucidates complex microstructures with multiple crossing fibers and their probability distributions and is believed to provide richer and more complete information of diffusion directionality.

In this study, ODF is used to parcel amygdala subfields that have similar microstructural characteristics. Specifically, ODF is first decomposed to a combination of spherical harmonics, from which features of the ODF surface will be extracted. Similar to Fourier basis functions (i.e., a series of sinusoidal functions), the spherical harmonic basis functions are orthogonal with each other, and their coefficients describe distinctive features of the ODF surface. Coefficients of spherical harmonics have been used to segment the brain into different levels of microstructural complexity [19, 20]. Herein, we use the spherical harmonic coefficients to assess similarity between imaging voxels within the amygdala. Amygdala subfields are identified via similarity matrices using spectral k-mean clustering [21]. We tested our approach on healthy volunteers who received high angular and high spatial resolution diffusion imaging.

2   Material and Methods

2.1   Data Acquisition

MRI scans were performed on 32 healthy volunteers at a 3.0T Phililps Achieva INTERA scanner with a 32-channel head coil. Written informed consent was obtained from all participants in accordance with ethical approval from the Dartmouth College Internal Review Board.

High spatial resolution dMRI sequence was acquired with a single-shot spin-echo echo-planer imaging sequence at an isotropic voxel size of 1.6 mm with four repetitions (TE/TR = 79/3382 ms, FOV = 230 mm × 230 mm × 35.2 mm, in-plane matrix size = 114 × 114, and 22 slices). Diffusion-weighted (DW) images were acquired with one volume at b-value = 0 s/mm^2 (b0) and 61 noncollinear DW directions at b-value = 1000 s/mm^2 with a total acquisition time of 45 min. Other imaging protocols included: A matched field-of-view (FOV) gradient-echo sequence with 2-echo times (TE = 7 and 8 ms) to generate fieldmap to correct for dMRI geometric distortion; and a whole brain T1W image using a magnetization-prepared rapid acquisition gradient echo sequence (MP-RAGE) with TE/TR = 3.72/8.18 ms, FOV = 224 mm × 224 mm × 220 mm, and isotropic voxel size of 1 mm^3.

2.2   Post-processing

Motion correction, eddy current correction and susceptibility distortion correction were applied to each volume of the DW images before averaging over the four repetitions using the toolbox in FSL (FMRIB Software Library, University of Oxford, http://fsl.fmrib.ox.ac.uk/fsl/). Motion and eddy current distortions were corrected using a linear registration to the b0 image (eddy_correct, FSL) for each volume within each repetition. Susceptibility distortion was corrected by calculating

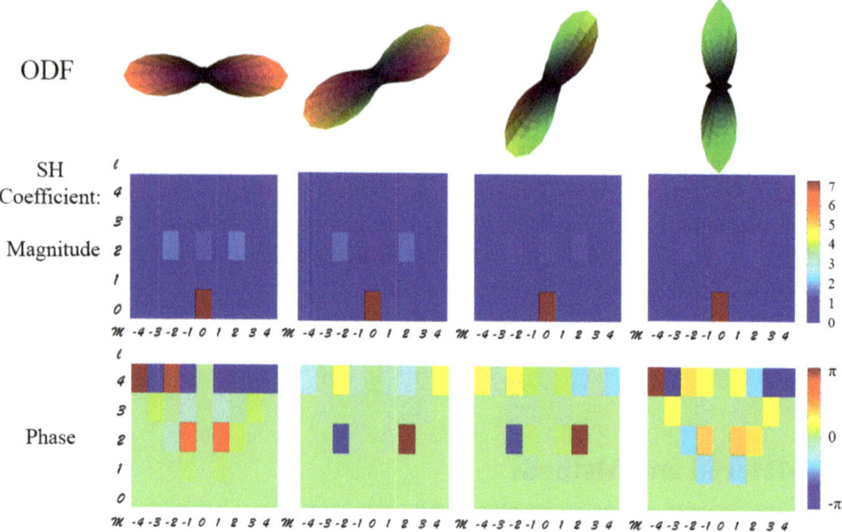

Fig. 1 The *top panel* shows simulated ODFs of a single fiber orientation (0°, 30°, 60°, 90°). The ODFs were simulated with a single tensor with axial diffusivity of 1200 mm²/s and radial diffusivity of 250 mm²/s at b = 2500 s/mm². The *middle panel* shows magnitude components of SH coefficients. The *bottom panel* shows phase components of SH coefficients. l and m are orders of Legendre function in the spherical harmonic bases. For illustrating purpose, SH coefficients of $l = 0$ to 4 and $m = -l$ to l are shown here

the geometric distortion and signal loss from the field map and was compensated in the DW images (fudge, FSL). A final motion correction was applied to all four repetitions by rigidly registering the b0 images from each repetition before averaging.

In the diffusion space, the averaged DW images were then used to calculate the structural ODF profiles of the amygdala using in-house MATLAB programs [22] with a Q-ball Imaging (QBI) algorithm [14]. Spherical Harmonics (SH) coefficients of each ODF profile were extracted up to an order of 6, i.e., $l_{max} = 6$. As a symmetric ODF was assumed and odd orders contain only noise information, only coefficients of even orders were kept [19, 20]. A total of 28 SH coefficient pairs (i.e., magnitude and phase) that represent the shape and orientation of ODF in each voxel were entered into the subsequent spectral clustering. Figure 1 shows simulated ODFs of a single fiber orientation (0°, 30°, 60°, 90°) and their SH coefficients. Figure 2 shows simulated ODFs for crossing fibers with a rotating 2nd fiber (0°, 30°, 60°, 90°) and their SH coefficients. Consistent with observations described in [19], the shape (e.g., number of crossing fibers) and the orientation (e.g., rotation angle) of the ODFs are described by the combination of magnitude and phase components of the SH coefficients.

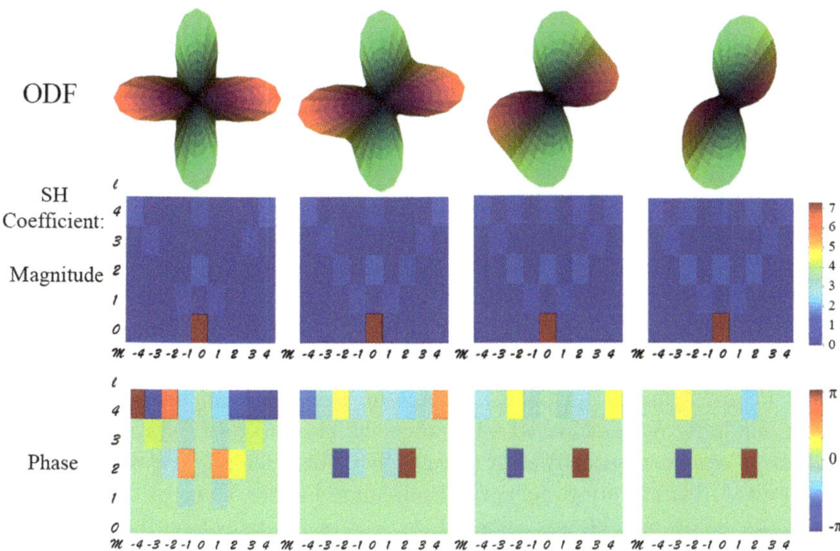

Fig. 2 The *top panel* shows simulated ODFs for crossing fibers with a rotating 2nd fiber (0°, 30°, 60°, 90°). The ODFs were simulated with two tensors at b = 2500 s/mm². Each tensor has axial diffusivity of 1200 mm²/s and radial diffusivity of 250 mm²/s. The *middle panel* shows the magnitude components of the SH coefficients. The *bottom panel* shows the phase components of the SH coefficients. l and m are orders of Legendre function in the spherical harmonic bases; and the SH coefficients of $l = 0$ to 4 and $m = -l$ to l are shown here

2.3 Amygdala Segmentation

A amygdala probability mask was first obtained from the Harvard-Oxford sub-cortical structural atlas provided in FSL in the MNI 152 standard space. The mask was then warped to the subject diffusion space through the transformation achieved by aligning T1W of each subject to the T1W in MNI space using a nonlinear registration algorithm (fnirt, FSL). A threshold of 50% was then applied to the probability mask to exclude extraneous tissue. The resulting masks were conservatively away from the edge to avoid alignment errors and partial voluming effects.

2.4 Amygdala Parcellation: K-mean Spectral Clustering

For each voxel, 28 SH coefficient pairs ($l_{max} = 6$, even orders) were extracted to describe the diffusion characteristics that reflect the underlying tissue microstructure. Voxels within the mask of the amygdala would be grouped together according to the similarity of their SH coefficients.

To prepare for the subsequent Laplacian transformation of Spectral Clustering, the graph similarities (S_{ij}) between two voxels i,j were computed by converting the weighted pair-wise Pearson's correlation coefficient, i.e., C_{ij} of the SH coefficients according to their spherical distance [21]. The weighting, W_{ij}, is to adjust physical (Euclidean) distance between voxels i,j. The dimension of the S matrix, $M \times M$, equals to the number of voxels within the segmented amygdala.

$$S_{ij} = \exp\left(-\sin^2\left(\frac{\cos^{-1}\left(W_{ij} \cdot C_{ij}\right)}{2}\right) / sigma^2\right) \tag{1}$$

Sigma is a threshold parameter that deems the importance of cells in C where values below sigma are penalized. Therefore, S is a sparser matrix than C, as higher similarity S_{ij} is achieved only when the two voxels i,j have similar SH coefficients and are physically close to each other. The value of *sigma* was optimized by iteratively incrementing *sigma* until minimum Fiedler Value of the Laplacian matrix (see below or [21]) was achieved.

The graph similarity matrix (S) of each subject was then transformed into a normalized symmetric graph Laplacian matrix, on which eigen decomposition was performed. According to spectral clustering theory [21], the first few ordered eigen values contain critical structural information regarding the data. To determine the number of eigen values that best reflect the underlying structure, we tested the eigen values against those generated from unstructured data. The unstructured data were generated by randomizing the SH coefficients. The randomization process was bootstrapped for 1200 iterations to create a null distribution of eigenvalues of the unstructured Laplacian matrices. For each subject, eigenvalues of original "structured" Laplacian matrix were tested against the null distribution using z-scoring, and the number of significant eigenvalues were determined as the number of clusters, denoted as N.

To perform k-mean clustering to classify the voxels within the amygdala, we picked the N eigenvectors corresponding to the N eigenvalues starting from Fiedler Value. Each eigen-vector has M elements that equals to the dimension of the Laplacian and S matrix. Note that M also denotes the number of voxels within the segmented amygdala. The N eigen-vectors were stacked up to form a $N \times M$ matrix. Thus, the $N \times M$ matrix described N distinct features for M voxels. K-mean clustering was performed across M voxels to yield a cluster label for each voxel. The clustering would then be complete and yield N amygdala subfields for each subject in the native space. In order to check the inter-subject variability, the individual results were transformed to the template brain. Individual clusters were averaged across subjects to generate a consistency map.

3   Results

Consistently three eigenvalues of the Laplacian transformed similarity matrix were found to be statistically significant across 32 subjects with p < 0.001. Such significance indicated a consistent pattern whose optimal solution was related to the three eigenvalues. Therefore, N = 3 was the optimal cluster number found for this study. In addition, we found that this N was independent from the sigma during the iterative optimization process where we found *sigma* = 0.55 gives minimal Fiedler Value.

The ODF profiles of the right amygdala with various orientations, shapes, and peaks are shown in Fig. 3. The ODFs were overlaid on the clustering results of one subject on an axial slice. It can be seen that groups of amygdala voxels show characteristically different orientations and shapes of the ODFs that were associated with fiber structures.

The similarity matrix (S) calculated from the SH coefficients of the ODF profiles of the same subject in Fig. 3 is shown in Fig. 4. Red suggests high similarity. Three clusters are noticeable, which correspond to three regions with distinct ODF characteristics. As the similarity matrix also contains voxel correspondence, it demonstrates consistent region separations as well.

The 3D scatter plot of the center of masses of each cluster across subjects is shown in Fig. 5. The coordinates are in voxels and were oriented to match with the image in coronal view (top-left) in Fig. 6. The spatial distribution of the center of masses may be a measure of across subject consistency. Alternatively, Fig. 6 shows the consistency map of clusters across subjects overlaid on the T1W images for the left amygdala. It clearly shows three clusters as the following subfields: medial (red), posterior-superior-lateral (green), anterior-inferior-lateral (blue).

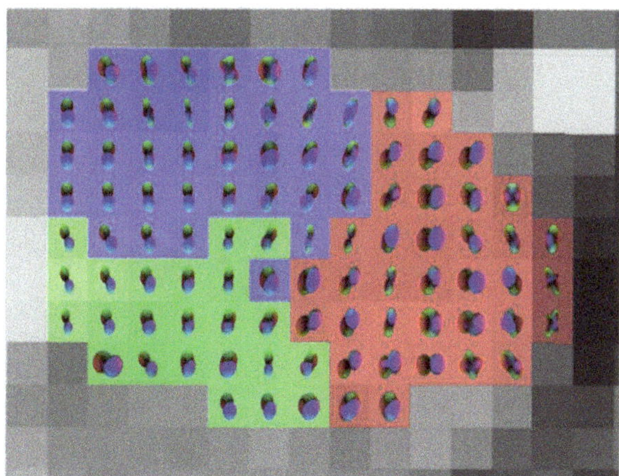

Fig. 3 Right amygdala (axial view) with ODF overlaid on T1W for one subject

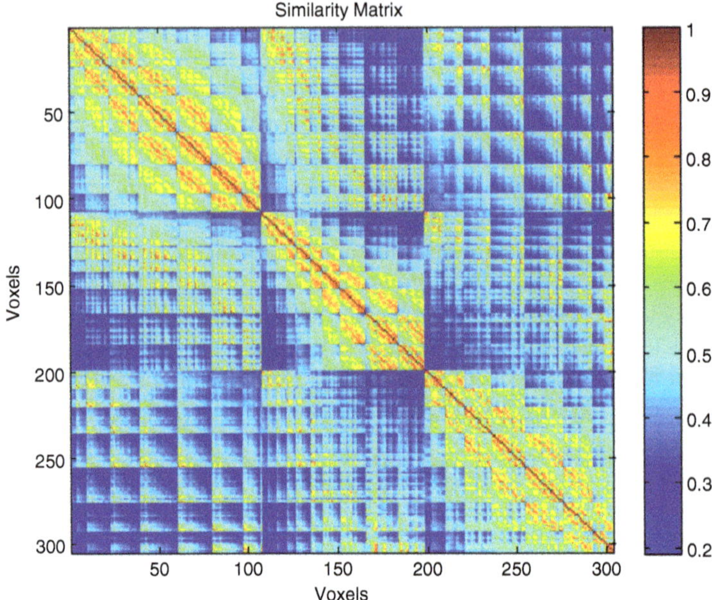

Fig. 4 The similarity matrix, S (300 × 300), of a subject's amygdala with 300 voxels for cluster number N = 3. Three distinct regions are noticeable. *Red* suggests high similarity

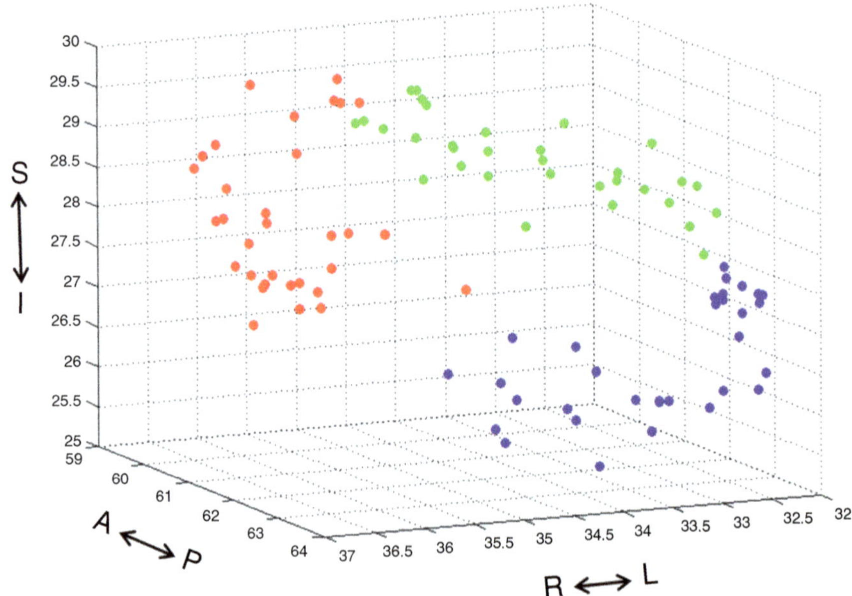

Fig. 5 3D scatter plot of cluster center of masses across subjects. Coordinates are by image voxels in the standard MNI space. The color code and orientation of the scatter plot match with the image in coronal view (*top-left*) in Fig. 6

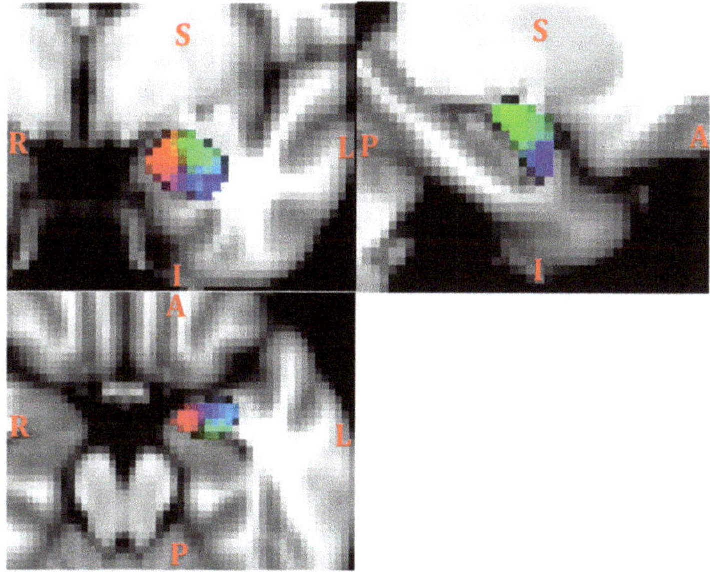

Fig. 6 Consistency map of the three clusters in the left amygdala across subjects in coronal (*top-left*), axial (*bottom*), and sagittal (*top-right*) views

4 Discussion and Conclusions

This study demonstrates that with high angular and spatial resolution diffusion imaging, the amygdala can be parceled into three subfields. The automated clustering uses only microstructural information within the amygdala and does not require prior knowledge of histology or cortical functional projections of amygdaloid subnuclei. The physical locations of the three subfields infer three subnuclei including lateral, basolateral, and centromedial nuclei. However, further study is warranted to validate their cortical projections by incorporating dMRI tractography to link each cluster to functionally relevant cortical regions and to compare with histologically defined subnuclei.

Acknowledgements Supported in part by Dartmouth Synergy, Indiana Alzheimer Disease Center pilot grant, NIH R01 MH080716, R01 EB022574, R01 LM011360, R01 AG19771 and P30 AG10133.

References

1. Aggleton, J.P.: The Amygdala: Neurobiological Aspects of Emotion, Memory, and Mental Dysfunction, xii, 615 p. Wiley-Liss., New York; Chichester (1992)
2. Barr, M.L., Kiernan, J.A.: The Human Nervous System: An Anatomical Viewpoint, 6th edn, vii, 451 p. Lippincott, Philadelphia (1993)

3. Pitkanen, A., Savander, V., LeDoux, J.E.: Organization of intra-amygdaloid circuitries in the rat: an emerging framework for understanding functions of the amygdala. Trends Neurosci. **20**(11), 517–523 (1997)
4. Whalen, P.J., et al.: Functional neuroimaging studies of the amygdala in depression. Semin. Clin. Neuropsychiatry. **7**(4), 234–242 (2002)
5. Entis, J.J., et al.: A reliable protocol for the manual segmentation of the human amygdala and its subregions using ultra-high resolution MRI. Neuroimage. **60**(2), 1226–1235 (2012)
6. Saygin, Z.M., et al.: Connectivity-based segmentation of human amygdala nuclei using probabilistic tractography. Neuroimage. **56**(3), 1353–1361 (2011)
7. Bach, D.R., et al.: Deep and superficial amygdala nuclei projections revealed in vivo by probabilistic tractography. J. Neurosci. **31**(2), 618–623 (2011)
8. Balderston, N.L., et al.: Functionally distinct amygdala subregions identified using DTI and high-resolution fMRI. Soc. Cogn. Affect. Neurosci. **10**(12), 1615–1622 (2015)
9. Solano-Castiella, E., et al.: Diffusion tensor imaging segments the human amygdala in vivo. Neuroimage. **49**(4), 2958–2965 (2010)
10. Basser, P.J., Mattiello, J., LeBihan, D.: MR diffusion tensor spectroscopy and imaging. Biophys. J. **66**(1), 259–267 (1994)
11. Wu, Y.C.: Diffusion MRI: Tensors and Beyond in Medical Physics, p. 150. University of Wisconsin-Madison, Madison (2006)
12. Tournier, J.D., Mori, S., Leemans, A.: Diffusion tensor imaging and beyond. Magn. Reson. Med. **65**(6), 1532–1556 (2011)
13. Alexander, D.C.: Multiple-fiber reconstruction algorithms for diffusion MRI. Ann. N. Y. Acad. Sci. **1064**, 113–133 (2005)
14. Tuch, D.S.: Q-ball imaging. Magn. Reson. Med. **52**(6), 1358–1372 (2004)
15. Tournier, J.D., et al.: Direct estimation of the fiber orientation density function from diffusion-weighted MRI data using spherical deconvolution. Neuroimage. **23**(3), 1176–1185 (2004)
16. Hess, C.P., et al.: Q-ball reconstruction of multimodal fiber orientations using the spherical harmonic basis. Magn. Reson. Med. **56**(1), 104–117 (2006)
17. Wedeen, V.J., et al.: Mapping complex tissue architecture with diffusion spectrum magnetic resonance imaging. Magn. Reson. Med. **54**(6), 1377–1386 (2005)
18. Rathi, Y., et al.: Directional functions for orientation distribution estimation. Med. Image Anal. **13**(3), 432–444 (2009)
19. Frank, L.R.: Characterization of anisotropy in high angular resolution diffusion-weighted MRI. Magn. Reson. Med. **47**(6), 1083–1099 (2002)
20. Alexander, D.C., Barker, G.J., Arridge, S.R.: Detection and modeling of non-Gaussian apparent diffusion coefficient profiles in human brain data. Magn. Reson. Med. **48**(2), 331–340 (2002)
21. von Luxburg, U.: A tutorial on spectral clustering. Stat. Comput. **17**(4), 395–416 (2007)
22. Wu, Y.C., Field, A.S., Alexander, A.L.: Computation of diffusion function measures in q-space using magnetic resonance hybrid diffusion imaging. IEEE Trans. Med. Imaging. **27**(6), 858–865 (2008)

Sparse Representation for White Matter Fiber Compression and Calculation of Inter-Fiber Similarity

Gali Zimmerman Moreno, Guy Alexandroni, Nir Sochen, and Hayit Greenspan

Abstract Recent years have brought about impressive reconstructions of white matter architecture, due to the advance of increasingly sophisticated MRI based acquisition methods and modeling techniques. These result in extremely large sets of streamelines (fibers) for each subject. The sets require large amount of storage and are often unwieldy and difficult to manipulate and analyze. We propose to use sparse representations for fibers to achieve a more compact representation. We also propose the means for calculating inter-fiber similarities in the compressed space using a measure, which we term: Cosine with Dictionary Similarity Weighting (CWDS). The performance of both sparse representations and CWDS is evaluated on full brain fiber-sets of 15 healthy subjects. The results show that a reconstruction error of slightly below 2 mm is achieved, and that CWDS is highly correlated with the cosine similarity in the original space.

1 Introduction

Recent advances in the field of magnetic resonance (MR) based imaging of white matter (WM) have brought about the means to create extremely detailed 3D representations of WM architecture. These include advanced imaging techniques such as High Angular Resolution Imaging (HARDI) as well as sophisticated modeling and tractography algorithms. Tractography creates sets of "fibers" (3D streamlines), which represent the major pathways of neural connections. A full brain fiber set often contains half a million or more fibers and results in extremely large file (of the order of 1 GB). The storage problem is further exacerbated by the need to save fiber-sets for multiple brain scans, as is often the case in many studies and databases. There are several possible ways to approach this problem: smart coding of the original data to optimize bit allocations, omission of part of the fibers to minimize redundancies, which is a form of smart down-sampling of the dataset, or

G.Z. Moreno (✉) • G. Alexandroni • N. Sochen • H. Greenspan
Tel Aviv University, Tel Aviv, Israel
e-mail: galizimmor@gmail.com

A. Fuster et al. (eds.), *Computational Diffusion MRI*, Mathematics and Visualization, DOI 10.1007/978-3-319-54130-3_11

finding an alternative representation for the fibers themselves. Ultimately all three elements need to be combined to create a complete compression scheme for WM fiber sets. In recent years several works have addressed the issue of reducing the number of fibers [1, 2]. A complete compression pipeline with fiber representation and coding was presented in a work by Presseau et al. [3].

In this paper, we address the issue of compressing the fibers, or in other words we seek a fiber representation that requires less storage, while still providing a good approximation to the original fibers. This "compressed" representation is intended to serve as part of a lossy compression scheme. In addition, we strive to provide the means to evaluate similarities between fibers without explicitly returning to the original, uncompressed format. Calculation of inter-fiber distances or similarities is one of the frequently performed tasks in many algorithms for fiber clustering, classification, or registration. Allowing such calculations to be completed using the compressed representation will facilitate reduction in storage space and computational complexity. We propose to use sparse representations for fibers in a high dimensional space defined by overcomplete dictionary. This method of signal decomposition was shown to be beneficial to compression in various applications [4]. Inter-fiber similarity can then be calculated directly in the compressed space, using sparse representations [5] and a specially tailored similarity measure— Cosine with Dictionary Similarity Weighting (CWDS), which we define below. The proposed method is shown in Sect. 2, followed by experimental validation in Sect. 3 and discussion and conclusions in Sect. 4.

2 Methods

A signal $f \in \Re^d$ can be represented as a sparse linear combination of prototype signals from an overcomplete dictionary , $D \in \Re^{d \times K}$, $K > d$. These prototype signals are the columns of D, usually termed "atoms", and designated $\{a_j\}_{j=1}^K$. The representation coefficients constitute the vector $x \in R^K$, so that for exact signal representation $f = Dx$. We seek the sparsest representation of f, using the dictionary D. This sparsest representation is the solution to the problem in Eq. (1). The solution of Eq. (1) is an NP-hard problem. However as long as sparse enough solution exists, its uniqueness can be verified [5].

The overcomplete dictionary D that leads to sparse representation can be chosen in advance, or especially adapted to fit a training set of signal examples. This latest approach is adopted here. The dictionary is trained using K-SVD algorithm [5], which minimizes the following objective function [Eq. (2)].

$$\min_x \|x\|_0 \ s.t. \ f = Dx \tag{1}$$

$$\min_{D,x} \|F - DX\|_F^2 \ s.t. \ \forall i \ \|x_i\|_0 \leqslant T_0 \tag{2}$$

where T_0 is a predetermined number of non-zero entries in a coefficient vector and F is a matrix of the size $d \times N$, containing N original data points $f_i \in R^d$, as its columns. X is a matrix of the size $K \times N$, containing N coefficients vectors $x_i \in R^K$, as its columns. The notation $\|A\|_F$ stands for Frobenius norm, given by $\|A\|_F = \sqrt{\sum_{ij} A_{ij}^2}$. K-SVD iteratively minimizes the function in Eq. (2), in two stages: first D is fixed and the best coefficient matrix X is found using Orthogonal Matching Pursuit (OMP [6]). This stage is termed the sparse coding stage. The second stage is the codebook update stage. It searches for a better dictionary, by fixing all the columns of D but one, and finding a new column and its updated coefficients such that the mean square error, $\|F - DX\|_F^2$, is reduced.

In case of fibers, the matrix $F_{d \times N}$ contains the original fibers as its columns and $X_{K \times N}$ contains the sparse representations of the fibers as its columns. N is the number of fibers, d is the length of original fiber representation and K is the length of the sparse representation. A fiber, f, is represented as a sequence of m points in a 3D space, sampled equidistantly: $f = \{x_1, y_1, z_1, , x_m, y_m, z_m\}$, where $m = 20$ for all fibers ($d = 60$). This choice of m was found to be a good compromise between the representation length and representation precision [7]. Once the dictionary is finalized, the fibers can be sparsely represented as a combination of dictionary atoms. This step is termed sparse coding, or atom decomposition. The representation coefficients x are found based on the given signal f and the dictionary D. It requires solving the problem in stated in Eq. (1). OMP algorithm that is used is a greedy algorithm that selects at each step the atom with the highest correlation to the current residual. The signal is then orthogonally projected to the span of the previously selected atoms and the residual is iteratively recomputed [5]. The compressed fibers set will consist of the matrix X containing the new sparse representations as its columns, and of the dictionary D. An approximate reconstruction of original representation is achieved by

$$\tilde{F} = D \cdot X \tag{3}$$

Instead of learning the dictionary on an entire fiber set, a representative sub-set of fibers is used in order to reduce the learning time. Simple down-sampling of the fiber set may compromise the outcome by randomly excluding parts of the fiber-set that may be important. Here, we propose to employ the coreset concept [8] in order to select a meaningful sub-set of fibers for learning the dictionary. Coresets are an innovative paradigm in data science, useful in tasks requiring large computation time and/or memory [8]. Selective reduction of large fiber-sets using coresets was explored in our previous work [9]. A novel algorithm called Density Coreset (DS) was proposed, that selects a subset of fibers using an iterative non-uniform sampling process. In DS, the effective sampling rate is set to be inversely proportional to the fibers density in brain space. This reduction process tends to choose representative fibers, while omitting redundancies (which are the fibers nearly identical to the ones selected). Feigin et al. [10] have shown that the optimization problem of learning D can be solved on a coreset, which is much smaller, without sacrificing too much accuracy.

2.1 Inter-Fiber Similarity and Sparse Representation

There exist numerous similarity measures that can be used with fibers. Here we focus on the cosine similarity measure which was shown in an earlier work to be advantageous for fibers [10]:

$$sim^{cos}\left(f_i, f_j\right) = \frac{\langle f_i, f_j \rangle}{\|f_i\|\,\|f_j\|} \tag{4}$$

where $\langle \cdot \rangle$ stands for inner product and $\|\cdot\|$ for L_2 norm. Since the new representation basis is not orthogonal, we cannot use this measure directly with sparse vectors. We propose to address the issue by modifying a cosine similarity measure in a way that takes into account the non-orthogonality of the sparse basis. Assuming that the reconstructed fibers $\tilde{f}$ are similar enough to the originals, we can write

$$sim^{cos}\left(f_i, f_j\right) \cong sim^{cos}\left(\tilde{f}_i, \tilde{f}_j\right) \tag{5}$$

Since reconstructed fibers are found by multiplication of the sparse representation x with the dictionary (3), the following relationship holds

$$sim^{cos}\left(f_i, f_j\right) \cong sim^{cos}\left(Dx_i, Dx_j\right) \tag{6}$$

Using the definition of cosine similarity Eq. (4) we get

$$sim^{cos}\left(f_i, f_j\right) \cong \frac{\langle Dx_i, Dx_j \rangle}{\|Dx_i\|\,\|Dx_j\|} = \frac{(Dx_i)^T \cdot Dx_j}{\|Dx_i\|\,\|Dx_j\|} = \frac{x_i^T D^T Dx_j}{\|Dx_i\|\,\|Dx_j\|} \tag{7}$$

We define S as a $K \times K$ matrix, such that s_{ij} contains a similarity measure between the atom a_i and the atom a_j in D. Since all atoms in D have a unit norm, this can be written as

$$S = D^T D \quad ; \quad s_{ij} = \langle a_i, a_j \rangle \tag{8}$$

rewriting Eq. (7) using Eq. (8) we have

$$sim^{cos}\left(f_i, f_j\right) \cong \frac{x_i^T S x_j}{\|Dx_i\|\,\|Dx_j\|} \tag{9}$$

Notice that the norms in the denominator are in fact the norms of the fibers that can be reconstructed using their sparse representation. However, we seek here to perform the similarity computation without going back to the original space. We therefore propose to substitute these norms by the norms of the original fibers, which can be saved before the sparse coding phase and later saved as part of the compressed data. That step would add one additional value to the representation, which will not have significant impact on the representation length, while allowing to use the original fiber norm for similarity approximation. The modified compressed representation $\widehat{x}$ will contain the value: $norm_i = \|f_i\|$, concatenated to the sparse coefficients vector x_i.

$$\widehat{x} = \{x_i, norm_i\} \tag{10}$$

Based on the above, we propose to use the following similarity measure in order to calculate fiber similarities using compressed representations, termed Cosine With Dictionary Similarity Weighting (CWDS):

$$sim^{CWDS}\left(\widehat{x_i}, \widehat{x_j}\right) = \frac{x_i^T S x_j}{\|norm_i\| \|norm_j\|} \tag{11}$$

Algorithm

- *Find a coreset C that contains a subset of N fibers from the original set F.*
- *Learn sparse dictionary $D_{d \times K}$ from that coreset using K-SVD, where K is the length of the new sparse representation and d is the original length of fiber representation.*
- *Find sparse representations x_i for all fibers (OMP). Calculate $\|f_i\|$ for each fiber. The compressed representation of f_i is given by $\widehat{x_i} = \{x_i, norm_i\}$.*
- *Calculate the feature similarity matrix S, Eq. (8), where s_{ij} represents how similar is the dictionary word a_i to dictionary word a_j.*
- *Calculate the similarity between two compressed representations using CWDS similarity, Eq. (11).*

The dictionary can be learned for each fiber-set and saved along with the compressed representation, or it can be learned from co-registered multiple fiber sets. The latter is more computationally efficient and is in fact necessary for calculating similarities between fibers originating from different brains.

3 Performance Evaluation

The proposed method was evaluated on MRI datasets of 15 healthy volunteers from the Human Connectome Project (HCP), Wu-Minn[1] database . The acquisition protocol included three shells (b-values of 1000, 2000, 3000), 96 unique directions for each, isotropic resolution of 1.25 mm and imaging matrix of $144 \times 168 \times 111$ pixels [11]. The diffusion data were preprocessed using the HCP diffusion pipelines [12], which included susceptibility, eddy-current and motion distortions correction,

---

[1]http://www.humanconnectome.org.

and registration to a common space. WM fibers were obtained using Q-Space Diffeomorphic Reconstruction (QSDR) reconstruction and tractography by DSI-Studio.[2] Tractography was terminated upon reaching 1 M fibers. In this section we evaluate the performance of the proposed scheme. There are three main aspects we would like to explore: how well does the sparse representation approximate the original fibers; how well is the original similarity measure approximated by CWDS; and is it possible to use a common dictionary for different fiber-sets. The experiments that are described next shed some light on these questions.

3.1 How Well Do the Sparse Representations Approximate the Original Fibers

For each of the fiber-sets F, a dictionary D was learned as described in Sect. 2. The dictionary learning was performed on a subset C of the fibers, which constitute a coreset of F. The coreset size was set to 20,000 for all the experiments (reduction by 50), in order to shorten the dictionary building times in Matlab. Dictionary sizes of 500, 600, and 700 atoms were evaluated. The sparsity constraint, T_0, was set to: 3, 5, 7. The complexity of calculating cosine similarity on the original space is $O(D_1)$, D_1 being the dimension of the original representation. The complexity of CWDS is $O(D_2^2)$, where D_2 is T_0. Therefore in order not to increase the computational requirements of CWDS, T_0 needs to be kept below $\sqrt{D_1}$, or in our case $T_0 < 7.7$ (as $D_1 = 60$).

First, we calculate the representation error relatively to the coreset fibers, which were used to train each dictionary. For each original coreset fiber, the reconstructed fiber is found using Eq. (3) and a L_2 distance is evaluated between the original and the reconstructed fibers. Figure 1 presents the mean distance for all 15 brains for different values of K and T_0. The mean values over all 15 fiber-sets are summarized in Table 1. In addition, we check whether the quality of sparse approximation remains the same for the fibers in the sets which are not part of the coreset. Here the reconstruction error is calculated for 10,000 fibers randomly selected from the full fiber set. Mean values over all sets are summarized in Table 1.

As expected, the reconstruction error becomes smaller for higher T_0. $T_0 = 7$ achieves the lowest error which is stable around 2 mm. It is also important to note that the error for random fibers is only a slightly higher than that of the coreset fibers. The difference is of the order of magnitude of the standard deviations. This can be seen as evidence that the coreset is a good enough subset for training the dictionary.

---

[2]Developed by Fang-Cheng Yeh from the Advanced Biomedical MRI Lab, National Taiwan University Hospital, Taiwan, and made available at http://dsi-studio.labsolver.org/Download/.

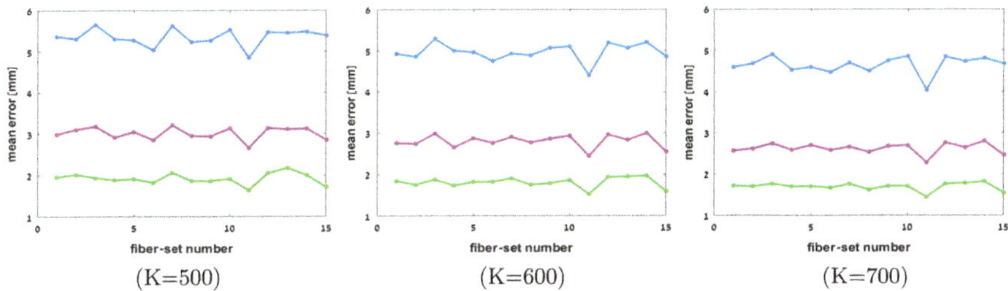

(K=500)   (K=600)   (K=700)

Fig. 1 Mean reconstruction errors for coreset fibers; *blue*-T0=3, *purple*-T0=5, *green*-T0=7

Table 1 Mean reconstruction errors in mm and standard deviations (in parentheses)

$Mean\left(|f - \tilde{f}|\right)$	$T_0 = 3$	$T_0 = 5$	$T_0 = 7$
Coreset, $K = 500$	9 (0.2)	3.01 (0.15)	1.92 (0.13)
Random set, $K = 500$	5.65 (0.24)	3.31 (0.16)	2.18 (0.15)
Coreset, $K = 600$	4.97 (0.2)	2.81 (0.15)	1.81 (0.12)
Random set, $K = 600$	5.28 (0.25)	3.09 (0.18)	2.05 (0.14)
Coreset, $K = 700$	4.65 (0.2)	2.62 (0.13)	1.7 (0.0.09)
Random set, $K = 700$	4.97 (0.23)	2.91 (0.15)	1.94 (0.11)

Figure 2 illustrates the reconstruction quality for one of the fiber sets. The original and reconstructed fibers are shown in row 1. Rows (2–4) show examples of single fibers and their reconstructed versions for different error magnitudes (zoomed in).

3.2 How Well is the Original Similarity Measure Approximated by CWDS

Our CWDS similarity measure is evaluated by comparing the distances between the fibers in their original representation (measured by cosine similarity [Eq. (4)]) and the distances between the same fibers as calculated in the sparse representation space using CWDS [Eq. (11)]. The distances were calculated using 10,000 randomly selected fibers from each brain. Figure 3 presents plots of the original cosine vs. CWDS for one of the brains and K = 500.

Mean differences between the two similarity measures were calculated for all fiber-sets and different values of K and T_0. The results are presented in Table 2.

Both Fig. 3 and Table 2 show that the differences in similarity measures are very small for all tested values of K and T_0, with the smallest being for $T_0 = 7, K = 700$.

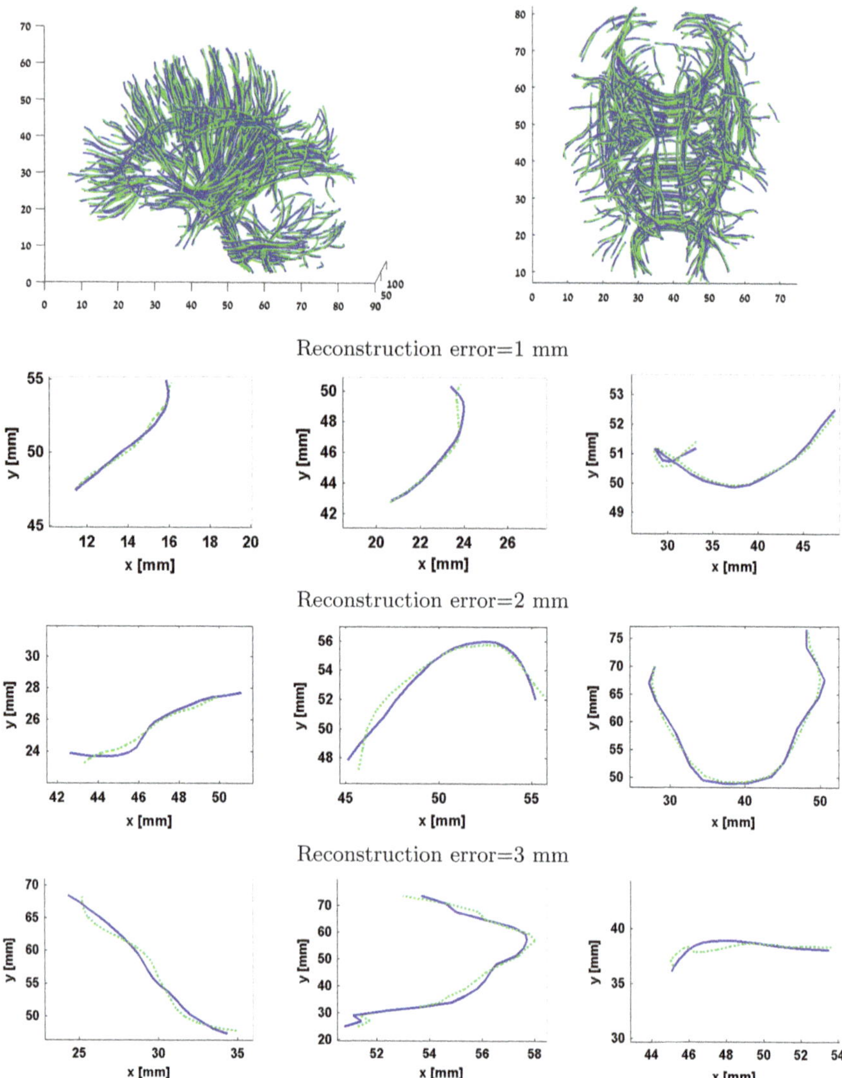

Fig. 2 Reconstruction of fibers from their sparse representations (arbitrary chosen fiber set). Here K = 700, T0 = 7. *Row* (1) two views of the same fiber set; *blue*-original fibers, *green*—reconstructed. *Rows* (2), (3), (4) each shows three examples of fibers reconstructed with the error of 1 mm, 2 mm, 3 mm, respectively

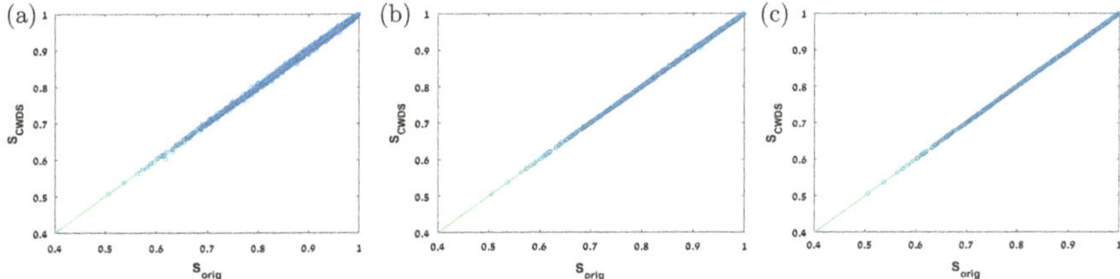

Fig. 3 Original vs. CWDS similarities for one of the brains. K = 500; *green* is an identity line. (**a**) $T_0 = 3$, (**b**) $T_0 = 5$, (**c**) $T_0 = 7$

Table 2 Mean differences between the two similarity measures

$Mean\left(|S_{orig} - CWDS|\right)$	$T_0 = 3$	$T_0 = 5$	$T_0 = 7$
$K = 500$	$0.0016\left(0.08 \cdot 10^{-3}\right)$	$0.0004\left(0.04 \cdot 10^{-3}\right)$	$0.00013\left(0.02 \cdot 10^{-3}\right)$
$K = 600$	$0.0015\left(0.08 \cdot 10^{-3}\right)$	$0.00037\left(0.04 \cdot 10^{-3}\right)$	$0.00013\left(0.02 \cdot 10^{-3}\right)$
$K = 700$	$0.0014\left(0.08 \cdot 10^{-3}\right)$	$0.000035\left(0.03 \cdot 10^{-3}\right)$	$0.000011\left(0.01 \cdot 10^{-3}\right)$

Table 3 Performance with common dictionary: mean reconstruction errors and mean differences between the two similarity measures

	$T_0 = 3$	$T_0 = 5$	$T_0 = 7$
Mean rec. error	$6.5\,(0.23)$	$3.85\,(0.18)$	$2.49\,(0.12)$
$Mean\left(|S_{orig} - CWDS|\right)$	$0.0018\left(0.07 \cdot 10^{-3}\right)$	$0.00048\left(0.03 \cdot 10^{-3}\right)$	$0.00014\left(0.01 \cdot 10^{-3}\right)$

3.3 *Representation of Different Fiber-Sets with Common Dictionary*

For this experiment, the coresets of all 15 brains were pooled into one huge mixed set. This is possible due to the fact that the original brains are all preregistered to a common space. The mixed set was downsampled by 3 to speed up the calculation and a common dictionary was learned with $K = 500$, $T_0 = 3, 5, 7$. The mean reconstruction errors and mean differences between cosine similarity in original space and CWDS in compressed space are shown in Table 3.

Here too, the lowest reconstruction error occurs at $T_0 = 7$ and is only slightly higher than the error received for individual dictionaries. The distances differences remain as small as before.

4 Discussion and Conclusions

The results indicate that it is possible to use a sparse representation for fibers, with mean reconstruction error slightly above 1.5 mm when using seven non-zero coefficients per fiber. Furthermore, the size of the dictionary has much less impact on the reconstruction quality than T_0. In addition, one common dictionary can be used for a group of fiber-sets, which is more efficient and only slightly increase the reconstruction error. The transition from initial 60 dimensional representation to sparse representation with $T_0 = 7$ reduces the number of non-zero values by 87% (this includes the norm value saved for each fiber) and thus presents significant reduction in memory requirements. If the fiber set is further compressed, for example using Huffman coding, the sparse sets can achieve much higher compression ratio than the original set, due to much lower entropies of the sparse representations.

A very significant difference of our method from other fiber compression techniques [3] is that it enables the estimation of inter-fiber similarity directly in the compressed space, using our proposed CWDS measure. The calculation of similarities (which can be converted into distances) is a necessary part of many common analysis schemes (comparisons, classifications, etc.) often applied to fiber sets. CWDS allows to perform these tasks without "decompression" of the data.

We have demonstrated the performance of the CWDS measure for both individual dictionaries learned for each fiber-set and for a common dictionary, which allows for inter-set similarity calculations. The value of T_0 was constrained to 7 in order to achieve the same computational complexity as one can get using cosine similarity in the original space. If more accuracy is needed, it may be achieved with higher T_0, of course with additional computational cost. The dictionary learning, although a computationally intensive procedure in itself is performed offline and only once for a group of fiber sets. The computational burden is reduced further by learning from a corset and not the full fiber set.

Future work includes incorporating the presented concept into a full compression pipeline, together with elimination of redundant fibers and additional coding with adaptive bit allocation. We will also endeavor to lower the reconstruction error by incorporating an error constraint into the sparsity framework and by addressing the different fiber lengths during the dictionary learning process.

References

1. Guevara, P., Poupon, C., Riviére, D., Cointepas,Y., Descoteaux, M., Thirion, B., Mangin, J.F.: Robust clustering of massive tractography datasets. NeuroImage **54**, 1975–1993 (2011)
2. Garyfallidis, E., Brett, E., Morgado Correia, M., Williams, G.B., Nimmo-Smith, I.: Quickbundles, a method for tractography simplification. Front. Neurosci. **6**, Article 175 (2012)
3. Presseau, C., Jodoin, P.M., Houde, J.C., Descoteaux, M.: A new compression format for fiber tracking datasets. NeuroImage **109**, 73–83 (2015)
4. Aharon, M., Elad, M., Bruckstein, A.: K-SVD: an algorithm for designing overcomplete dictionaries for sparse representation. IEEE Trans. Signal Process. **54**(11), 4311–4322 (2006)
5. Bruckstein, A.M., Donoho, D.L., Elad, M.: From sparse solutions of systems of equations to sparse modeling of signals and images. SIAM Rev. **51**(1), 34–81 (2009)
6. Rubinstein, R., Zibulevsky, M., Elad, M.: Efficient implementation of the K-SVD algorithm using batch orthogonal matching pursuit. Technical Report—CS Technion (April 2008)

7. Zvitia, O., Mayer, A., Shadmi, R., Miron, S., Greenspan, H.: Co-registration of white matter tractographies by adaptive-mean-shift and Gaussian mixture modeling. IEEE Trans. Med. Imaging **29**(1), 132–145 (2010)
8. Agarwal, P.K., Har-Peled, S., Varadarajan, K.R.: Geometric approximation via coresets. In: Goodman, J.E., Pach, J., Welzl, E. (eds.) Combinatorial and Computational Geometry, pp. 1–30. Cambridge University Press, Cambridge (2005)
9. Alexandroni, G., Zimmerman-Moreno, G., Sochen, N., Greenspan, H.: Coresets vs clustering: comparison of methods for redundancy reduction in very large white matter fiber sets. In: SPIE Medical Imaging, San Diego (2015)
10. Feigin, M., Feldman, D., Sochen, N.: From high definition image to low space optimiza-tion. In: Scale Space and Variational Methods in Computer Vision, pp. 459–470. Springer, Berlin, Heidelberg (2012)
11. Andersson, J.L., Sotiropoulos, S.N.: An integrated approach to correction for off-resonance effects and subject movement in diffusion MR imaging. NeuroImage **125**, 1063–1078 (2015)
12. Glasser, M.F., Sotiropoulos, S.N., Wilson, J.A., Coalson, T.S., Fischl, B., Andersson, J. L., Van Essen, D.C.: The minimal preprocessing pipelines for the Human Connectome Project. Neuroimage **80**, 105–124 (2013)

An Unsupervised Group Average Cortical Parcellation Using Diffusion MRI to Probe Cytoarchitecture

Tara Ganepola, Zoltan Nagy, Daniel C. Alexander, and Martin I. Sereno

Abstract Cortical parcellations provide valuable localisation resources for other neuroimaging modalities such as fMRI as well as insight into the structure-function relationship of the brain. The venerable but now dated ex vivo Brodmann map is currently being superseded by in vivo techniques that can better take into account intersubject variability. One popular in vivo method focusses on myeloarchitecture by measuring T1. This, however, probes only one aspect of cortical microstructure and is less useful in regions of low myelination. In contrast, diffusion MRI (dMRI) is sensitive to several additional microstructural features and can potentially provide a richer set of information regarding the architecture of grey matter microcircuitry. The following study used 3T HARDI data of multiple subjects to produce an entirely unsupervised, hemisphere-wide, group-average, parcellation. A qualitative assessment of the resulting cortical parcellation demonstrates several spatially coherent clusters in areas corresponding to well known functional anatomical areas. In addition, it exhibits some cluster boundaries that correlate with independently derived myelin mapping data for the same set of subjects, whilst also providing distinct clusters in areas (e.g., within MT+) where myelination is a less informative measurement.

T. Ganepola (✉)
Department of Cognitive, Perceptual and Brain Sciences, University College London, London, UK

Department of Computer Science, Centre for Medical Image Computing, University College London, London, UK
e-mail: tganepola@gmail.com

Z. Nagy
Laboratory for Social and Neural Systems ResearchUniversity of Zurich, Zurich, Switzerland

Wellcome Trust Centre for Neuroimaging, UCL Institute of Neurology, London, UK

D.C. Alexander
Department of Computer Science, Centre for Medical Image Computing, University College London, London, UK

M.I. Sereno
Department of Cognitive, Perceptual and Brain Sciences, University College London, London, UK

© Springer International Publishing AG 2017

A. Fuster et al. (eds.), *Computational Diffusion MRI*, Mathematics and Visualization, DOI 10.1007/978-3-319-54130-3_12

1 Introduction

The cytoarchitecture of the cerebral cortex in humans and many other mammalian species was first investigated in the early 1900s using histological sections of post-mortem brains stained for cell bodies or myelinated fibers. Pioneers of this era [1–3] discovered that the microstructure of the cortex was organised into six layers, the columnar appearance of which varies throughout the cortical sheet. Roughly homogeneous modules of variable size were observed and attributed to functional specificity, starting with striate cortex whose border with V2 is easily visible to the naked eye in hand-cut unfixed tissue. The hypothesis of a mosaic of internally homogeneous areas prevails today and these classical parcellations have been widely adopted in modern studies, for example, to localise activation foci in functional imaging studies.

Despite their pervasiveness, it is evident that traditional cortical maps suffer many methodological limitations. One limitation is observer dependant bias, [4]. Another problem is that histological methods are often restricted to a single cell stain per specimen, thus requiring the observer to combine identified boundaries across differently distorted adjacent sections. These limitations may explain the variability in size, location and number of cortical areas reported by different such methods [4–7]. The labour-intensive process of histological sectioning enforces further limits on the sample size used to generate such cortical maps. Subsequent studies have demonstrated a large degree of intersubject variability with regards to the exact location and extent of several well-defined cortical areas. Given this, classical maps derived from a small sample of cadaver brains, are unlikely to accurately reflect boundary definitions for the entire population. Other considerations include the introduction of artefacts from histological sectioning (e.g., including unique nonlinear distortions in each section due to slide mounting and outright tears in the tissue), which complicate registration of data back into undistorted 3D space.

Despite their lower resolution, in vivo methods have the potential to overcome some of these limitations—in vivo analysis provides observer independent image processing, much larger samples sizes, the possibility of multi-modal studies, and completely avoids histology artefacts. Thus far, in vivo investigations of cortical microstructure have focussed predominantly on myeloarchitectonics, via quantitative T1 [8] and R1 (1/T1) mapping [9–11] mapping using multiple flip angles, the ratio of T1-weighted over T2-weighted images [12, 13], and multiple inversion times (MP2RAGE). However, myelination density provides only a partial picture of cortical microstructure. More recently, Glasser et al. extended their T1-weighted/T2-weighted methods into a multi-modal framework for cortical mapping [14]. This approach combined myelin maps , resting state, and task-based functional MRI measures of approximately 200 subjects with expert anatomical knowledge and a complex processing pipeline to produce a semi-automated, group-average, full-hemisphere, cortical parcellation. Nevertheless, the datasets in that paper do not directly measure the fine-grained structural information that is associated with the cyto- and myeloarchitecture of the cortex. For investigators wishing to acquire a detailed understanding of the structure-function relationship in the cortex, it may be desirable to include measurements of additional features that characterise grey matter (GM) micro-environments.

There is a growing body of evidence [15–22] to support the use of diffusion MRI in cortical imaging facilitated by recent technological advancements, such as multi-band excitation, magnetic field probes [23], and ultra high field imaging. In particular, investigators have demonstrated changes in the dominant diffusion direction between the primary somatosensory and motor cortices, via a measure of radiality [20]. Others have shown the relationship between cortical gyrencephaly and diffusion tensor metrics [21]. Nagy et al. demonstrated the in vivo individualised discriminative power of a feature set derived from high angular resolution diffusion imaging data by testing distinct fMRI-based regions of interest [22]. These findings suggest that dMRI in grey matter may provide an additional informative modality for replicating and possibly refining/redefining the boundary definitions of existing cortical parcellation approaches.

The dMRI signal is sensitive to several microstructural features, including but not limited to axon diameter, neurite density, and dominant fibre direction and hence may offer additional structural information beyond bulk myelination density alone. To test the idea that grey matter dMRI might provide a richer description of cortical microenvironments, we used unsupervised, surface-normal-based, group-average cortical parcellation derived from dMRI-based measures of cytoarchitecture. We applied and refined the framework initially developed by Nagy et al. [22] to a large group of subjects using surface-based and surface-referenced cross-subject averaging of dMRI to obtain a hemisphere-wide map of grey matter diffusion patterns from high resolution, 3T data. The resultant parcellation exhibits several coherent clusters that correspond closely with the locations of well-known cortical areas, despite the classifier having no prior information or non-local spatial constraints of any kind.

2 Methods

2.1 Data and Pre-Processing

Imaging datasets for 17 unrelated subjects (10m, 7f aged 22–35) were randomly selected from the minimally pre-processed, 500-Subjects release of the Human Connectome Project (HCP). For a thorough description of the protocols and pre-processing pipelines refer to the HCP documentation [24–26]. In brief, data were collected on a Siemens 3T Skyra system. Each diffusion dataset comprised of 270 gradient directions, acquired evenly across three interleaved b-shells, b = 1000, 2000 and 3000 s/mm^2. An additional eighteen b=0 images were interleaved throughout the acquisition. The high angular and spatial (1.25 mm isotropic) resolution of the HCP datasets lends itself to investigations of grey matter diffusion where, partial volume effects and low anisotropy values are limiting factors.

The HCP pre-processing steps conducted prior to data release, include eddy current and motion correction, providing diffusion weighted images with good alignment and without major distortions. Therefore, further corrections to this end were not performed; however, HCP diffusion datasets suffer from subject specific gradient nonlinearities that were corrected for during the fitting procedure of the tissue model below.

2.2　Surface Reconstruction

In order to utilise the high resolution (0.7 mm isotropic) of the available structural data we chose the HCP FreeSurfer pipeline over the standard recon-all pipeline to generate cortical surface reconstructions for each subject. This improved pipeline does not down-sample the T1w images to 1 mm isotropic resolution, and incorporates the additional information available in the T2w scans to reduce surface placement errors [25].

Following cortical surface reconstruction the diffusion datasets of each subject were sampled at the midpoint between the white/grey matter (WM/GM) boundary and the pial surface so as to reduce the likelihood of either WM or CSF contamination [20, 22].

2.3　Feature Space

In a similar procedure to that of Nagy et al. [22], a sixth order spherical harmonic series (SHS) was fit to the dMRI signal in order to characterise the apparent diffusion coefficient (ADC) profile of the cortical tissue. A SHS was fit separately in each b-shell for each surface vertex of the right hemisphere of each subject. A subset of the features presented in [22] were calculated from the ADC to obtain a [1×5] feature vector per vertex, per b-shell. The features, as detailed below, characterise the ADC profile in relation to the local surface normal, and therefore describe the GM tissue irrespective of the orientation differences that result from cortical folding.

1. The value of the ADC profile along the surface normal.

$$f(\mathbf{n})$$

2. The mean of the ADC profile in the plane perpendicular to the surface normal, i.e. parallel to the cortical sheet. $C(\mathbf{n})$ is the unit circle perpendicular to n.

$$\bar{f}_{\perp} = (2\pi)^{-1} \int_{C(\mathbf{n})} f(x)dx$$

3–5. The k=2,3 and 4 moments, respectively, of the ADC in the plane perpendicular to the surface normal.

$$M_{k,\perp} = \int_{C(\mathbf{n})} [f(x)]^k dx$$

The group average of each of the 15 features was computed in turn using sulcus-based surface averaging [27]. This approach allows an individual's folding pattern to be aligned to an average folding pattern, in this case on the `fsaverage` surface. With this method, any given `fsaverage` vertex will combine data from individual subject vertices that have surface normals in different directions. This makes it possible to detect local-surface-geometry-dependent diffusion signatures of cortical areas even though their local normal directions might differ from subject to subject. This information would be compromised if the diffusion data were to be directly averaged in 3D (folded) space. The transformation between each subject's cortical surface and the target brain space was applied to each of the cortical features in turn. The mean across all subjects of each feature was then calculated for each vertex of the `fsaverage` surface. Finally, the averaged features were recombined into a [1×15] group average feature space for classification.

2.4 Classification

The unsupervised classification algorithm, k-means [28], was implemented to parcellate the group average feature set. Several values of k were tested on a trial and error basis, starting with $k = 40$, approximately the number of Brodmann areas. At lower values, the parcellation produces large smooth clusters, and doesn't provide additional structural information to the myelin density map (see below). Results are shown for a value of $k = 150$. At this value the parcellation displayed many more area-like clusters than for lower values, whereas, increasing beyond this value did not provide additional information in initial qualitative assessments. Furthermore, $k = 150$ was the value after which decreases in the sum of total distances for the clustering solution began to plateau, and the total runtime began to increase rapidly (Fig. 1).

Since the clusters are numbered arbitrarily by the algorithm, we included an additional ordering step whereby clusters were reordered by the similarity of cluster centres, starting with the pairing which had the highest affinity. Here, similarity was defined as the Euclidean distance between the mean feature vector of each cluster. This additional ordering stage acts to smooth to the results when viewed on the surface, compared to a completely randomised cluster order.

The resulting group average cortical parcellation was qualitatively compared to a group average myelin map, estimated from the T1w/T2w ratio of the same set of HCP subjects.

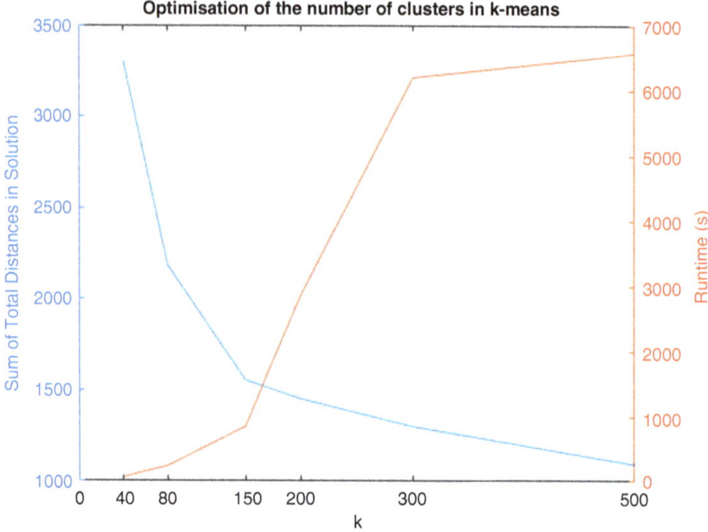

Fig. 1 The tested values of k for the k-means algorithm against the best sum of total distances for each clustering solution (*blue*) and the total runtime of the algorithm in seconds (*orange*)

3 Results

Figure 2 shows the lateral view of the group average diffusion MRI based parcellation (right) alongside the group average myelin map (T1w/T2w) for the same set of subjects (left) on the inflated `fsaverage` surface. Figure 4 shows the medial view of the same. Figure 3 shows the distribution of myelin measurements within regions of interest (ROI) selected from the dMRI parcellation.

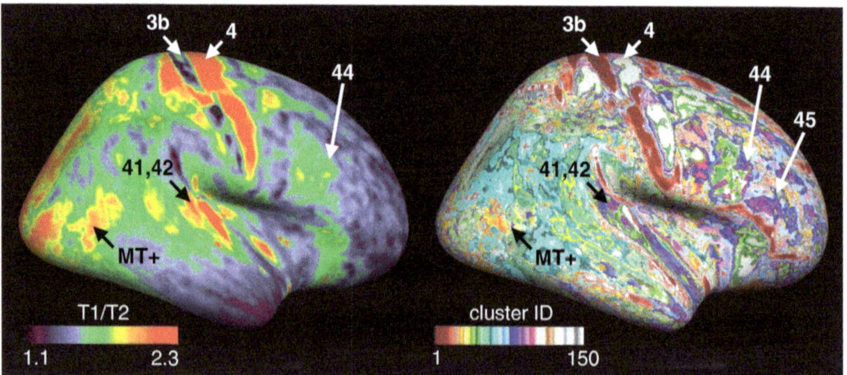

Fig. 2 The lateral view of the diffusion-based parcellation (*right*) and the group average myelin map (*left*)

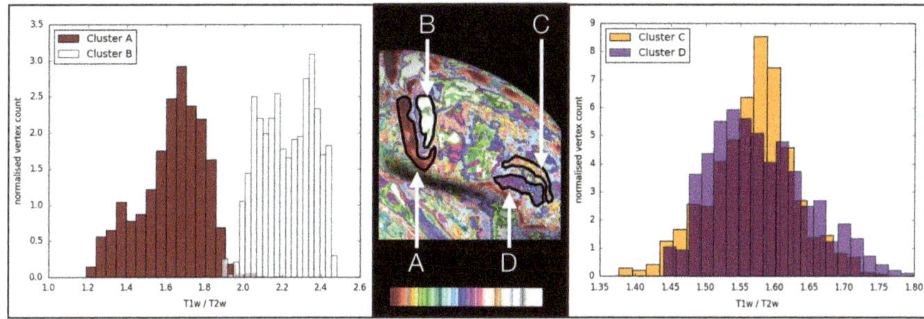

Fig. 3 The distributions of myelin measurements corresponding to regions of interest from the dMRI parcellation result. The histograms on the *left* show T1w/T2w distribution from regions A and B within the central sulcus and are distinct in both modalities. The histograms on the right correspond to regions C and D which appear distinct in the parcellation but have closely overlapping myelin distributions. The outlines of the regions of interest from which the histogram data were extracted are shown in the centre image

3.1   Central Sulcus

The most salient feature of the parcellation is the emergence of distinct and spatially coherent clusters along the anterior (white cluster) and posterior (red cluster) banks of the central sulcus. These have been provisionally labelled 3b and 4 due to their consistency with the location and extent of Brodmann areas 3b and 4. These cortical areas correspond to part of primary somatosensory cortex (S-I) and to primary motor cortex (M-I), respectively. Comparison with the myelin map (left) indicates that the white cluster ID correlates with an area of high myelination, whereas, the red cluster correlates with a drop in myelination. Figure 3 confirms that both the myelin and diffusion measurements discriminate these regions. However, the independently derived diffusion based parcellation produces a more spatially coherent area along the posterior bank of the central sulcus, when compared to the variability of the myelin map in Fig. 2.

There are several factors that may have lead to the group average parcellation exhibiting the closest agreement to the Brodmann map within the central sulcus. The boundary between S-I and M-I represents one of the most prominent transitions within the cortex [20, 29]. The input layers of S-I possess many small cell bodies giving it a granular appearance. In contrast, long cortico-spinal projections in M-I result in large pyramidal cell bodies known (in the foot representation) as Betz Cells, giving an agranular appearance. S-I also exhibits highly myelinated tangential bands of Baillarger, which are less prominent in M-I. Furthermore, in vivo studies at 7T support the hypothesis that differences in the laminar composition between these two regions are manifested in dMRI signal [20].

Another factor which may have improved the detection of these areas is that they demonstrate relatively low intersubject variability. S-I occupies the posterior bank of the central sulcus and extends back into the postcentral gyrus and M-I occupies anterior bank of the central sulcus, extending forwards into the precentral gyrus, with their transition consistently located at the fundus of the central sulcus [5, 29] near the location of area 3a, which receives predominant input from muscle receptors. This is consistent with the location and extent of the red and white clusters in the parcellation. Therefore, it is likely that architectural changes in these regions, as characterised by their feature vectors, are reinforced by averaging across multiple subjects.

3.2 Broca's Region

Areas 44 and 45 are collectively referred to as Broca's region , which has long been implicated in the production and recognition of speech. We note that both the parcellation and myelin map exhibit a distinct region that is consistent with the location of area 44. This area emerged as a coherent patch despite it not having a consistent relation to macroscopic landmarks in the majority of subjects [6].

In addition, anterior to area 44, we note the presence of a spatially coherent purple/blue cluster, provisionally labelled area 45. It seems that area 45 has no counterpart in the myelin map, supporting the notion that diffusion based cortical imaging may be able to provide additional information to myelin mapping, particularly in areas of lower myelination such as the premotor and prefrontal cortex. This notion is further supported in Fig. 3 where it is clear that the distribution of myelin values between area 45 and the adjacent ROI are very similar. In contrast, these two regions could be differentiated in the diffusion based feature set. The frontal lobe of the diffusion-based parcellation appears more like a patchwork of distinct clusters, whereas the myelin map in this region appears more homogenous.

3.3 Auditory Areas

On the temporal lobe we note that both the myelin map and diffusion-based parcellation exhibited distinct patches that roughly coincide with primary auditory core and belt areas (BA 41 and 42). This suggests that some structural information in the dataset is maintained despite Heschl's gyrus exhibiting a markedly variable folding pattern across subjects [30].

3.4 Occipital Areas

On the right hand side of Fig. 4 the posterior occipital lobe contained prominent purple, blue, and red clusters, giving it a distinct appearance compared to much of the rest of the medial cortical sheet, which was assigned predominantly to green and

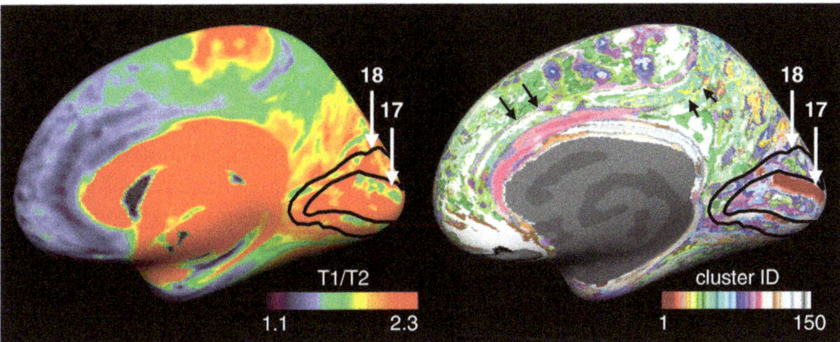

Fig. 4 The medial view of the diffusion-based parcellation (*right*) and the group average myelin map (*left*)

white clusters. This generally correlates with the high myelination of this region, seen in the T1/T2 data at the left of Fig. 4; however it is worth noting that the region of apparent heavy myelination in V2 just below the tip of the "18" arrowhead projected further in the superior direction than the purple region in the diffusion-based result.

The black contours outline the inner and outer extents of area 18 from the FreeSurfer probabilistic atlas, i.e the secondary visual area V2. The inner boundary of this contour corresponds to the neighbouring primary visual cortex, V1 (area 17), within the calcarine sulcus. Despite V1 possessing a prominent tangential band in layer 4B that is lacking in extrastriate area V2 [5, 17], we did not observe distinct coherent clusters corresponding to the full extent of these two areas in either the T1/T2 data or the diffusion data. Instead the most salient feature of this region was the red cluster, which is located near the upper vertical meridian of V1. It is unclear why the boundary of V1 was characterised uniquely by the dMRI feature set, rather than the entire region. However, the myelin map showed a significant decrease in myelination in the same location that is not consistent with the underlying anatomy. This suggests the presence of a systematic surface placement error that my have resulted in CSF partial voluming in both data sets, which resulted in a region near the upper and lower vertical meridian border between V1 and V2 standing out.

Finally, returning to the lateral surface (see Fig. 2) in the middle of the myelin-dense region of MT+ it is possible to distinguish a border between a posterior orange cluster and an anterior white/tan cluster. A study examining the relation between quantitative T1 and retinotopy [11] surprisingly showed that the heavily myelinated oval in the lateral occipital cortex does not directly correspond to MT; instead, MT proper only accounts for the posterior part of that oval. The anterior part may correspond to FST, which represents parts of the visual field already mapped in MT, and which responds to the ipsilateral visual field unlike MT. Once again, this suggests that diffusion data may help distinguish regions not easily separated by using myelin density alone.

3.5   Gyrification

The unlabeled black arrows on the right of Fig. 4 indicate curvature-like features in the parcellation. These lines follow the fundus and crown of the cingulate sulcus and gyrus respectively. The emergence of these macroscopic landmarks could be associated with sampling errors at areas of high curvature, where partial voluming is more prevalent. Alternatively, it may reflect a relationship between gyrification and diffusion anisotropy, as suggested by several groups—e.g., [21]. Deeper cortical layers appear to thin in sulci, which has been suggested to be a way of maintaining equal local volume by folding-induced tangential stretching [31, 32]. By contrast, upper cortical layers appear to puff out and become more myelinated on gyri. These systematic folding-correlated effects may give rise to detectable differences in grey matter diffusion patterns. The initial detection of a correlation between gyrification and T1 was similarly initially dismissed as a depth-sampling artifact, but then subsequently suggested to be partly due to real myelination differences between sulcal and gyral cortex. An additional complication is that partial volume errors may be detecting systematic differences in fiber direction near the grey/white matter border; for example, the dominant diffusion direction is expected to be highly radial in areas of high curvature, such as gyral crowns, and more tangential in along the banks of gyri due to the angle at which u-fibres project into the cortex [20, 21].

4   Conclusion

We presented a parcellation result using dMRI data, demonstrating areal definitions that reflect some well known architectonically defined regions without the use of a training stage or any non-local spatial constraints. The population average feature set is most discriminative in primary areas that are consistently located across subjects, such as S-I and M-I, and heavily myelinated regions. However, we also observe clusters that may correspond to non-primary areas such as area 44 and 45. Our results demonstrate that the higher-order, diffusion-based, feature set may be distinguishing local differences in the texture and geometry of the myelinated meshwork of the neocortex not all of which are visible in myelin density maps. Incorporating this information is likely to improve the performance of non-supervised multimodal parcellation schemes for cortical areas.

References

1. Brodmann, K.: Vergleichende Lokalisationslehre der Grosshirnrinde in ihren Prinzipien dargestellt auf Grund des Zellenbaues. Barth, Leipzig (1909)
2. Vogt, C., Vogt, O.: Allgemeine ergebnisse unserer hirnforschung, vol. 25. JA Barth (1919)

3. von Economo, C.F., Koskinas, G.N., Triarhou, L.C.: Atlas of Cytoarchitectonics of the Adult Human Cerebral Cortex. Karger, Basel (2008)
4. Zilles, K., Amunts, K.: Centenary of Brodmann's map - conception and fate. Nat. Rev. Neurosci. **11**(2), 139–145 (2010)
5. Amunts, K., Malikovic, A., Mohlberg, H., Schormann, T., Zilles, K.: Brodmann's areas 17 and 18 brought into stereotaxic space – where and how variable? Neuroimage **11**(1), 66–84 (2000)
6. Amunts, K., Schleicher, A., Bürgel, U., Mohlberg, H., Uylings, H., Zilles, K.: Broca's region revisited: cytoarchitecture and intersubject variability. J. Comp. Neurol. **412**(2), 319–341 (1999)
7. Zilles, K., Schleicher, A., Langemann, C., Amunts, K., Morosan, P., Palomero-Gallagher, N., Schormann, T., Mohlberg, H., Bürgel, U., Steinmetz, H., et al.: Quantitative analysis of sulci in the human cerebral cortex: development, regional heterogeneity, gender difference, asymmetry, intersubject variability and cortical architecture. Hum. Brain Mapp. **5**(4), 218–221 (1997)
8. Fischl, B., Salat, D.H., van der Kouwe, A.J.W., Makris, N., Ségonne, F., Quinn, B.T., Dale, A.M.: Sequence-independent segmentation of magnetic resonance images. Neuroimage **23**, S69–S84 (2004)
9. Sigalovsky, I.S., Fischl, B., Melcher, J.R.: Mapping an intrinsic MR property of gray matter in auditory cortex of living humans: a possible marker for primary cortex and hemispheric differences. Neuroimage **32**(4), 1524–1537 (2006)
10. Lutti, A., Dick, F., Sereno, M.I., Weiskopf, N.: Using high-resolution quantitative mapping of R1 as an index of cortical myelination. Neuroimage **93**, 176–188 (2014)
11. Sereno, M.I., Lutti, A., Weiskopf, N., Dick, F.: Mapping the human cortical surface by combining quantitative T1 with retinotopy. Cerebral Cortex **23**(9), 2261–2268 (2013)
12. Glasser, M.F., Van Essen, D.C.: Mapping human cortical areas in vivo based on myelin content as revealed by T1-and T2-weighted MRI. J. Neurosci. **31**(32), 11597–11616 (2011)
13. Glasser, M.F., Goyal, M.S., Preuss, T.M., Raichle, M.E., Van Essen, D.C.: Trends and properties of human cerebral cortex: correlations with cortical myelin content. Neuroimage **93**, 165–175 (2014)
14. Glasser, M.F., Coalson, T., Robinson, E., Hacker, C., Harwell, J., Yacoub, E., Ugurbil, K., Anderson, J., Beckmann, C.F., Jenkinson, M., et al. A multi-modal parcellation of human cerebral cortex. Nature **536**, 171–178 (2016)
15. Leuze, C.W.U., Anwander, A., Bazin, P.-L., Dhital, B., Stüber, C., Reimann, K., Geyer, S., Turner, R.: Layer-specific intracortical connectivity revealed with diffusion MRI. Cerebral Cortex **24**(2), 328–339 (2014)
16. Anwander, A., Pampel, A., Knosche, T.R.: In vivo measurement of cortical anisotropy by diffusion-weighted imaging correlates with cortex type. Proc. Int. Soc. Magn. Reson. Med **18**, 109 (2010)
17. Aggarwal, M., Nauen, D.W., Troncoso, J.C., Mori, S.: Probing region-specific microstructure of human cortical areas using high angular and spatial resolution diffusion MRI. Neuroimage **105**, 198–207 (2015)
18. Deoni, S.C., Jones, D.K.: Time-series analysis of diffusion signal as a model-free approach to segementing tissue. In: *Proceedings of the 14th Annual Meeting of ISMRM*, p. 2734 (2006)
19. Haroon, H.A., Binney, R.J., Parker, G.J.: Probabilistic quantification of regional cortical microstructural complexity. Proc. Intl. Soc. Mag. Reson. Med. **18**, 578 (2010)
20. McNab, J.A., Polimeni, J.R., Wang, R., Augustinack, J.C., Fujimoto, K., Stevens, A., Janssens, T., Farivar, R., Folkerth, R.D., Vanduffel, W., et al.: Surface based analysis of diffusion orientation for identifying architectonic domains in the in vivo human cortex. Neuroimage **69**, 87–100 (2013)
21. Kleinnijenhuis, M., van Mourik, T., Norris, D.G., Ruiter, D.J., van Cappellen van Walsum, A.-M., Barth, M.: Diffusion tensor characteristics of gyrencephaly using high resolution diffusion MRI in vivo at 7T. NeuroImage **109**, 378–387 (2015)
22. Nagy, Z., Alexander, D.C., Thomas, D.L., Weiskopf, N., Sereno, M.I.: Using high angular resolution diffusion imaging data to discriminate cortical regions. PloS ONE **8**(5), e63842 (2013)

23. Wilm, B.J., Nagy, Z., Barmet, C., Johanna Vannesjo, S., Kasper, L., Haeberlin, M., Gross, S., Dietrich, B.E., Brunner, D.O., Schmid, T., et al.: Diffusion MRI with concurrent magnetic field monitoring. Magn. Reson. Med. **74**(4), 925–933 (2015)
24. Sotiropoulos, S.N., Jbabdi, S., Xu, J., Andersson, J.L., Moeller, S., Auerbach, E.J., Glasser, M.F., Hernandez, M., Sapiro, G., Jenkinson, M., et al.: Advances in diffusion MRI acquisition and processing in the human connectome project. Neuroimage **80**, 125–143 (2013)
25. Glasser, M.F., Sotiropoulos, S.N., Anthony Wilson, J., Coalson, T.S., Fischl, B., Andersson, J.L., Xu, J., Jbabdi, S., Webster, M., Polimeni, J.R., et al.: The minimal preprocessing pipelines for the human connectome project. Neuroimage **80**, 105–124 (2013)
26. Uğurbil, K., Xu, J., Auerbach, E.J., Moeller, S., Vu, A.T., Duarte-Carvajalino, J.M., Lenglet, C., Wu, X., Schmitter, S., Van de Moortele, P.F., et al.: Pushing spatial and temporal resolution for functional and diffusion MRI in the human connectome project. Neuroimage **80**, 80–104 (2013)
27. Fischl, B., Sereno, M.I., Tootell, R.B.H., Anders M Dale, et al. High-resolution intersubject averaging and a coordinate system for the cortical surface. Hum. Brain Mapp. **8**(4), 272–284 (1999)
28. Hartigan, J.A., Wong, M.A.: Algorithm as 136: a k-means clustering algorithm. Appl. Stat. **28**(1), 100–108 (1979)
29. White, L.E., Andrews, T.J., Hulette, C., Richards, A., Groelle, M., Paydarfar, J., Purves, D.: Structure of the human sensorimotor system. I: Morphology and cytoarchitecture of the central sulcus. Cerebral Cortex **7**(1), 18–30 (1997)
30. Leonard, C.M., Puranik, C., Kuldau, J.M., Lombardino, L.J.: Normal variation in the frequency and location of human auditory cortex landmarks. heschl's gyrus: where is it? Cerebral Cortex **8**(5), 397–406 (1998)
31. Bok, S.T.: Der einflu\ der in den furchen und windungen auftretenden krümmungen der gro\ hirnrinde auf die rindenarchitektur. Zeitschrift für die gesamte Neurologie und Psychiatrie **121**(1), 682–750 (1929)
32. Waehnert, M.D., Dinse, J., Weiss, M., Streicher, M.N., Waehnert, P., Geyer, S., Turner, R., Bazin, P.-L.: Anatomically motivated modeling of cortical laminae. Neuroimage **93**, 210–220 (2014)

Using Multiple Diffusion MRI Measures to Predict Alzheimer's Disease with a TV-L1 Prior

Julio E. Villalon-Reina, Talia M. Nir, Boris A. Gutman, Neda Jahanshad, Clifford R. Jack Jr, Michael W. Weiner, Ofer Pasternak, Paul M. Thompson, and for the Alzheimer's Disease Neuroimaging Initiative (ADNI)

Abstract Microstructural measures from diffusion MRI have been used for classification purposes in neurodegenerative and psychiatric conditions. Novel diffusion reconstruction models can lead to better and more accurate measures of tissue properties: each measure provides different information on white matter microstructure in the brain, revealing different signs of disease. The diversity of computable measures makes it necessary to develop novel classification procedures to capture all of the available information from each measure. Here we introduce a multichannel regularized logistic regression algorithm that classifies individuals' diagnostic status based on several microstructural measures, derived from their diffusion MRI scans. With the aid of a TV-L1 prior, which ensures sparsity in the classification model, the resulting linear models point to the most classifying brain regions for each of the diffusion MRI measures, giving the method additional descriptive power. We apply our regularized regression approach to classify Alzheimer's disease patients and healthy controls in the ADNI dataset, based on their diffusion MRI data.

J.E. Villalon-Reina (✉) • T.M. Nir • B.A. Gutman • N. Jahanshad • P.M. Thompson
Imaging Genetics Center, University of Southern California, Marina del Rey, CA, USA
e-mail: julio.villalon@ini.usc.edu

C.R. Jack
Department of Radiology, Mayo Clinic and Foundation, Rochester, MN, USA

M.W. Weiner
Department of Radiology, UCSF School of Medicine, San Francisco, CA, USA

O. Pasternak
Laboratory of Mathematics in Imaging, Brigham and Women's Hospital, Harvard Medical School, Boston, MA, USA

© Springer International Publishing AG 2017
A. Fuster et al. (eds.), *Computational Diffusion MRI*, Mathematics and Visualization, DOI 10.1007/978-3-319-54130-3_13

1 Introduction

Diffusion MRI (dMRI) reveals a number of properties of white matter (WM) microstructure. Its sensitivity to water diffusion in living tissue allows us to compute numerous summary measures that relate to neural fiber integrity and architecture in the brain. Based on certain assumptions, each can quantify different aspects of WM microstructure. One of the most basic measures—fractional anisotropy (FA)—is based on the diffusion tensor model (DTI) [1], and continues to be popular despite its known limitations, which include its ambiguity at fiber crossings. Other models overcome some limitations of DTI, including multi-tensor models, such as the tensor distribution function (TDF) [2], q-ball imaging and the orientation distribution function (ODF) [3], constrained spherical deconvolution [4], neurite orientation dispersion and density imaging (NODDI) [5], and freewater index (FW) [13] among others. Each model leads to its own set of scalar microstructural measures and many offer a richer understanding of WM microstructure than FA does. Which combination of measures best characterizes brain disease remains an open question, and depends on the disease examined, and the spectral and angular resolution of the available data. This question may have a different answer in different parts of the brain depending on the underlying changing pathology (e.g., pathological changes in gray/white matter interfaces or more central white matter tracts).

At the time of writing, around 20 microstructural measures have been proposed for single-shell dMRI. Microstructural measures derived from new dMRI models may carry even more information on WM microstructure including the geometry of diffusion anisotropy, diffusivity, complexity, estimated number of distinguishable fiber compartments, number of crossing fibers and neurite dispersion. Combining these in a classification task is challenging, and requires proper regularization. Here, we use a Total Variation-Lasso or TV-L1 regularization as a prior term in a logistic regression framework. The channel-wise TV term leads to linear models that are approximately spatially piecewise constant, giving the weight maps descriptive power to suggest both the regions and measures that are helpful in a disease classification task, while considering *multiple measures together*. We build on prior work with TV-L1 regularizers in neuroimaging; they have been used successfully for fMRI decoding and in electrophysiological studies [6].

The classification task examined here is to discriminate Alzheimer's disease patients (AD) and healthy aging controls (NC), based on their dMRI data, by merging information from a range of complementary indices. A discriminative model in this setting may be useful as a disease biomarker, for drug trial enrichment and to help identify those most likely to decline in the future. In view of this, many studies describe WM microstructural differences between AD and NC [7], and some exploit WM metrics for classification [8–10]. By combining several measures in a classification task, we hope to generate a biomarker of disease that is "greater than the sum of its parts."

2 Methods

2.1 Data Acquisition and Preprocessing

Baseline MRI, dMRI, and clinical data were downloaded from the ADNI database (adni.loni.usc.edu). Here we performed an analysis of dMRI data from 102 participants: 53 healthy controls (CN; mean age: 72.4 ± 6.0 years; 24 M/29 F), and 49 AD patients (mean age: 74.9 ± 8.7 years; 29 M/20 F).

All subjects underwent whole-brain MRI scanning on 3T GE Medical Systems scanners at 14 acquisition sites across North America. Anatomical T1-weighted SPGR (spoiled gradient echo) sequences (256 × 256 matrix; voxel size = 1.2 × 1.0 × 1.0 mm^3; TI = 400 ms; TR = 6.98 ms; TE = 2.85 ms; flip angle = 11°), and dMRI (128 × 128 matrix; voxel size: 2.7 × 2.7 × 2.7 mm^3; TR = 9000 ms; scan time = 9 min were acquired; 46 separate images were acquired for each dMRI scan: 5 images with no diffusion sensitization (b_0 images) and 41 diffusion-weighted images (DWI; $b = 1000$ s/mm^2).

Images were preprocessed as in [7]. To summarize, raw dMRI images were corrected for motion and eddy current distortions, and T1-weighted images underwent inhomogeneity normalization. Extra-cerebral tissue was removed from both scan types. Each T1-weighted anatomical image was linearly aligned to a standard brain template (the down-sampled Colin27 [11]): 110 × 110 × 110, with 2-mm isotropic voxels). The diffusion images were linearly and then elastically registered [12] to their respective T1-weighted structural scans to correct for echo-planar imaging induced susceptibility artifacts. The gradient tables were corrected to account for the linear registration of the DWI images to the structural T1-weighted scan.

2.2 DMRI Reconstruction Models, Scalar Maps, and Spatial Normalization

For each subject, dMRI microstructural measures were computed from four different reconstruction models: DTI, TDF, NODDI and FW. Five measures were extracted from these models: FA and mean diffusivity (MD) from DTI, fractional anisotropy from TDF (FA-TDF), the orientation dispersion index (OD) from NODDI and the free water index (FW). We will not describe the well known DTI based FA and MD here, but will briefly describe the other three models:

The **Tensor Distribution Function (TDF)** represents the diffusion profile as a probabilistic mixture of tensors [2] allowing the reconstruction of multiple underlying fibers per voxel, together with a distribution of weights. We compute the voxel-wise TDF as the probability distribution function $P(\mathbf{D})$ defined on all feasible 3D Gaussian diffusion processes in tensor space $\mathbf{D}$:

$$S(\mathbf{q}) = P(\mathbf{D}) \, e^{\left(-\tau \mathbf{q}^T \mathbf{D}\mathbf{q}\right)} d\mathbf{D}, \tag{1}$$

where S is the measured intensity signal, $\mathbf{q} = r\delta G$, where r, δ, and G are the gyromagnetic ratio, the duration of the diffusion sensitization, and the applied magnetic gradient vector, respectively. The number of detected peaks is estimated by examining the local maxima of the tensor orientation distribution (TOD), defined in the unit sphere along directions θ:

$$\mathrm{TOD}\,(\theta) = \int_{\lambda} P\,(\mathbf{D}\,(\theta, \lambda))\,d\lambda, \tag{2}$$

where λ are the eigenvalues. The TDF-averaged eigenvalues of each fiber were calculated by computing the expected values along the principal direction of the fiber. From these eigenvalues a scalar TDF anisotropy (FA-TDF) is calculated as an extension of the standard FA formula:

$$\mathrm{FA\ TDF} = \int \mathrm{TOD}\,(\theta) * \mathrm{FA}\,(\theta)\,d\theta$$

$$= \sqrt{\frac{\left(\lambda_1'(\theta)-\lambda_2'(\theta)\right)^2+\left(\lambda_1'(\theta)-\lambda_3'(\theta)\right)^2+\left(\lambda_2'(\theta)-\lambda_3'(\theta)\right)^2}{2\left[\lambda_1'(\theta)^2+\lambda_2'(\theta)^2+\lambda_3'(\theta)^2\right]}}$$

$$\lambda_i'(\theta) = \frac{\int P\,(\mathbf{D}\,(\theta, \lambda))\,\lambda_i d\lambda}{\int P\,(\mathbf{D}\,(\theta, \lambda))\,d\lambda} \tag{3}$$

The **Neurite Orientation Dispersion and Density Imaging (NODDI)** is a composite model that takes into account three compartments that affect water diffusion in the brain: the intracellular compartment, the extracellular compartment, and the cerebrospinal fluid (CSF) [5]. The intracellular compartment is modeled as cylinders with a radius of zero that represent the axons and dendrites of the brain tissue, which are jointly called neurites. The ODF of the intracellular compartment is modeled as a Watson distribution that can capture the dispersion orientation of coherent central white matter bundles as well as the incoherent neurites of the grey matter. The normalized intracellular compartment A_{ic} is modeled as:

$$A_{ic} = \int_{\mathbb{S}^2} f\,(\mathbf{n})\,e^{-bd_{\parallel}(\mathbf{q}\cdot\mathbf{n})^2}\,d\mathbf{n} \tag{4}$$

Here, $\mathbf{q}$ represents the gradient directions, b the b-value of the diffusion weighting, $\mathbf{n}$ are the orientations of the cylinders with parallel diffusivity $d_{\parallel}$ along which the signal is attenuated and $f\,(\mathbf{n})$ is the Watson distribution, which has two parameters $(\boldsymbol{\mu}, \mathcal{K})$ and is defined as:

$$f\,(\mathbf{n}) = M\left(\frac{1}{2}, \frac{3}{2}, \mathcal{K}\right)^{-1} e^{\mathcal{K}(\boldsymbol{\mu}\cdot\mathbf{n})^2} \tag{5}$$

Here, the distribution tends to be symmetric around the mean orientation $\boldsymbol{\mu}$, and M is Kummer's confluent hypergeometric function. $\mathcal{K}$ is called the concentration parameter. For $\mathcal{K} > 0$, as $\mathcal{K}$ increases the density along $\boldsymbol{\mu}$ tends to concentrate.

Once $\mathcal{K}$ is estimated the orientation dispersion index (OD) is calculated as:

$$OD = \frac{1}{\pi} \arctan\left(\frac{1}{\mathcal{K}}\right) \tag{6}$$

OD goes from 0 to 1, the higher the value the more dispersed the neurites in a particular voxel. In our analyses below we used only the OD maps. The intracellular and extracellular volume fractions as well as the isotropic CSF volume fraction are not taken into account in our analyses. Zhang et al. demonstrated that the latter measures require more than one shell in order to be reliable, whereas the OD can be computed reliably with single shell data even with standard clinical acquisition b-values of $b = 1000$ s/mm^2 [5]. OD may be more informative than DTI, in areas with less organized patterns such as areas of multiple fiber crossings as well as towards the gray/white matter boundaries.

Free-Water Imaging (FW) estimates the contribution of freely diffusing water molecules to the diffusion signal with a bi-tensor model [13]. The first component of the model is the so-called *tissue* compartment that represents either grey matter or a bundle of the white matter. The second component reflects the free-water compartment, which is said to be proportional to the amount of CSF contamination, especially in areas of the white matter that are close to the ventricles. The free-water component is also expected to increase with neuroinflammation due to edema. The full model is defined as:

$$S_{\mathbf{q}}\left(\mathbf{D}, f\right) = f e^{\left(-b\mathbf{q}^T \mathbf{D}\mathbf{q}\right)} + (1 - f)\, e^{(-bd_w)}, \tag{7}$$

where S is the attenuated signal, $\mathbf{q}$ are the applied diffusion gradient directions, b is the b-value of the diffusion weighting, $\mathbf{D}$ is the diffusion tensor and f is the fractional volume of the *tissue* compartment $(0 < f \le 1)$. The second term is a fully isotropic tensor, where d_w is the bulk diffusivity of water, which is constant at body temperature $(3 \times 10^{-3}$ mm^2/s$)$.

Voxel-wise maps of all five measures—FA, MD, FA-TDF, OD, and FW—were created for all 102 subjects; all subjects' maps were spatially normalized to a custom ADNI- derived minimal deformation template (MDT). Template creation and spatial normalization was performed according to previously published voxelwise ADNI-DTI analyses [7].

2.3 Regularized Logistic Regression Classification

In general, the linear logistic regression model has the following classification function

$$y = f\left(\mathbf{X}, w, b\right) = F\left(\mathbf{X}w + b\right) \tag{8}$$

Here $\mathbf{X} \in \mathfrak{R}^{n \times p}$, n is the number of samples (subjects) and p is the number of features. As all the computations were performed within the MDT mask (193,586 $\sim$200,000 voxels), p is the number of voxels times the number of diffusion measures (five in this case). The parameters to be estimated are w and b, where $w \in \mathfrak{R}^p$ is a p-dimensional vector, $b \in \mathfrak{R}_n$ is the intercept and $y \in \{-1, 1\}$ is the class label, in our case, to be the subject diagnosis. The regularized cost to be optimized is:

$$\widehat{w} = \arg\min \mathcal{L}\left(y, F\left(\mathbf{X}w + b\right)\right) + \lambda \mathfrak{J}\left(w\right), \quad \lambda \geq 0 \tag{9}$$

where $\mathcal{L}$ is the logistic loss function, $\mathfrak{J}\left(w\right)$ is the regularization term and λ is the Lagrange multiplier. The intercept b is not regularized, and only depends on the loss function. We will simplify $\mathcal{L}\left(y, F\left(\mathbf{X}w + b\right)\right)$ to $\mathcal{L}\left(w\right)$. In our case, the standard TV-L1 norm cost becomes:

$$\mathfrak{J}\left(w\right) = (1 - \alpha)\left\|w\right\|_1 + \alpha \sum_{j=1}^{N_m} \mathrm{TV}\left(w_j\right), \quad \mathrm{TV}(y) = \left\|\nabla y\right\|, \tag{10}$$

where the first term is the LASSO or L1 cost, TV is the Total Variation penalty [6], w_j is the weight map of a microstructural measure j, N_m ($=5$ here) is the number of measures used and α is a constant that sets the desired tradeoff between L1 and TV terms. The L1 penalty encourages sparsity in the model, by setting most coefficients to zero. This penalty function suffers from some limitations when there is a large number of parameters p to fit, and few observations n, as LASSO selects at most n variables before it saturates. Further, if there is a group of highly correlated variables, then LASSO tends to select one variable from a group and ignores the others. On the other hand, the TV is defined as the L1 norm of the image gradient, which allows for sharp edges, encouraging the recovery of a smooth, piecewise constant weights map. This in turn allows us to interpret the weight maps as they may highlight clusters that can resemble anatomical regions.

We used the FISTA procedure [6] to find $\widehat{w}$ (the estimated value for w). As the L1 terms are not smooth, a naïve gradient descent may not always converge to a good minimum. For this convex optimization, smooth and non-smooth terms are considered separately. The logistic loss and the logistic gradient are the smooth terms:

$$\mathcal{L}\left(w\right) = \frac{1}{n} \sum_{i=1}^{n} \log\left(1 + e^{-y_i\left(\mathbf{X}_i^T w\right)}\right) \tag{11}$$

$$\nabla \mathcal{L}\left(w\right) = -\frac{1}{n} \sum_{i=1}^{n} \frac{y_i \mathbf{X}_i}{1 + e^{y_i\left(\mathbf{X}_i^T w\right)}} \tag{12}$$

We used an eightfold nested cross-validation to tune the parameters α and λ.

3   Results

We were able to classify individuals into diagnostic groups (AD vs. NC) with an accuracy of 76.2%. We ran a parallel test by using only one measure (FA-DTI) and the prediction accuracy was 50%. As expected, the resulting maps of significant predictors showed cohesive regional patches of stable coefficients, a property that is favored by the TV regularization term. Figure 1 shows the resulting map for each of the five measures.

FW and MD showed similar predictive properties, with large regions of negative coefficients in the frontal lobes (both hemispheres). FA-DTI and FA-TDF also showed a similar pattern, but FA-TDF showed larger and more cohesive regions in the frontal white matter, especially in areas with fiber crossings. OD showed some similarities with the MD map although the regions with the larger coefficients (both positive and negative) tended to be smaller and more widespread. Many of these observations are in line with what is expected for each measure. The direction of the coefficients is also important to note. It is expected that the anisotropy of the white matter tends to decrease in AD compared to healthy aging controls, but MD, FW and OD on the other hand tend to increase with white matter disruption.

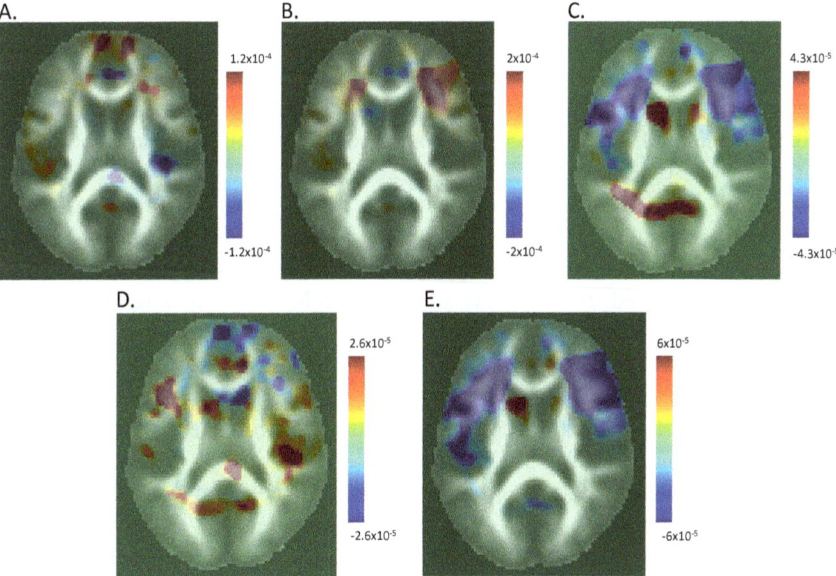

Fig. 1 Regularized maps of useful diagnostic predictors, based on measures computed from diffusion MRI. (**a**) FA-DTI, (**b**) FA-TDF, (**c**) MD-DTI, (**d**) OD, (**e**) FW. Color bars show the value of the coefficients, from negative (*blue*) to positive (*red*), with zero in *green*

4 Discussion

In this article, we evaluated the utility of the TV-L1 prior logistic regression to assess the ability of multiple dMRI reconstruction methods to simultaneously distinguish alterations in WM microstructure between people with AD and matched healthy controls. We computed five dMRI derived microstructural measures from four different reconstruction models that were used together in a regularized classification framework and we were able to successfully classify AD from healthy controls and to derive spatially coherent discrimination patterns across the entire brain for each measure.

AD pathology includes disturbances in the brain's WM pathways including loss of axons, myelin sheaths, and oligodendroglial cells, which may not all be detected by using DTI based descriptors alone. Machine learning for classification based on dMRI features has been focused mainly on DTI derived measures; although HARDI derived measures have also been explored [19, 20]. Volumetric measures, including hippocampal volume, gray matter volume from voxel-based morphometry, and cortical thickness [14–16, 18], have effectively classified AD patients, but few studies have used dMRI-derived biomarkers for classification purposes. Most of these studies have used DTI based measures: several used voxel-wise features from DTI maps, using methods such as Pearson correlation and ReliefF for feature reduction [8–10], reporting classification accuracies of >90%. In [17], tractography-based connectivity metrics based on fiber count, FA-DTI, and diffusivity were used for SVM classification, reporting an accuracy of 88%. Clearly, these accuracies depend on the problem and dataset used, and are not directly comparable with one another. Spatial and anatomical regularization for classification purposes have also been tested on AD discrimination against controls by Cuingnet et al. [18]. Here they achieved improved classification accuracies by using this type of regularization on cortical features and producing discriminatory parcellated maps of the cortex highlighting the brain regions traditionally compromised in AD.

Here we evaluated 102 subjects and were able to reach a relatively high classification accuracy for a white matter study of AD. Although our approach did not necessarily "beat" prior classification results, our goal was to compare the relative utility of multiple metrics for classification, which leads to some insight on how the disease may affect different fiber properties. Moreover, it was important to see if these measures might complement and add to the information provided by DTI measures—particularly in regions outside the coherent WM. Many dMRI measures are correlated with each other to some extent, but each captures the microstructure slightly differently, and at the various spatial locations, there may be greater sensitivity to detecting subtle changes with one measure versus another.

In conclusion, different reconstruction models and their respective scalar descriptors provide distinct micro-anatomical features, which differ in classification value by brain region. Together these estimates may improve brain-wide classification and may overcome the need to compute localized statistically determined regions of interest, and allow us to observe microstructural changes in the entirety of the brain. We made use of the main functionality of the TV prior, namely its denoising and smoothing capabilities across the image. This is essential in this context since single voxels prove to be very noisy and neighboring anatomy is presumably similar. Future work should compare other classification methods and improve estimates by incorporating tissue volume differences. We will also test if dMRI metrics can contribute to leading classification approaches based on biomarkers such as hippocampal volume, amyloid deposition, and tensor-based morphometry.

Acknowledgment This work is partially supported by an NIH U54 grant to the ENIGMA Center for Worldwide Medicine, Imaging & Genomics.

References

1. Basser, P.J., et al.: MR diffusion tensor spectroscopy and imaging. Biophys. J. **66**(1), 259–267 (1994)
2. Leow, A.D., et al.: The tensor distribution function. Magn. Reson. Med. **61**(1), 205–214 (2009)
3. Tuch, D.S.: Q-ball imaging. Magn. Reson. Med. **52**(6), 1358–1372 (2004)
4. Tournier, J.D., et al.: Direct estimation of the fiber orientation density function from diffusion-weighted MRI data using spherical deconvolution. Neuroimage. **23**, 1176–1185 (2004)
5. Zhang, H., et al.: Axon diameter mapping in the presence of orientation dispersion with diffusion MRI. Neuroimage. **56**(3), 1301–1315 (2011)
6. Gramfort, A., et al.: Identifying predictive regions from fMRI with TV-L1 prior. In: 3rd International Workshop on Pattern Recognition in Neuroimaging, Philadelphia, PA, 2013, pp. 17–20 (2013)
7. Nir, T., et al.: Effectiveness of regional DTI measures in distinguishing Alzheimer's disease, MCI, and normal aging. Neuroimage Clin. **3**, 180–195 (2013)
8. Graña, M., et al.: Computer aided diagnosis system for Alzheimer disease using brain diffusion tensor imaging features selected by Pearson's correlation. Neurosci. Lett. **502**(3), 225–229 (2011)
9. Haller, S., et al.: Individual prediction of cognitive decline in mild cognitive impairment using support vector machine-based analysis of diffusion tensor imaging data. J. Alzheimers Dis. **22**(1), 315–327 (2010)
10. O'Dwyer, L., et al.: Using support vector machines with multiple indices of diffusion for automated classification of mild cognitive impairment. PLoS One. **7**(2), e32441 (2012)
11. Holmes, C.J., et al.: Enhancement of MR images using registration for signal averaging. J. Comput. Assist. Tomogr. **22**(2), 324–333 (1998)
12. Leow, A.D., et al.: Statistical properties of Jacobian maps and the realization of unbiased large-deformation nonlinear image registration. IEEE Trans. Med. Imaging. **26**(6), 822–832 (2007)
13. Pasternak, O., et al.: Free water elimination and mapping from diffusion MRI. Magn. Reson. Med. **62**(3), 717–730 (2009)
14. Klöppel, S., et al.: Automatic classification of MR scans in Alzheimer's disease. Brain. **131**(3), 681–689 (2008)
15. Lerch, J.P., et al.: Automated cortical thickness measurements from MRI can accurately separate Alzheimer's patients from normal elderly controls. Neurobiol. Aging. **29**(1), 23–30 (2008)
16. Magnin, B., et al.: Support vector machine-based classification of Alzheimer's disease from whole-brain anatomical MRI. Neuroradiology. **51**(2), 73–83 (2009)
17. Wee, C.Y., et al.: Enriched white matter connectivity networks for accurate identification of MCI patients. Neuroimage. **54**(3), 1812–1822 (2011)

18. Cuingnet, R., et al.: Spatial and anatomical regularization of SVM: a general framework for neuroimaging data. IEEE Trans. Pattern Anal. Mach. Intell. **35**(3), 682–696 (2013)
19. Bloy, L., et al.: HARDI based pattern classifiers for the identification of white matter pathologies. Med. Image Comput. Comput. Assist. Interv. **14**(2), 234–241 (2011)
20. Nagy, Z., et al.: Using high angular resolution diffusion imaging data to discriminate cortical regions. PLoS One. **8**(5), e63842 (2013)

Accurate Diagnosis of SWEDD vs. Parkinson Using Microstructural Changes of Cingulum Bundle: Track-Specific Analysis

Farzaneh Rahmani, Somayeh Mohammadi Jooyandeh, Mohammad Hadi Shadmehr, Ahmad Shojaie, Farsad Noorizadeh, and Mohammad Hadi Aarabi

Abstract SWEDD (scans without evidence of dopaminergic deficit) patients often are misdiagnosed as having Parkinson disease (PD) but later prove to have distinct features from PD. A commonly found symptom of these patients being focal and unilateral dystonia. SWEDD patients do not respond to dopaminergic therapy and may in turn benefit from management of adult onset dystonia, therefore early differential diagnosis from PD is important in order to avoid over diagnosis of PD and mismanagement of these patients. Along with a different pattern of tremor from PD, SWEDD patients do not show the non-motor symptoms associated with different stages of PD, do not exhibit cognitive deficit and depict a and task specificity of the motor symptoms without any deterioration along time. We hypothesized that the cingulum which is both functional in cognitive control and task set performance and is structurally affected in early stages of PD and is implicated in other non-motor symptoms of PD might be differentially affected in PD and SWEDD group. The diffusion imaging data from 39 PD, 28 SWEDD and 21 normal subjects were reconstructed in the MNI space using q-space diffeomorphic reconstruction (QSDR) to assess association of quantitative anisotropy (QA) and generalized fractional anisotropy (GFA) of left and right cingulum with the PD and SWEDD groups in the baseline level (diagnosis of PD or SWEDD) and age-sex matched controls. We found significant difference between GFA and QA of the left cingulum and QA of the right cingulum in SWEDD and control group versus the PD group. These results suggest a diagnostic value for the cingulum in early

F. Rahmani • M.H. Shadmehr
Students' Scientific Research Center, Tehran University of Medical Sciences, Tehran, Iran

Neuroimaging Network (NIN), Universal Scientific Education and Research Network (USERN), Tehran, Iran

S. Mohammadi Jooyandeh
Department of Psychiatry and Psychotherapy, University of Regensburg, Regensburg, Germany

A. Shojaie • F. Noorizadeh • M.H. Aarabi (✉)
Basir Eye Health Research Center, Tehran, Iran
e-mail: Mohammadhadiarabi@gmail.com

© Springer International Publishing AG 2017

A. Fuster et al. (eds.), *Computational Diffusion MRI*, Mathematics and Visualization, DOI 10.1007/978-3-319-54130-3_14

PD/SWEDD and also reveal that the diffusion metric parameters of cingulum that are not necessarily sensitive to axonal loss (GFA) might be a better indicator of microstructural changes in early PD/SWEDD.

1   Introduction

SWEDD or (scans without evidence of dopaminergic deficit) are a group of clinically diagnosed patients with Parkinson symptoms who reveal no evidence of dopaminergic deficit on [123I] FP-CIT Single Photon Emission Computerized Tomography (SPECT) which is identified as marker of disease progression [1, 2]. The true entity of patients with Parkinsonism as with SWEDD is still unknown. While SWEDD patients were first identified following entrance and follow up DAT Scanning of patients with assumed Parkinson disease (PD), there is propensity to classify SWEDD patients as a distinct disorder in that they do not show imaging progress toward PD and do not respond to classical levodopa treatment [3]. Additionally studies have shown that PD is clinically over diagnosed in uncertain cases therefore misdiagnosis of this group might expire a golden time for initiation of a proper treatment. In fact a longitudinal follow up of patients with DAT imaging within normal range has revealed that in up to 44% of these patients the initial diagnosis changes to other disorders not associated with DAT deficit or PD. These patients also exhibit lower Unified Parkinson's Disease Rating Scale (UPRDS) score which remain relatively constant during the course of disease [4]. Another study demonstrated that the arm tremor pattern in SWEDD group as well as their response to PMS conditioning along with their minimal responsiveness to dopaminergic therapy can clinically discriminate between them and PD patients [5]. The occurrence of focal or segmental dystonia and task specificity of dystonia. Lack of true bradykinesia and absence of the non-motor symptoms of PD also favors the diagnosis of SWEDD rather than PD [6]. Furthermore emerging evidence of differential DAT scan quantification parameters and patterns in PD group vs. normal and SWEDD group [7] are being provided whereas little data exist on the specific regional involvement of extranigral or cortical areas that might help determine the true nature of SWEDD group and facilitate clinical judgment between SWEDD and PD group and adult onset dystonia which often exhibits overlapping clinical and experimental features with SWEDD [5].

The cingulate gyrus is a major white matter tract with implications in emotion formation and executive function and also plays a major role in cognitive control of limbic lobe functions such as response initiation. Cingulate gyrus also works in close functional and structural relation with prefrontal cortex and its adjacent dorsal anterior cingulate cortex to maintain an intact executive function [8] and connecting sites with known role in cognitive control. Decreased FA is observed in cingulum of PD patients in both demented and early-stage non-demented patients. Contrary to FA, the increase in mean diffusivity in early stages of PD compared to normal controls is associated with better performance in semantic fluency and other cognitive tasks in newly diagnosed PD patients [9, 10]. The anterior and posterior cingulum microstructure and function differ in which each convey different cortical connections to the prefrontal and parieto-occipital cortices respectively [8]. This can explain their role in task set/verbal memory loss (rostral part of cingulum) and visuospatial memory impairment (parahippocampal Cingulum) in PD [11].

2 Procedure

2.1 Participants

Participants involved in this research were recruited from Parkinson's Progression Markers Initiative (PPMI) [12]. Participants were tested and confirmed negative for any neurological disorders apart from PD. The participants' PD status was confirmed by Movement Disorder Society-Unified Parkinson's Disease Rating Scale (MDS-UPDRS) and the loss of dopaminergic neurons were observed in DaTscans. Every participant involved in this research has signed informed written consents in order to share their unidentified clinical data to investigators. DWI images were obtained for 39 PD, 28 SWEDD and 21 normal age and sex matched were available from the baseline visit (Table 1).

2.2 Data Acquisition

Data used in the preparation of this paper was obtained from Parkinson's Progression Markers Initiative (PPMI) database (www.ppmi-info.org/data/) [12]. This dataset was acquired on a 3 Tesla Siemens scanner, producing 64 DWI (repetition time = 7748 ms, echo time = 86 ms; voxel size: $2.0 \times 2.0 \times 2.0$ mm^3; field of view = 224×224 mm) at b = 1000 s/mm^2 and one b0 image along with a 3D T1-weighted structural scan (repetition time = 8.2 ms, echo time = 3.7 ms; flip angle = 8°, voxel size: $1.0 \times 1.0 \times 1.0$ mm^3; field of view = 240 mm, acquisition matrix = 240×240).

Table 1 Baseline characteristics and clinical features in control and PD and SWEDD

	Parkinson	SWEDD	Control
Sex ratio (male/female)	23/13	18/10	15/6
Age (years± SD)	63.11±8.74	61.28±9.73	61.38±7.11
UPRDS score (± SD)	20.27±8.87	15.51±7.08	–
Hoehn & Yahr score (± SD)	1.66±0.47	1.59±0.50	–
MOCA score (± SD)	27.33±2.05	26.82±2.55	28.14±1.1

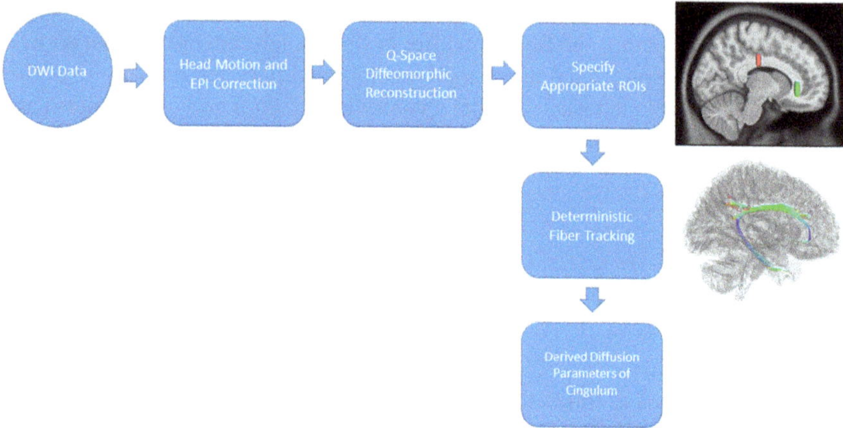

Fig. 1 Overview of method

2.3 *Diffusion MRI Data Processing, Fibers Tractography and Group Analysis*

Diffusion MRI data were corrected for subject motion, eddy current distortions, and susceptibility artefacts due to the magnetic field inhomogeneity using ExploreDTI toolbox [13]. The diffusion data were reconstructed in the MNI space using q-space diffeomorphic reconstruction to obtain the spin distribution function. A diffusion sampling length ratio of 1.25 was used, and the output resolution was 2 mm [14]. A seeding region was placed at whole brain. An ROI was placed in exactly the same location as the rostral ROI and the second ROI was placed in the subgenual part of the cingulum [15, 16]. The anisotropy threshold was 0.15. The angular threshold was 30°. The step size was 1 mm. Tracks with length less than 300 mm were discarded. A total of 1,000,000 seeds were placed. Quantitative anisotropy (QA) and generalized fractional anisotropic (GFA) were derived for each participant. The analysis was conducted using publicly available software DSI Studio (http://dsi-studio.labsolver. org). Figure 1 shows the overview of method. Quantitative statistical comparison of anisotropic parameters cingulum was conducted using analysis of variance (ANOVA) (SPSS version 15: SPSS, Chicago, IL, USA).

3   Result

Herein we used Diffusion Tensor Imaging study to reveal changes in brain connectivity associated with SWEDD or Parkinson group compared to control group.

One way ANOVA analysis revealed significant difference between QA and GFA of left cingulum and QA of the right cingulum between groups. Tukey post-hoc test

Table 2 Result of quantitative measurements of diffusion MRI in control, PD and SWEDD

	PD	SWEDD	Normal
GFA of the left cingulum (mean±SD)	0.55±0.085	0.47±0.091	0.45±0.051
QA of left cingulum (mean±SD)	0.102±0.005	0.096±0.006	0.101±0.008
GFA of the right cingulum (mean±SD)	0.49±0.078	0.52±0.102	0.51±0.064
QA of the right cingulum (mean±SD)	0.098±0.006	0.102±0.004	0.107±0.007

Table 3 ANOVA and post hoc multiple comparisons of diffusion parameters of left and right cingulum

Diffusion parameter of a fibers	ANOVA *P-value*	Post hoc multiple comparisons	*P-value* after Bonferroni correction
GFA of the left cingulum	0.000	Controls vs. PD	< 0.001
		SWEDD vs. PD	0.002
QA of the left cingulum	0.007	SWEDD vs. PD	0.011
QA of the right cingulum	0.038	SWEDD vs. PD	0.031
		Controls vs. PD	< 0.001
		SWEDD vs. Control	0.049

was used to analyses between groups difference. The mean ± SD for each diffusion parameter in each group is depicted in Table 2. Homogeneity of variances was met for all tested variables using Leven's test of homogeneity of variances, except for QA of right cingulum which was further analyzed by the Welch ANOVA and post-hoc Games-Howel test. For the ANOVA, a non-corrected p-value of < 0.05 was considered significant. Conditional on a significant F-value, post hoc pairwise t-tests were used and controlled with Bonferroni correction for multiple comparisons. Table 3 shows significant results of analysis of QA and GFA of cingulum between groups.

4 Conclusion

After the cingulum is implicated in many aspects of early PD manifestations including attention deficit, verbal and episodic memory impairment and depression which can also emerge as late consequences of PD [11]. Results of our study showed that SWEDD and control group shared similar diffusion metric parameters which were significantly different from those with Parkinson disease (Table 2). As demonstrated by a previous study [4] the baseline severity of parkinsonian symptoms was lower in SWEDD group compared to PD group (T-test P-value=0.03). Meanwhile the H & Y stage of PD patients and SWEDD group were not statistically different (T-test P-value=0.55), both implicating minimal unilateral motor involvement. The MOCA score demonstrates absence of any detectable cognitive decline in any of the three groups. In fact all patients were enrolled from drug-naïve recently diagnosed PD and SWEDD patients of the PPMI database whose PD or SWEDD status had been confirmed by DAT SCAN. This difference in microstructural changes of cingulum in PD and SWEDD group is in line with the absence of cognitive decline and non-motor symptoms of any kind in SWEDD group. The difference in microstructural parameter of Cingulum can be considered as novel biomarker for early differential diagnosis of SWEDD from PD patients. The preponderance of GFA association but not the QA of cingulum might suggest that nondegenerative processes not involving axonal loss can better define or determine specific structural changes of PD vs. SWEDD group in newly diagnosed patients.

Acknowledgements This work was funded by grants from the Michael J Fox Foundation for Parkinson's Research, the W Garfield Weston Foundation, and the Alzheimer's Association, the Canadian Institutes for Health Research, and the Natural Sciences and Engineering Research Council of Canada. We thank Christian Beckmann and Simon Eickhoff for their advice on data analysis. Data used in this article were obtained from the Parkinsons Progression Markers Initiative (PPMI) database (www.ppmi-info.org/data). For up-to-date information on the study, visit www.ppmi-info.org. PPMI is sponsored and partially funded by the Michael J Fox Foundation for Parkinsons Research and funding partners, including AbbVie, Avid Radiopharmaceuticals, Biogen, Bristol-Myers Squibb, Covance, GE Healthcare, Genentech, GlaxoSmithKline (GSK), Eli Lilly and Company, Lundbeck, Merck, Meso Scale Discovery (MSD), Pfizer, Piramal Imaging, Roche, Servier, and UCB (www.ppmi-info.org/fundingpartners).

References

1. Marek, K., Jennings, D., Seibyl, J.: Single-photon emission tomography and dopamine transporter imaging in parkinson's disease. Adv. Neurol. **91**, 183–191 (2002)
2. Whone, A.L., Moore, R.Y., Piccini, P.P., Brooks, D.J.: Plasticity of the nigropallidal pathway in parkinson's disease. Ann. Neurol. **53**(2), 206–213 (2003)
3. Marshall, V.L., Patterson, J., Hadley, D.M., Grosset, K.A., Grosset, D.G.: Two-year follow-up in 150 consecutive cases with normal dopamine transporter imaging. Nucl. Med. Commun. **27**(12), 933–937 (2006)
4. Marek, K., Seibyl, J., Eberly, S., Oakes, D., Shoulson, I., Lang, A.E., Hyson, C., Jennings, D., Investigators, P.S.G.P., et al.: Longitudinal follow-up of SWEDD subjects in the precept study. Neurology **82**(20), 1791–1797 (2014)
5. Schwingenschuh, P., Ruge, D., Edwards, M.J., Terranova, C., Katschnig, P., Carrillo, F., Silveira-Moriyama, L., Schneider, S.A., Kägi, G., Palomar, F.J., et al.: Distinguishing SWEDDs patients with asymmetric resting tremor from parkinson's disease: a clinical and electrophysiological study. Mov. Disord. **25**(5), 560–569 (2010)
6. De Rosa, A., Carducci, C., Carducci, C., Peluso, S., Lieto, M., Mazzella, A., Saccà, F., Morra, V.B., Pappatà, S., Leuzzi, V., et al.: Screening for dopa-responsive dystonia in patients with scans without evidence of dopaminergic deficiency (SWEDD). J. Neurol. **261**(11), 2204–2208 (2014)
7. Prashanth, R., Roy, S.D., Ghosh, S., Mandal, P.K.: Shape features as biomarkers in early parkinson's disease. In: 2013 6th International IEEE/EMBS Conference on Neural Engineering (NER), pp. 517–520. IEEE, New York (2013)
8. Metzler-Baddeley, C., Jones, D.K., Steventon, J., Westacott, L., Aggleton, J.P., O'Sullivan, M.J.: Cingulum microstructure predicts cognitive control in older age and mild cognitive impairment. J. Neurosci. **32**(49), 17612–17619 (2012)

9. Duncan, G.W., Firbank, M.J., Yarnall, A.J., Khoo, T.K., Brooks, D.J., Barker, R.A., Burn, D.J., O'Brien, J.T.: Gray and white matter imaging: a biomarker for cognitive impairment in early parkinson's disease? Mov. Disord. **31**(1), 103–110 (2016)
10. Gattellaro, G., Minati, L., Grisoli, M., Mariani, C., Carella, F., Osio, M., Ciceri, E., Albanese, A., Bruzzone, M.: White matter involvement in idiopathic parkinson disease: a diffusion tensor imaging study. Am. J. Neuroradiol. **30**(6), 1222–1226 (2009)
11. Munhoz, R.P., Moro, A., Silveira-Moriyama, L., Teive, H.A.: Non-motor signs in parkinson's disease: a review. Arq. Neuropsiquiatr. **73**(5), 454–462 (2015)
12. Marek, K., Jennings, D., Lasch, S., Siderowf, A., Tanner, C., Simuni, T., Coffey, C., Kieburtz, K., Flagg, E., Chowdhury, S., et al.: The parkinson progression marker initiative (PPMI). Prog. Neurobiol. **95**(4), 629–635 (2011)
13. Leemans, A., Jeurissen, B., Sijbers, J., Jones, D.: ExploreDTI: a graphical toolbox for processing, analyzing, and visualizing diffusion MR data. In: 17th Annual Meeting of International Society for Magnetic Resonance in Medicine, vol. 209, p. 3537 (2009)
14. Yeh, F.C., Tseng, W.Y.I.: NTU-90: a high angular resolution brain atlas constructed by q-space diffeomorphic reconstruction. Neuroimage **58**(1), 91–99 (2011)
15. Jones, D.K., Christiansen, K., Chapman, R., Aggleton, J.: Distinct subdivisions of the cingulum bundle revealed by diffusion MRI fibre tracking: implications for neuropsychological investigations. Neuropsychologia **51**(1) , 67–78 (2013)
16. Yeh, F.C., Verstynen, T.D., Wang, Y., Fernández-Miranda, J.C., Tseng, W.Y.I.: Deterministic diffusion fiber tracking improved by quantitative anisotropy. PLoS One **8**(11), e80713 (2013)

Colocalization of Functional Activity and Neurite Density Within Cortical Areas

Achille Teillac, Sandrine Lefrance, Edouard Duchesnay, Fabrice Poupon, Maite Alaitz Ripoll Fuster, Denis Le Bihan, Jean-Francois Mangin, and Cyril Poupon

Abstract In this work, we investigated the link between the blood-oxygen-level dependant (BOLD) effect observed using functional magnetic resonance imaging (fMRI) and the neurite density inferred from the Neurite Orientation Dispersion and Density Imaging (NODDI) model in some well-known lateralized cortical areas. We found a strong colocalization between those two parameters in lateralized areas such as the primary motor cortex, the language network, but also the primary visual cortex, which might indicate a strong link between microstructure and functional activity.

1 Introduction

Since the early twentieth century, neuroanatomists aim at disentangling the link between the functional organization of the brain and the tissue microstructure at the cellular scale. Brodmann was among the first to publish his cytoarchitectonic atlas built from the observation of cortical histological slices using optical microscopy, that is debated but still remains used today. Its construction relying on very few subjects is a strong limitation since it prevents from investigating the inter-subject variability and gives limited confidence about the boundaries separating the established cortical areas. In addition, it prevents from any comparison with brain functioning. Recently, the emergence of diffusion-based MR microscopy providing quantitative features of the tissue microstructure such as the axon diameter and density [1, 2] may open an avenue to the establishment of novel atlas of the brain cytoarchitecture. It relies on in-vivo acquisition and therefore enables to look at the variability of these features between subjects and to correlate them with brain functions investigated using functional MRI. Moreover, the access to such

A. Teillac (✉) • M.A. Ripoll Fuster • D. Le Bihan • C. Poupon
NeuroSpin/UNIRS, I^{2}BM, CEA, Gif-sur-Yvette, France
e-mail: achille.teillac@cea.fr

S. Lefrance • E. Duchesnay • F. Poupon • J.-F. Mangin
NeuroSpin/UNATI, I^{2}BM, CEA, Gif-sur-Yvette, France

A. Fuster et al. (eds.), *Computational Diffusion MRI*, Mathematics and Visualization, DOI 10.1007/978-3-319-54130-3_15

quantitative features of the ultrastructure may bring valuable imaging markers of brain diseases since most pathological mechanisms occur at the cellular level.

For this study, the NODDI model [3] has been chosen because of its relatively easy use in clinical routine involving a multiple-shell diffusion-weighted MRI protocol and because the underlying modeling of the tissue relies on the definition of three compartments: a compartment corresponding to the CSF characterized by a fast isotropic diffusion process mainly used to account for partial volume effects, a restricted cylinder compartment corresponding to the part of water constrained within the intra-dendritic and intra-axonal spaces represented by sticks, an hindered compartment corresponding to the extracellular space characterized by a Gaussian diffusion model. This extracellular model might not reflect the anatomical complex organization because of the Gaussian assumption for all the components in the extracellular compartment. However, the NODDI model has proven to be a useful tool to explore the cortex in some pathological diseases such as the focal cortical dysplasia as detailed in [4]. It comes with several metrics of interest such as the intracellular fraction (f_{intra}) representing the local neurite density or the orientation dispersion index (ODI) being very small in white matter where fibers present a high degree of alignment and closer to 1 in the cortical ribbon where dendrites are almost arbitrarily oriented in space.

In this work, we investigate the relation between microarchitectural features measured using the NODDI model and the underlying functional activities observed using fMRI. The Materials and methods section describes the acquisition protocol, the preprocessing and computation of the NODDI maps, the pipeline to obtain the intracellular fraction and how it has been correlated with the z-score maps stemming from the fMRI; the Results section presents the obtained maps and describes more explicitly the relationship between the neurite density and the functional activity for cortical regions; the Discussion section summarizes the contribution and presents the potential of the tools addressed in this paper.

2 Material and Methods

2.1 Acquisition

73 right-handed healthy volunteers were scanned on a 3T MRI (Siemens MAGNETOM Trio, Tim system) using a dedicated protocol [5] including: a MPRAGE sequence for the T1-weighted anatomy (1 mm isotropic; TE=2.98 ms; TR=2.3 s), a multiple-shell diffusion-weighted SE-EPI sequence (1.7 mm isotropic; TE=117 ms; TR=14 s; 10 b-values from 300 to 3000 s/mm² along 20 directions and 10 scans at b=0 s/m²), an echo-planar sequence for the BOLD signal (3 mm isotropic; TE=2.4 ms; TR=30 ms) and a fieldmap calibration to remove distorsions. This protocol originally designed in the frame of the CONNECT project remains relevant according to the protocols presented in the NODDI paper by Zhang et al. [3]

as the restricted number of directions has been counterbalanced with the high number of shells. Moreover, the restricted number of direction was not a problem to study the dendrites within the grey matter as they are isotropically distributed. The experimental fMRI protocol [6] is freely accessible for a set of subjects (http:// brainomics.cea.fr/localizer). This localizer protocol is a 5-min fMRI sequence that captures the cerebral bases of auditory and visual perception, motor actions, reading, language comprehension and mental calculation at an individual level. In this work, the functional contrasts which have been considered are: "right hand click minus left hand click" and "left hand click minus right hand click" for hands motor activations, "phrase video minus checkerboard" for reading activations and a visual contrast combining "right video click, left video click, video calculation, video sentence minus right audio click, left audio click, audio calculation, audio sentence".

2.2 *Individual NODDI Maps*

Individual diffusion-weighted dataset were preprocessed using Connectomist [5] to remove imaging artifacts (motion, eddy current, susceptibility...), thus enabling accurate matching of DW and T1-weighted data using rigid registration. Individual NODDI maps were computed using an inhouse command included in the Connectomist software as depicted on Fig. 1: the intracellular fraction (f_{intra}) referring to the space bounded by the membranes of neurites, their orientation dispersion index (ODI) which represents the angular variation of neurite orientation, the CSF fraction (f_{iso}) which quantifies the CSF volume fraction and the Watson concentration parameter (κ evolving at the opposite of the ODI). We verified that the ODI values were close to 0 in the white matter where the axons orientation are parallel and close to 1 in the grey matter where the dendrites distribution is more arbitrary.

Figure 1 shows all the individual NODDI maps merged with the corresponding anatomical T1-weighted image for a better anatomical colocalization.

The NODDI model can be easily described using the three compartments Eq. (1) below:

$$A = (1 - f_{iso}) * [f_{intra}A_{intra} + (1 - f_{intra})A_{extra}] + f_{iso}A_{iso} \tag{1}$$

where A is the normalized diffusion attenuation resulting from the contribution of the three compartments: the CSF (A_{iso}), the intracellular space (A_{intra}) and the extracellular space (A_{extra}). f_{iso} denotes the volume fraction of the isotropic diffusion compartment and f_{intra} denotes the volume fraction of the intracellular compartment.

The intra-axonal or intra-dendritic compartment was mathematically modeled using a cylinder geometry. The initial parallel diffusivity was set to $1.7 \times 10^{-3} \text{m}^2\text{s}^{-1}$ and the orientation dispersion of the cylinder direction was modeled using a Watson distribution, the isotropic diffusivity was set to $3.0 \times 10^{-3} \text{m}^2\text{s}^{-1}$ and the normalized noise standard attenuation was measured equal to 0.03.

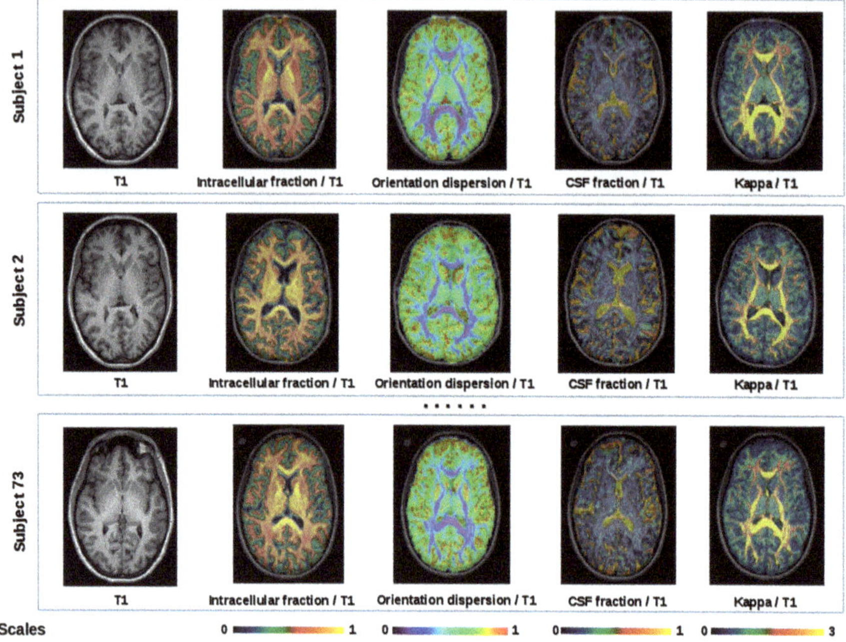

Fig. 1 Individual NODDI quantitative maps merged with T1-weighted MRI

2.3 Pial and White Surfaces

Extraction of T1-weighted MR scans were processed using FreeSurfer [7] to obtain individual pial and white matter surfaces. Homologue vertices between pial/white surfaces and between individuals allow to easily navigate between subjects. Cortex parcellation was done using the aparc.a2009s Destrieux's atlas [8] defining 152 regions shown on Fig. 2 detailed in the next section.

2.4 Individual Quantitative Maps of Neurite Density

As displayed on Fig. 2, the correspondence of vertices allowed to extract a distribution of f_{intra} for each vertex by sampling the matched f_{intra} map along the segment defined by each pair of corresponding (pial, white) vertices. Maps of local distributions of f_{intra} were computed and statistics were inferred to build maps of average, standard deviation (stddev) and median of f_{intra} at the vertex level. In order to get f_{intra} distributions at the scale of cortical areas, the vertex-wise distributions included in the considered area were merged together providing a microstructural signature of this area per subject. Figure 2 summarizes the cortical sampling pipeline developed to extract quantitative features on the cortex at the individual level.

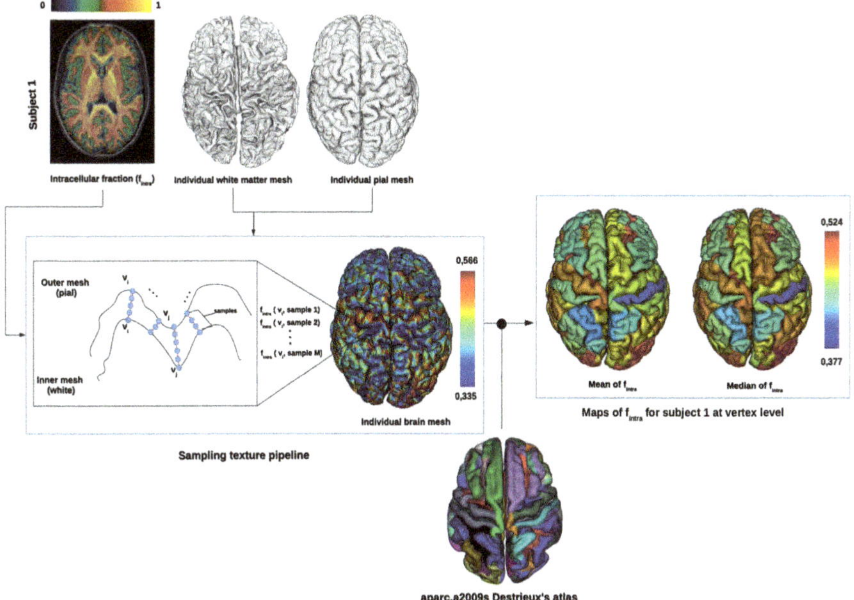

Fig. 2 Cortical sampling pipeline for one subject

2.5 Co-localization of Neurite Density and Functional Activity

We used the same approach to map the z-scores stemming from BOLD fMRI data of each individual onto its cortical surface. The z-scores were computed voxel-wise and integrated at the scale of the cortical region. So, at the end of the two pipelines, we get for each subject and for each vertex of the pial mesh, the integral of the neurite density over the cortical thickness, as well as, for each functional contrast, the integral of its z-scores over the same cortical thickness. A Gaussian smoothing was then applied onto the pial surface in order to enhance the peaks of neurite density and the peaks of functional activity. All the individual surface maps were finally averaged together to better visualize the colocalization of those peaks at the group level (see Fig. 3).

2.6 Sørensen–Dice Coefficient

In order to characterize the overlap between the f_{intra} and z-score maps, we chose the Sørensen–Dice coefficient defined by the Eq. (2).

$$DiceIndex = \frac{2|A.B|}{|A|^2 + |B|^2} \tag{2}$$

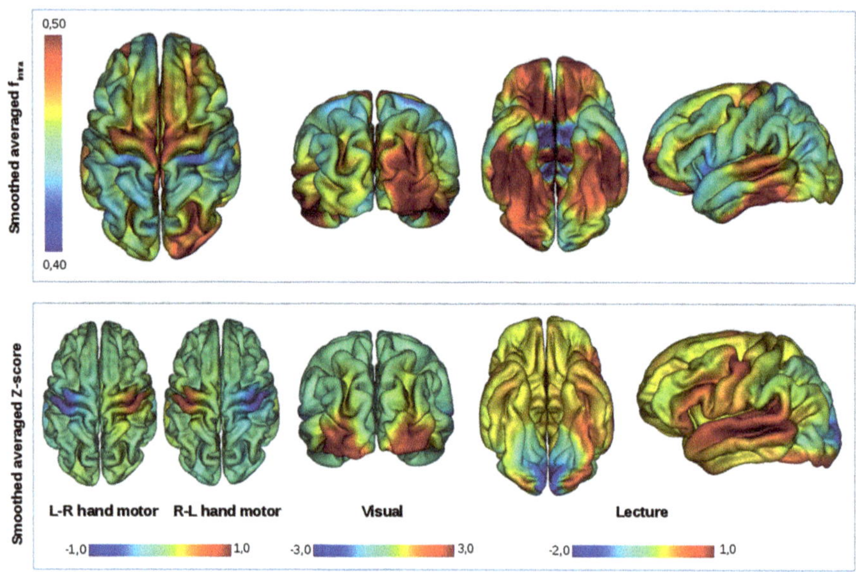

Fig. 3 Group level average z-scores and f_{intra} maps

For the computation of the binary textures A and B in the Eq. (2), we took the individual smoothed maps of f_{intra} and z-scores for each contrast. For the f_{intra}, we set the threshold to half of the standard deviation (ie, $threshold = mean - 0.5 * stddev$) and for the z-scores, as it can be negative, we limited the threshold to one standard deviation (ie, $threshold = mean + stddev$). The two maps have their own range of values and we had to adapt each threshold independently: it has been done empirically but would benefit from an automatized process in the future. Then, we used Eq. (2) to compute the Dice index for each cortical area defined by the Destrieux's parcellation at the subject level.

3   Results and Discussion

3.1   Statistical Evaluation of Left-Right Neurite Density Asymmetries

First of all, we checked the gaussianity of the f_{intra} distributions using the Shapiro-Wilcoxon test. Then, for all the cortical regions taken from the Destrieux's atlas [8], the signed differences of mean f_{intra} between the left area and its associated right one were computed for all the subjects. A t-test was then applied on this list of left-right differences and finally, a False Discovery Rate (FDR) was computed to get rid of the false positives. We only represented on Fig. 4 brain areas depicting a significant

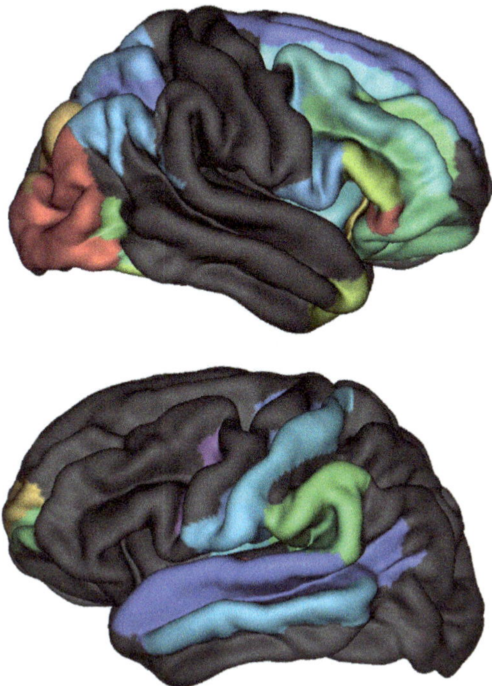

Fig. 4 Left-right difference of f_{intra} in cortical regions

difference between left and right hemispheres and the color of the area corresponds to the difference using a rainbow colormap (the higher difference is shown in red).

Among the cortical regions where $f_{intra}(LH) > f_{intra}(RH)$, we recognize the frontopolar cortex, the secondary motor area, the somatosensory primary cortex (central sulcus and postcentral gyrus but surprisingly not the left precentral gyrus), the auditory cortex and some areas involved in the language network (Broca's area, Wernicke's area, the inferior parietal lobule). As the language has been admitted to be left-lateralized in 80% of the right-handed population and about 75% of the left-handed population (cf. pioneer studies of language hemispheric lateralization using the Wada test [9] but also more recent corroboration of those numbers [10]), our findings seem to back up this cortical asymmetry. Furthermore, the link between handedness and language dominance for the right-handed volunteers is in adequation with the literature's statements from [11].

On the other hand, by looking at the regions where $f_{intra}(RH) > f_{intra}(LH)$, we can notice that a portion of the visual primary cortex is highlighted which seem to indicate a right lateralization in neurite density of this cortical region. A recent article [12] has studied the cerebral response to a simple visual stimulation and they suggest a right-hemispheric dominance of the concerned areas also in adequation with what we have found in our study; to be verified with the functional underlying activity in the next part.

To link the microstructure with the underlying functional activity, we guided our studies based on the Penfield homonculus [13] using a motor hand, a reading and a visual contrasts.

3.2 *Investigation of the Neurite Density in the Sensorymotor Cortex*

For the hand motor contrast, the first row of Fig. 5 shows an important activity in the primary motor and the sensorymotor cortex assessed by strong z-scores. For the "Left minus Right click" contrast, we highlight the right hemisphere and the left one for the "Right minus Left click" contrast as expected knowing the contralateral control of motor areas.

The second row of the Fig. 5 depicts Dice index values for each cortical region. We computed a t-test and found that the precentral gyrus, the central sulcus and the post central gyrus are significantly different in term of Dice index compared to the homologous cortical regions on the other hemisphere. The contralateral pattern of

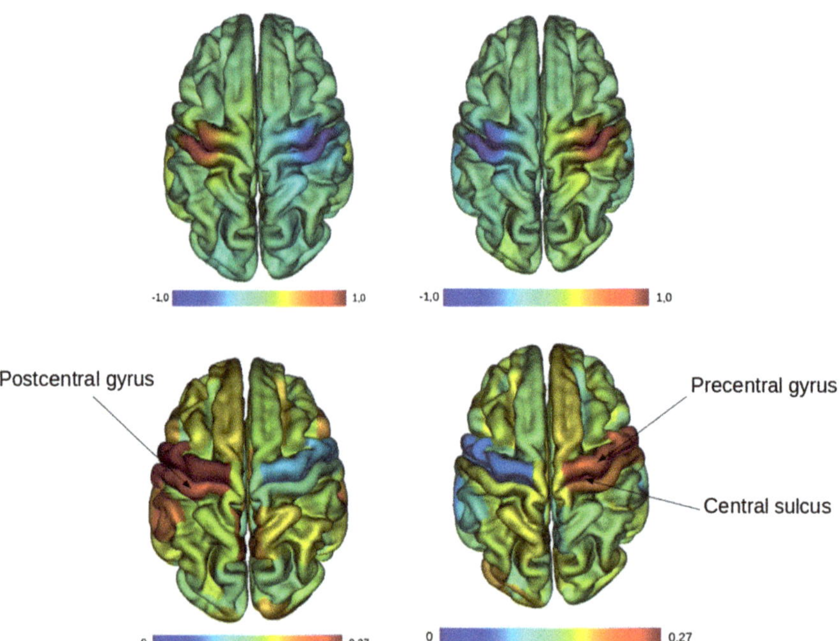

Fig. 5 Group level maps for the hand motor contrasts: (*top-left*) z-scores for the "Right-Left click" contrast at the vertex level; (*top-right*) z-scores for the "Left-Right click" contrast at the vertex level; (*bottom-left*) Dice index results for the "Right-Left click" contrast at the cortical area level; (*bottom-right*) Dice index results for the "Left-Right click" contrast at the cortical area level

the motor areas implies that for the right hand motor contrast, the left hemisphere regions show more activity and the other way around when it is the left hand motor contrast. The colocalization of peaks of neurite density and functional activity is thus assessed by the Dice index. A noteworthy fact is that the Dice index values in the mentioned cortical areas are higher while doing the "Right minus Left click" contrast than while performing the "Left minus Right click" contrast which is in good agreement with the fact that the volunteers are all right-handed.

3.3 *Investigation of the Neurite Density in Language Areas*

As for the language contrast, Fig. 6(top-left) depicts the group level neurite density map, Fig. 6(top-right) the group level z-scores map stemming from the reading contrast and Fig. 6(bottom) the corresponding group level Dice index map at the cortical area level (using the Destrieux's parcellation [8]). The language network has been widely studied and has been proven to be left-lateralized in most cases (right and left-handed). Figure 6 shows a high level of activation in the primary auditory cortex, the motor tongue area and more generally the temporal lobe.

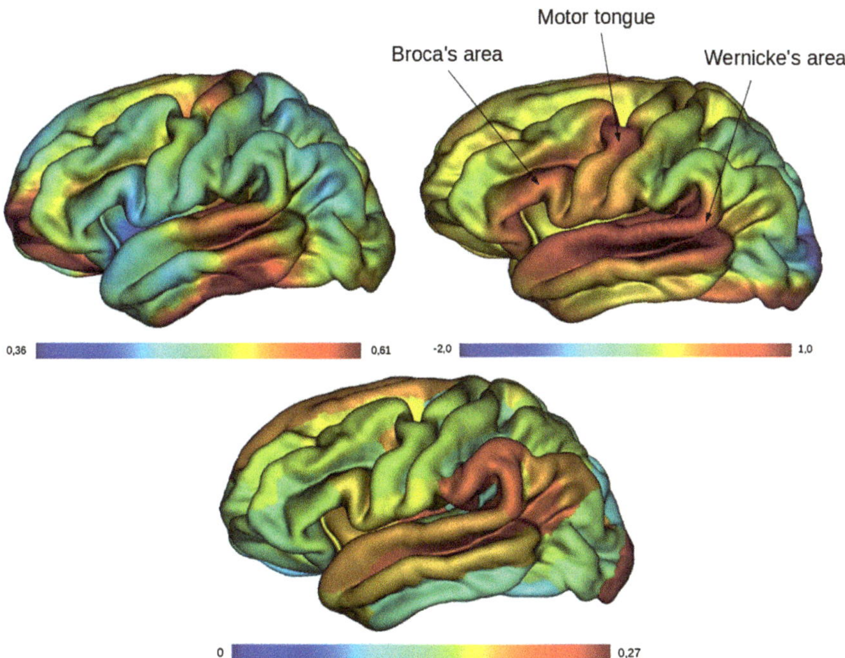

Fig. 6 Group level maps for the language contrast: (*top-left*) neurite density at the vertex level; (*top-right*) z-scores at the vertex level; (*bottom*) Dice index results at the cortical area level

As we did for the hand motor tasks, we computed a statistical t-test in order to characterize the significant asymmetrical areas involved in the reading paradigm used. More precisely, we can recognize the Broca's area, the Wernicke's area, the inferior parietal lobule and some parts of the primary auditory cortex to be the highest meaningful cortical regions for this paradigm. Thus, the Dice index corroborates the link between the neurite density and the functional activity in those areas.

3.4 Investigation of the Neurite Density in the Visual Cortex

For the visual activity, Fig. 7 (top-left) depicts the group level neurite density map, Fig. 7 (top-right) the group level z-scores map stemming from the visual contrast and Fig. 7 (bottom) the corresponding group level Dice index map at the cortical area level (using the Destrieux's parcellation [8]).

As we can see, the occipital lobe shows the highest values of the Dice indices and especially higher values on the right hemisphere compared to the left ones (the inferior occipital gyrus (O3) and associated sulcus, the lunate sulcus...). But

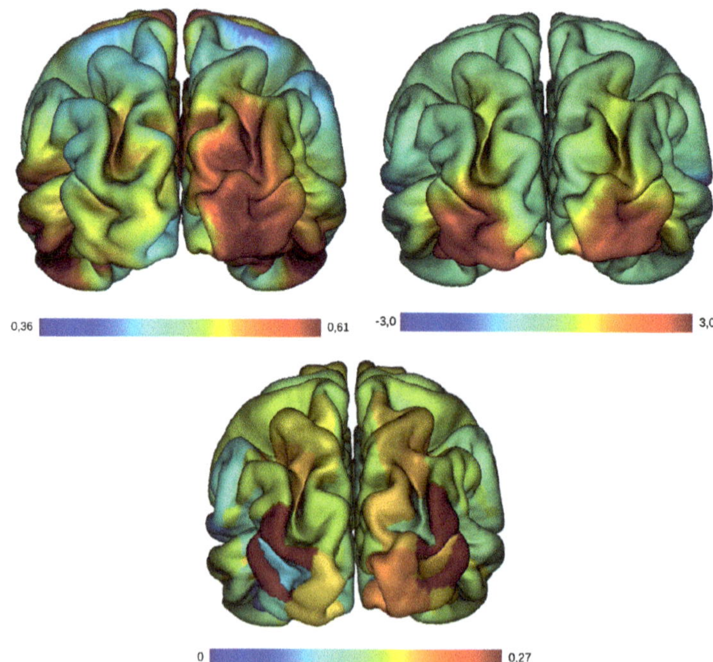

Fig. 7 Group level maps for the visual contrast: (*top-left*) neurite density at the vertex level; (*top-right*) z-scores at the vertex level; (*bottom*) Dice index results at the cortical area level

surprisingly, we found only few cortical areas significantly higher on the right hemisphere when we used a statistical t-test on the mean difference over all subjects (p-value $< 5\%$). This can be explained by the fact that regarding the occipital lobe, the neurite density is highly asymmetrical whereas the functional activity is not. A recent work [14] established the complementary specialization regarding the language dominance and the visuospatial attention. In our case, as the right-handed population seem to all have a left-lateralized language network and as we saw the right-lateralization of the occipital lobe neurite density, we could explain our cortical asymmetries by thinking the visual network as a high neuron-dense path.

4 Conclusion and Perspectives

To conclude, we saw that there are some strong asymmetries of neurite density in cortical regions representing a well-known lateralized underlying functional activity (such as the language network on the left hemisphere or the hand motor areas depending on the handedness of the volunteers population). The colocalization of neurite density and brain activation peaks may suggest that the level of local activation could be linked to the local neurite density. Of course, this remains an assumption that needs to be investigated more deeply in the future. More surprisingly, while the level of activation on the left and right visual cortical areas does not present any significant left-right asymmetry, we found a strong asymmetry of the neurite density in the visual cortex in favor of the right hemisphere. This could be linked to the known right localization of the visuospatial attention network described in [14]. This needs to be further investigated from a functional point of view in light of the study described in [15] mentioning the same trend on primates using visual block paradigm.

References

1. Assaf, Y., et al.: AxCaliber: a method for measuring axon diameter distribution from diffusion MRI. Magn. Reson. Med. **59**(6), 1347–1354 (2008)
2. Alexander, D.C. A general framework for experiment design in diffusion MRI and its application in measuring direct tissue microstructure features. Magn. Reson. Med. **60**(2), 439–448 (2008)
3. Zhang, H., et al.: NODDI: practical in vivo neurite orientation dispersion and density imaging of the human brain. Neuroimage **61**(4), 1000–1016 (2012)
4. Winston, G.P., et al.: Advanced diffusion imaging sequences could aid assessing patients with focal cortical dysplasia and epilepsy. Epilepsy Res. **108**(2), 336–339 (2014)
5. Assaf, Y., et al.: The CONNECT project: combining macro- and micro-structure. Neuroimage **80**, 273–282 (2013)
6. Pinel, P., et al.: Fast reproducible identification and large-scale databasing of individual functional cognitive networks. BMC Neurosci. **8**(1), 1 (2007)
7. Fischl, B.: FreeSurfer. Neuroimage **62**(2), 774–781 (2012)

8. Destrieux, C., et al.: Automatic parcellation of human cortical gyri and sulci using standard anatomical nomenclature. Neuroimage **53**(1) 1–15 (2010)
9. Wada, J., Rasmussen, T.: Intracarotid injection of sodium amytal for the lateralization of cerebral speech dominance: experimental and clinical observations. J. Neurosurg. **17**(2), 266–282 (1960)
10. Mazoyer, B., et al.: Gaussian mixture modeling of hemispheric lateralization for language in a large sample of healthy individuals balanced for handedness. PLoS One **9**(6), e101165 (2014)
11. Knecht, S., et al.: Handedness and hemispheric language dominance in healthy humans. Brain **123**(12), 2512–2518 (2000)
12. Hougaard, A., et al.: Cerebral asymmetry of fMRI-BOLD responses to visual stimulation. PLoS One **10**(5), e0126477 (2015)
13. Penfield, W., Boldrey, E.: Somatic motor and sensory representation in the cerebral cortex of man as studied by electrical stimulation. Brain J. Neurol. **60**(4), 389–443 (1937)
14. Cai, Q., Van der Haegen, L., Brysbaert, M.: Complementary hemispheric specialization for language production and visuospatial attention. Proc. Natl. Acad. Sci. **110**(4), E322-E330 (2013)
15. Collins, C.E., et al.: Neuron densities vary across and within cortical areas in primates. Proc. Natl. Acad. Sci. **107**(36), 15927–15932 (2010)

Comparison of Biomarkers in Transgenic Alzheimer Rats Using Multi-Shell Diffusion MRI

Rutger H.J. Fick, Madelaine Daianu, Marco Pizzolato, Demian Wassermann, Russell E. Jacobs, Paul M. Thompson, Terrence Town, and Rachid Deriche

Abstract In this study, we assessed the evolution of diffusion MRI (dMRI) derived markers from different white matter models as progressive neurodegeneration occurs in transgenic Alzheimer rats (TgF344-AD) at 10, 15 and 24 months. We compared biomarkers reconstructed from Diffusion Tensor Imaging (DTI), Neurite Orientation Dispersion and Density Imaging (NODDI) and Mean Apparent Propagator (MAP)-MRI in the hippocampus, cingulate cortex and corpus callosum using multi-shell dMRI. We found that NODDI's dispersion and MAP-MRI's anisotropy markers consistently changed over time, possibly indicating that these measures are sensitive to age-dependent neuronal demise due to amyloid accumulation. Conversely, we found that DTI's mean diffusivity, NODDI's isotropic volume fraction and MAP-MRI's restriction-related metrics all followed a two-step progression from 10 to 15 months, and from 15 to 24 months. This two-step pattern might be linked with a neuroinflammatory response that may be occurring prior to, or during microstructural breakdown. Using our approach, we are able to provide—for the first time—preliminary and valuable insight on relevant biomarkers that may directly describe the underlying pathophysiology in Alzheimer's disease.

R.H.J. Fick (✉) • M. Pizzolato • D. Wassermann (✉) • R. Deriche
Université Côte d'Azur, Inria, Valbonne, France
e-mail: rutger361988@gmail.com; demian.wassermann@inria.fr

M. Daianu • P.M. Thompson
Imaging Genetics Center, Mark & Mary Stevens Neuroimaging & Informatics Institute, University of Southern California, Marina del Rey, CA, USA

R.E. Jacobs
Division of Biology and Biological Engineering, Beckman Institute, California Institute of Technology, Pasadena, CA, USA

T. Town
Department of Physiology & Biophysics, Zilkha Neurogenetic Institute, University of Southern California, Los Angeles, CA, USA

© Springer International Publishing AG 2017
A. Fuster et al. (eds.), *Computational Diffusion MRI*, Mathematics and Visualization, DOI 10.1007/978-3-319-54130-3_16

187

1   Introduction

Diffusion MRI (dMRI) allows us to non-invasively study microstructural changes caused by neuropathology. Among these pathologies, gaining understanding of Alzheimer's disease (AD) is of particular importance, affecting over one in nine people age 65 and above in the U.S. alone [1]. Traditionally, dMRI studies have used Diffusion Tensor Imaging (DTI) [2] to model the grey and white matter structure abnormalities in AD patients. Only recently, more complex white matter models like Neurite Orientation Dispersion and Density Imaging (NODDI) [3] have been explored to classify AD, and have shown *greater* discriminative power than DTI [4]. This reinforces the importance of exploring white matter models that provide more detailed microstructural information than DTI.

In human studies, it is hard to relate dMRI derived metrics to corresponding microstructural changes for lack of histological validation. As a solution, animal models provide a way to gain understanding on the underlying pathophysiology of AD by allowing dMRI in addition to histological measurements. Mouse models of human tauopathy (rTg4510) have been previously studied at various time points using DTI [5, 6], and at a single time point comparing DTI with NODDI metrics [7]. In this latter study, NODDI derived metrics once again appeared more discriminative than those derived from DTI. Further efforts focusing on multi-shell dMRI analysis of transgenic Alzheimer rats (TgF344-AD) have shown that dMRI measurements at higher gradient strengths aid the classification of AD-like pathology [8]. However, only anisotropy measures of DTI and hybrid diffusion imaging (HYDI) [9] were explored.

In this study, we compare the evolution of dMRI-derived markers from different white matter models as progressive neurodegeneration occurs in transgenic Alzheimer rats (TgF344-AD). In particular, we study the patterns of alteration across three time points in the hippocampus, cingulate cortex and corpus callosum—areas known to be affected in AD. The two grey matter areas were previously shown to manifest age-dependent cerebral amyloidosis that precedes tauopathy, gliosis and apoptotic loss of neurons [10], making these cortical regions extremely relevant for understanding the underlying mechanisms in AD. We compare biomarkers derived from DTI, NODDI and Mean Apparent Propagator (MAP)-MRI [11] using multi-shell data. To the best of our knowledge, this is the first study that investigates multi-shell biomarkers at different time points in AD animal models.

The paper is structured as follows: we first describe the diffusion MRI data and the metrics we derive in Sect. 2. We provide the results in Sect. 3 and discuss them in Sect. 4. We finally provide our conclusions in Sect. 5.

2   Materials and Methods

In this section, we first detail the diffusion MRI data acquisition, preprocessing and region of interest selection of the AD rats. We then give a brief overview of the methods we use and their metrics of interest. We detail the fractional anisotropy (FA) and mean diffusivity (MD) of classical DTI, the orientation dispersion index (ODI), neurite density index (NDI) and isotropic volume fraction (IsoVF) of the multi-compartment NODDI model, and finally the formulation of several q-space indices of the MAP-MRI functional basis. We estimated the DTI and MAP-MRI metrics using the diffusion imaging in python (dipy) open source software [12] and the NODDI metrics using the NODDI toolbox [3].

2.1   Processing of Transgenic Alzheimer Rat Data Sets

We use multi-shell dMRI data of three *ex-vivo* transgenic Alzheimer rats (line TgF344-AD) [10], also previously analyzed by Daianu et al. [8]. The rats were euthanized at 10, 15 and 24 months, fixed brains were prepared as described in [8], and scanned using a 7 Tesla Bruker Biospin MRI scanner at California Institute of Technology. A high-resolution fast low angle magnetic shot (FLASH) anatomical image with a mix of T1 and T2 weighting ($375 \times 224 \times 160$ matrix; voxel size: $0.08 \times 0.08 \times 0.08\,\mathrm{mm}^3$) was used. The diffusion MRI data were sampled on 5 shells with b-values $\{1000, 3000, 4000, 8000, 12{,}000\}\,\mathrm{s/mm}^2$, all with the same 60 directions and 5 b0 measurements. Other parameters were $\delta/\Delta = 11/16\,\mathrm{ms}$ and $TE/TR = 34/500\,\mathrm{ms}$. The voxel dimensions were $0.15 \times 0.15 \times 0.25\,\mathrm{mm}^3$.

During preprocessing, extra-cerebral tissue was removed using the "skull-stripping" Brain Extraction Tool from BrainSuite (http://brainsuite.org/), for both the anatomical images and the DWIs. We corrected for eddy current distortions using the "eddy correct FSL" tool (www.fmrib.ox.ac.uk/fsl) for which a gradient table was calculated to account for the distortions. As an image processing step, DWIs were up-sampled to the resolution of the anatomical images (with isotropic voxels) using FSL's flirt function with 9 degrees of freedom; the gradient direction tables were rotated accordingly after each linear registration. For our study, we draw regions of interest (ROIs) in the cingulate cortex, hippocampus and corpus callosum as shown in Fig. 1.

2.2   DTI Metrics

The classical DTI model [2] assumes that the measured diffusion signal belongs to the set of Gaussian distributions. While DTI has well-known limitations with respect to the modeling of crossing tissue configurations and restricted diffusion,

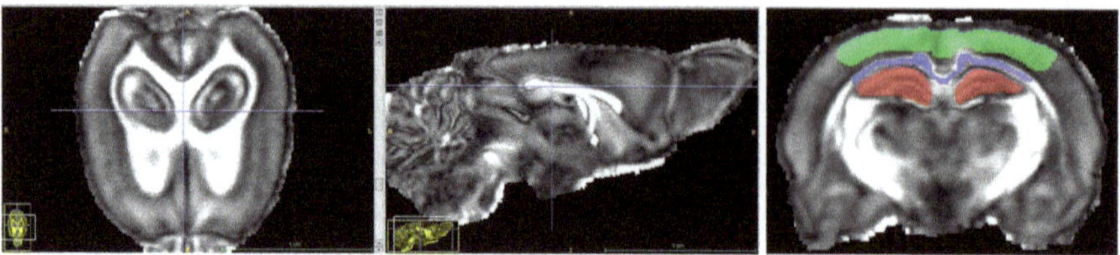

Fig. 1 Regions of interest for biomarker estimation on the registered FA map of rat 1. We mark the cingulate cortex (*green*), corpus callosum (*blue*) and hippocampus (*red*)

its derived metrics FA and MD have been found useful to classify AD patients [4]. Using signal attenuation $E(b) = S(b)/S(0)$, the DTI model describes the diffusion signal as $E(b) = \exp(-b\mathbf{g}^{\mathrm{T}}\mathbf{D}\mathbf{g})$ with $\mathbf{D}$ a 3×3 symmetric positive-definite matrix and $\mathbf{g}$ the gradient direction. Estimating the eigenvalues of $\mathbf{D}$ as $\{\lambda_1, \lambda_2, \lambda_3\}$ the FA and MD are given as

$$FA = \sqrt{\frac{1}{2}} \frac{\sqrt{(\lambda_1 - \lambda_2)^2 + (\lambda_2 - \lambda_3)^2 + (\lambda_3 - \lambda_1)^2}}{\sqrt{\lambda_1^2 + \lambda_2^2 + \lambda_3^2}} \quad MD = \frac{\lambda_1 + \lambda_2 + \lambda_3}{3} \quad (1)$$

In accordance with DTI's Gaussian diffusion assumption, we only use the b0 and $b = 1000\,\text{s/mm}^2$ data when fitting DTI. The FA and MD in our slice of interest are shown in Fig. 2.

2.3 NODDI Metrics

The more advanced multi-compartment NODDI model [3] separates the signal contribution of different tissues by fitting a combination of intra-cellular, extra-cellular and free-water models.

$$E = (1 - v_{iso})(v_{ic}E_{ic}(ODI) + (1 - v_{ic}) * E_{ec}) + v_{iso}E_{iso} \quad (2)$$

The intra-cellular signal E_{ic} is modeled as a set of dispersed sticks, i.e., cylinders of zero radius, to capture the highly restricted nature of diffusion perpendicular to neurites and unhindered diffusion along them. The amount of dispersion is given by the orientation dispersion index (ODI), which is defined by a Watson distribution. The extra-cellular signal E_{ec} is described as a dispersed mixture of Gaussian anisotropic diffusion, and an isotropic Gaussian compartment E_{iso} represents free diffusion. Similarly as in [7], we study the ODI, the neurite density index $NDI = (1 - v_{iso})v_{ic}$ and the isotropic volume fraction $IsoVF = v_{iso}$.

In accordance with NODDI's recommended acquisition scheme [3], we fit NODDI only using the b0 and $b = \{1000, 3000\}\,\text{s/mm}^2$ data. Furthermore, as water diffusivity changes in *ex-vivo* tissue, we set the intra-cellular and isotropic

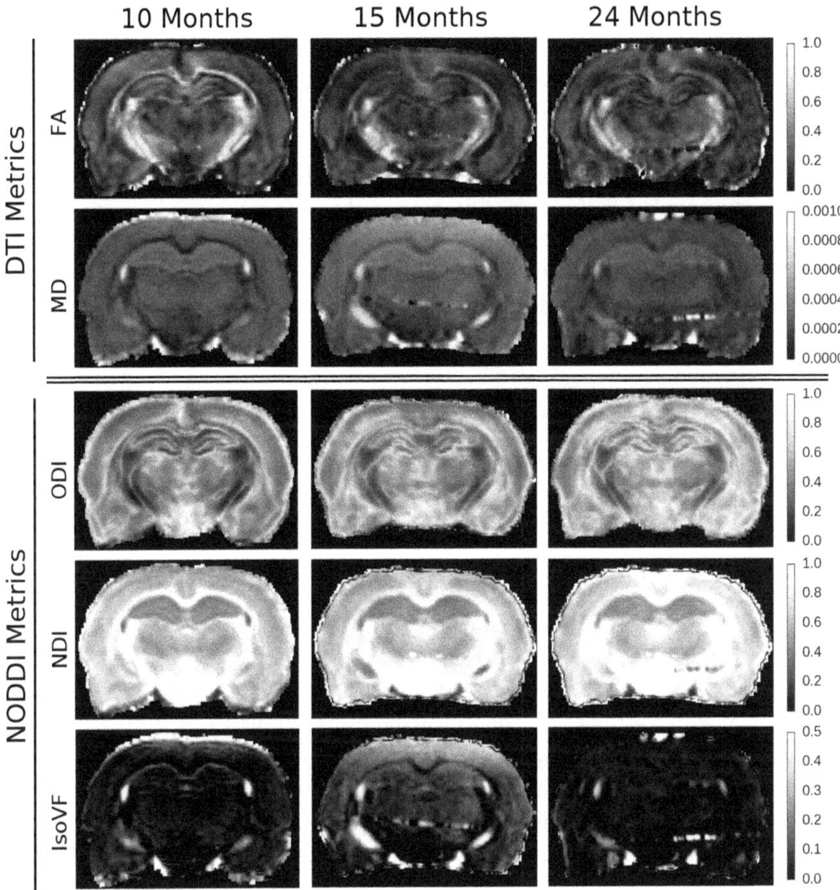

Fig. 2 Illustrations of a DTI and NODDI metrics in the same coronal slice for the three time points

diffusivity to $0.6\times10^{-9}\mathrm{m}^2\mathrm{s}^{-1}$ and $2.0\times10^{-9}\mathrm{m}^2\mathrm{s}^{-1}$ [13]. An illustration of the ODI, NDI and IsoVF can be seen in Fig. 2.

2.4 MAP-MRI Metrics

The MAP-MRI approach [11] uses a functional basis to represent the 3D diffusion signal with as little assumptions as possible. It then analytically reconstructs the 3D diffusion propagator by only assuming the short gradient pulse approximation ($\delta \approx 0$). In this way, it accurately estimates the diffusion propagator in the presence of both non-Gaussian diffusion and crossing tissue configurations.

MAP-MRI represents the discretely measured signal attenuation $E(\mathbf{q})$ using a set of *continuous* orthogonal basis functions representing the space $\hat{E}(\mathbf{q};\mathbf{c})$, where the signal is now represented in terms of basis coefficients $\mathbf{c}$ and the q-space wave vector $\mathbf{q} = |\mathbf{q}|\mathbf{g}$ with $\mathbf{g}$ the gradient direction is related to the b-value as $|\mathbf{q}| = \sqrt{b/(\Delta - \delta/3)}/2\pi$. Without going into the formulation of MAP-MRI's basis functions, we detail the estimation of basis coefficients $\mathbf{c}$ in Eq. (3). In short, we regularize the fitting of $\mathbf{c}$ such that $\hat{E}(\mathbf{q};\mathbf{c})$ smoothly interpolates between the measured q-space points by using Laplacian regularization [14], where regularization weight λ is set using voxel-wise generalized cross-validation. We also constrain the estimated diffusion Propagator $\hat{P}(\mathbf{R};\mathbf{c})$ to be positive using quadratic programming [11].

$$\text{argmin}_{\mathbf{c}} \overbrace{\int_{\mathbb{R}^3} \left[E(\mathbf{q}) - \hat{E}(\mathbf{q};\mathbf{c})\right]^2 d\mathbf{q}}^{\text{Data Fidelity}} + \lambda \overbrace{\int_{\mathbb{R}^3} \left[\nabla^2 \hat{E}(\mathbf{q};\mathbf{c})\right]^2 d\mathbf{q}}^{\text{Smoothness}} \tag{3}$$

$$\text{subject to } \hat{P}(\mathbf{R};\mathbf{c}) > 0 \quad \text{with} \quad \hat{P}(\mathbf{R};\mathbf{c}) = \text{IFT}\left(\hat{E}(\mathbf{q};\mathbf{c})\right)$$

Once $\mathbf{c}$ is known, the MAP-MRI basis simultaneously represents the 3D dMRI signal and 3D diffusion propagator. We estimate the q-space indices Return-To-Origin, Return-To-Axis and Return-To-Plane Probability (RTOP, RTAP and RTPP), which in theory are related to the volume, surface and length of a cylindrical pore [11]. We also estimate the non-Gaussianity (NG), which describes the ratio between the Gaussian and non-Gaussian volume of the signal. Finally we estimate the propagator anisotropy (PA), which is a normalized metric that describes the anisotropy of the 3D diffusion propagator. As MAP-MRI is designed to represent the entire 3D diffusion signal, we estimate all metrics using the entire 5 shell data up to a b-value of $12,000\,\text{s}/\text{mm}^2$, using a radial order of 6, resulting in 50 estimated coefficients. We illustrate these metrics in Fig. 3.

3   Results

In Fig. 4 we show the evolution of the mean with 0.5 standard deviation of all dMRI-derived metrics in the ROIs shown in Fig. 1. We use the same colors for the hippocampus (red), corpus callosum (blue) and cingulate cortex (green). The only metric that consistently increases over time is NODDI's ODI and consistently decreases is MAP-MRI's PA, with the exception of the cortex. It is also apparent that FA, NDI, RTOP, RTAP and RTPP follow a different, 2-step pattern, first decreasing and then slightly increasing. Inversely, for MD, IsoVF and NG we first find an increase and then a decrease. We provide the raw data values in Table 1. We also produce correlation plots for dispersion and anisotropy measures in Fig. 5 and for

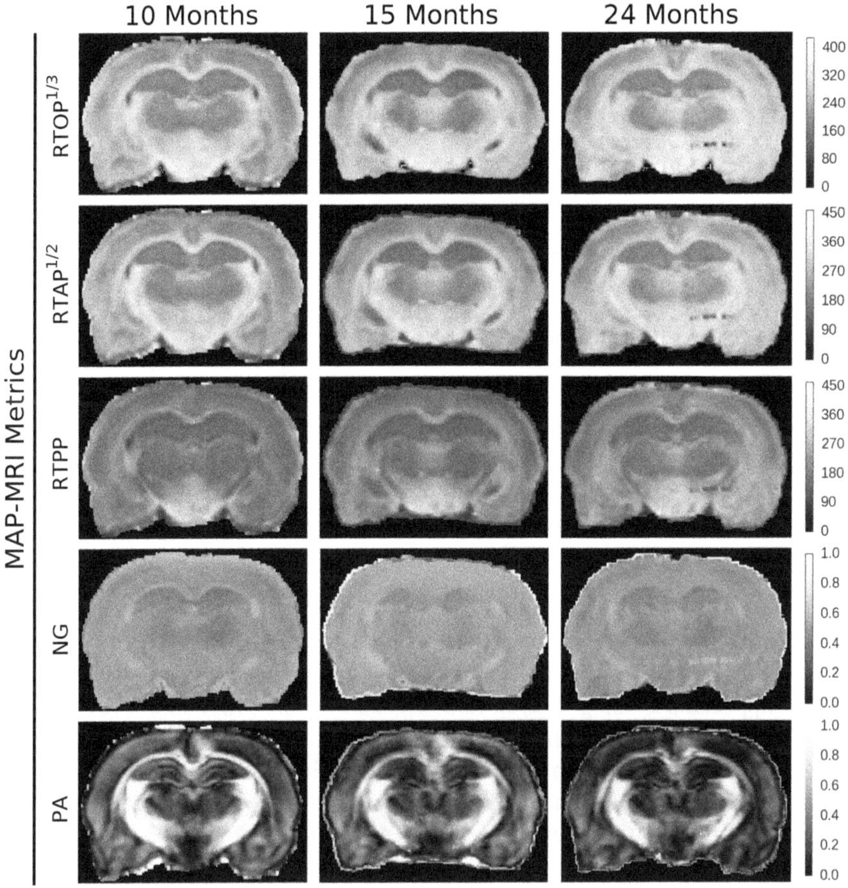

Fig. 3 Illustrations of MAP-MRI's q-space indices in the same coronal slice for the three time points. To visualize RTOP, RTAP and RTPP in the same unit (mm^{-1}) we show the cubed root of RTOP and squared root of RTAP

the 2-step metrics in Fig. 6. It can be seen that ODI is negatively correlated with FA and PA, and that IsoVF is positively correlated with MD and negatively with RTOP.

4 Discussion

In this work, we have shown that different metrics of DTI, NODDI and MAP-MRI appear to be sensitive to different processes as age-dependent cerebral amyloidosis manifests in both grey and white matter in the Alzheimer rats.

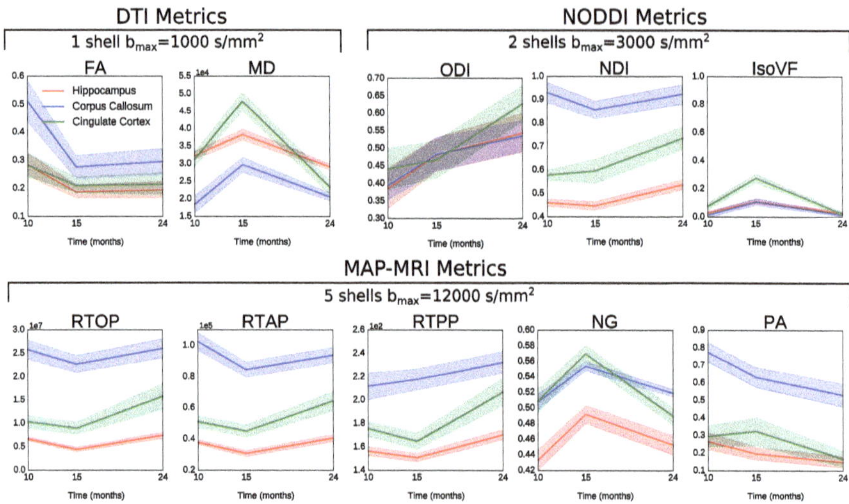

Fig. 4 DTI, NODDI and MAP-MRI metrics for the same time points in the hippocampus (*red*), corpus callosum (*blue*) and cingulate cortex (*green*)

DTI findings: We find a significant drop in FA in all ROIs from 10 to 15 months and a small increase from 15 to 24 months. This corresponds with previous findings in the hippocampus using data up to $b = 1000\,\text{s/mm}^2$ [8]. While a comparison of using different b-values in the DTI estimation was outside of the scope of this study, it was shown that when higher b-values are included, the FA trend consistently decreases over time [8]. Nonetheless, it has been argued that compared to FA, MD lends itself better to the assessment of cortical and subcortical grey matter, where net diffusion may not be expected to conform to any one specific direction [15]. When we assess MD, we consistently find an increase from 10 to 15 months and a decrease from 15 to 24 months. This may suggest that FA and MD are sensitive to different processes taking place in AD.

NODDI findings: Several studies have suggested that NODDI metrics, in particular ODI, have better AD classifying potential due to NODDI's ability to delineate signal contributions from different tissue compartments [4, 7]. While we cannot do a classification study using our data, we find that ODI consistently increases in areas where tau pathology increases in our rat model [10]; the hippocampus, cingulate cortex and corpus callosum. We also find that IsoVF shows an increase from 10 to 15 months and a decrease from 15 to 24 months in all areas, following the same trend as DTI's MD. Though, it should be mentioned that fitting NODDI requires presetting the intra-cellular and isotropic diffusivity, which influences obtained metric values. Fitting NODDI on the selected $b_{\max} = 3000\,\text{s/mm}^2$ or the full data does not significantly impact our findings.

MAP-MRI findings: To the best of our knowledge, this is the first study that estimates MAP-MRI metrics on data from an AD model. We find that all metrics

Table 1 Mean and standard deviation of DTI, NODDI and MAP-MRI metrics for the three time points in each region of interest

DTI metrics		Age		
Metric	ROI	10 months	15 months	24 months
FA	Hippocampus	0.29±0.08	0.19±0.05	0.20±0.06
	C. Callosum	0.51±0.15	0.27±0.08	0.30±0.09
	C. Cortex	0.28±0.08	0.20±0.05	0.22±0.08
MD ($\times 10^3$)	Hippocampus	0.32±0.02	0.39±0.03	0.29±0.02
	C. Callosum	0.19±0.05	0.30±0.05	0.21±0.02
	C. Cortex	0.31±0.04	0.49±0.06	0.23±0.04

NODDI metrics		Age		
Metric	ROI	10 months	15 months	24 months
ODI	Hippocampus	0.39±0.11	0.48±0.10	0.55±0.11
	C. Callosum	0.39±0.08	0.48±0.09	0.53±0.09
	C. Cortex	0.44±0.11	0.47±0.10	0.63±0.10
NDI	Hippocampus	0.46±0.03	0.45±0.04	0.54±0.05
	C. Callosum	0.93±0.09	0.86±0.07	0.93±0.08
	C. Cortex	0.58±0.04	0.60±0.10	0.74±0.10
IsoVF	Hippocampus	0.03±0.02	0.11±0.03	0.03±0.01
	C. Callosum	0.02±0.03	0.11±0.05	0.02±0.02
	C. Cortex	0.08±0.05	0.28±0.06	0.02±0.03

MAP-MRI Metrics		Age		
Metric	ROI	10 months	15 months	24 months
RTOP ($\times 10^7$)	Hippocampus	0.68±0.08	0.45±0.10	0.76±0.14
	C. Callosum	1.03±0.12	0.85±0.10	0.94±0.10
	C. Cortex	1.04±0.27	0.90±0.27	1.58±0.56
RTAP ($\times 10^5$)	Hippocampus	0.38±0.03	0.31±0.04	0.41±0.05
	C. Callosum	0.93±0.09	0.86±0.07	0.93±0.08
	C. Cortex	0.51±0.08	0.45±0.08	0.65±0.12
RTPP ($\times 10^3$)	Hippocampus	0.16±0.01	0.15±0.01	0.17±0.01
	C. Callosum	0.21±0.02	0.22±0.02	0.23±0.02
	C. Cortex	0.18±0.01	0.17±0.01	0.21±0.02
NG	Hippocampus	0.43±0.03	0.49±0.02	0.45±0.02
	C. Callosum	0.51±0.02	0.55±0.01	0.52±0.01
	C. Cortex	0.51±0.03	0.57±0.02	0.49±0.02
PA	Hippocampus	0.27±0.09	0.2±0.07	0.15±0.06
	C. Callosum	0.78±0.11	0.64±0.11	0.53±0.13
	C. Cortex	0.30±0.12	0.33±0.16	0.17±0.10

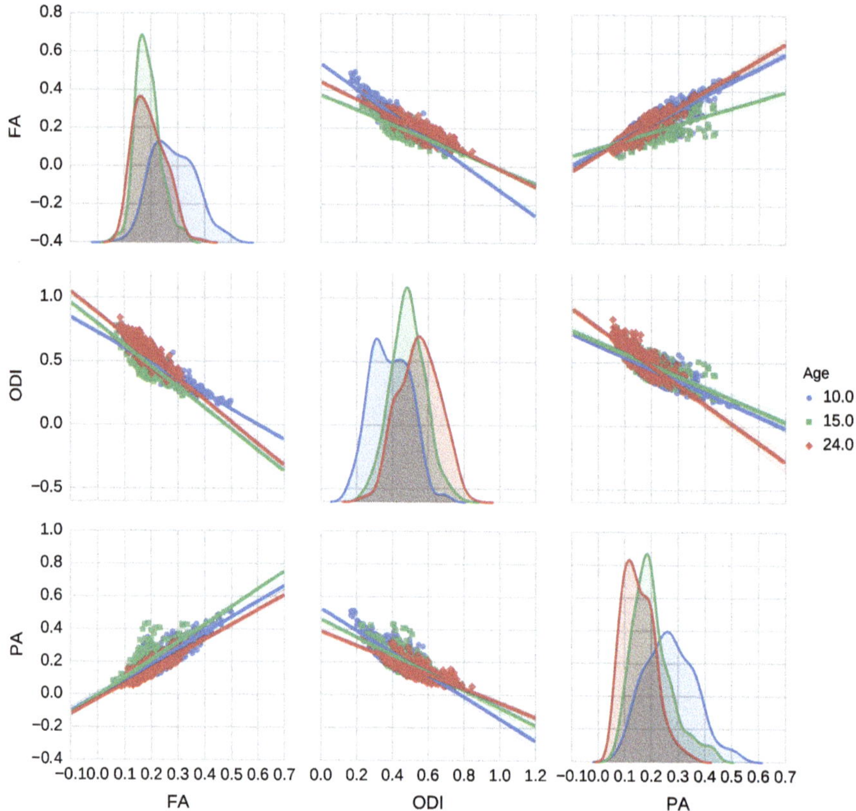

Fig. 5 Scatter plots of FA, ODI and PA for the rats of ages 10 months (*blue*), 15 months (*green*) and 24 months (*red*) in the hippocampus. It can be seen that ODI is negatively correlated with both FA and PA

except PA follow a two-stage progression pattern similar to DTI's MD. The decrease-increase of return-to-origin, return-to-axis and return-to-plane probability (RTOP, RTAP and RTPP) makes sense with the increase-decrease of MD, as an increased diffusivity means that spins are able to move away farther, reducing the chance they return to their origin, axis or plane. Interestingly, this does not make the signal more Gaussian, as the Non-Gaussianity follows an increase-decrease pattern in all ROIs. The exception to this trend is the RTPP in the corpus callosum, which increases monotonically, indicating a steady increase in restriction parallel to the axon direction. Finally, PA consistently decreases in all areas except the cortex, where a small increase is found, followed by a larger decrease. This decreasing trend in anisotropy measures when using higher gradients strengths was also reported with DTI's FA or HYDI's NQA [8]. We note that while we fitted MAP-MRI to the full data with 300 DWIs, it was shown that its metrics are stable under subsampling to

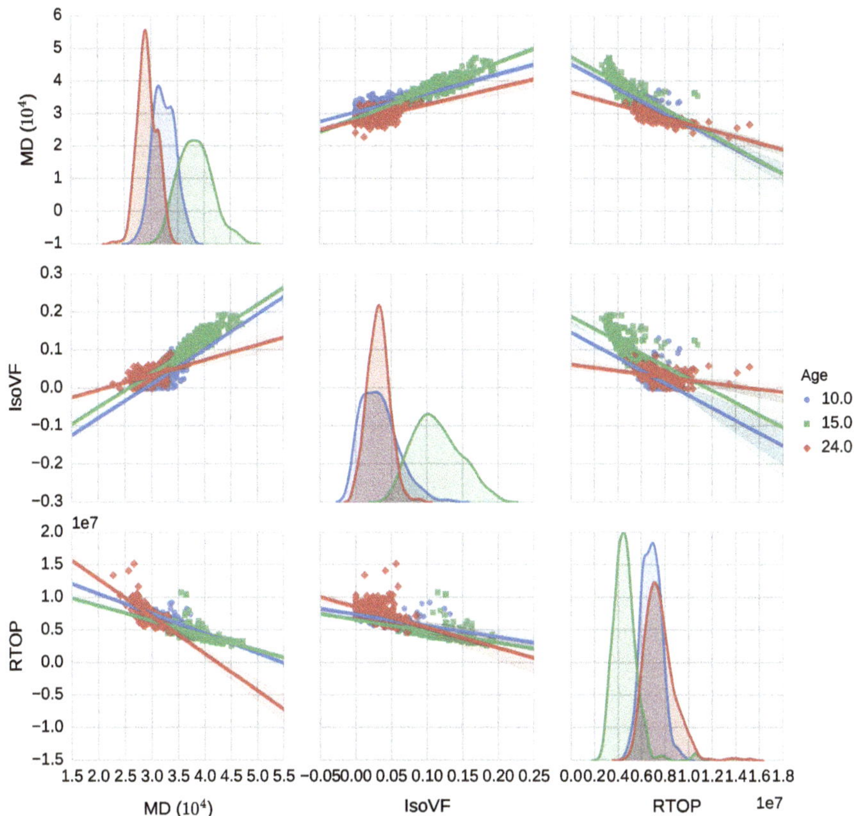

Fig. 6 Scatter plots of MD, IsoVF and RTOP for the rats of ages 10 months (*blue*), 15 months (*green*) and 24 months (*red*) in the hippocampus. It can be seen that IsoVF is positively correlated with MD and negatively with RTOP

less than 100 DWIs [14] or could even be fitted directly on a NODDI acquisition scheme.

Biological explanation for biomarker trends: The trends of all derived metrics can be divided into two groups: those that consistently decrease or increase and those that show a 'decrease-increase' or 'increase-decrease' pattern.

The first group could point towards the accelerating cerebral amyloidosis as age increases in these rats [10]. Over time, this "amyloid burden" results in age-dependent neuronal demise that is likely owed to oligomeric Aβ accumulation. In turn, this neuronal demise could result in a more dispersed, less anisotropic diffusion signal. This corresponds with the observed correlations between dispersion and anisotropy measures in Fig. 5.

The second group may indicate an inflammatory response to amyloid accumulation, occurring prior to (or coincident with and obscuring) the onset of microstructural breakdown and macrostructural atrophy [16]. At 15 months TgF344-AD rats have heavy plaque burden and strong neuroinflammation, whereas by 24 months most of the inflammatory reaction to the plaques has passed. This corresponds to what we see when MD and IsoVF increase-decrease and RTOP, RTAP and RTPP decrease-increase (except RTPP at corpus callosum). The correlations between MD, IsoVF and RTOP in Fig. 6 therefore makes sense. Though, the increase-decrease in NG indicates that while the inflammatory response increases diffusivity, it also increases the non-Gaussian portion of the signal at higher b-values.

Difficulties of comparing our findings with previous animal studies: There have been several previous dMRI studies using Alzheimer animal models. However, different species and disease expressions make comparisons of dMRI metrics difficult. For instance, our TgF344-AD rat model was made to drive cerebral amyloid and downstream tauopathy and neuronal loss, also known as the "amyloid cascade hypothesis" of John Hardy [17]. In contrast, the Tg4510 mouse model used by Colgan et al. [7] was developed to only assess tauopathy; and not the amyloid cascade hypothesis. For this reason, it is hard to make claims about differences in biomarker trends found between this study and theirs.

Limitations of the study: As we did not have healthy rats to statistically test for changes with disease progression—which means there is room for improvement— we used the youngest rat (10 months old) as a control subject to compare against suggestive changes at later time points. Another limitation is the low number of experimental subjects that also prevents us from statistically differentiating between the disease stages of the transgenic Alzheimer rat model.

5   Conclusion

We presented a unique study on transgenic Alzheimer rats at 10, 15 and 24 months, comparing DTI, NODDI and MAP-MRI-derived metrics, in grey and white matter areas known to manifest age-dependent cerebral amyloidosis that precedes neurofibrillary tangles and apoptotic loss of neurons. We found that NODDI's ODI and MAP-MRI's PA metrics uniformly changed over time, likely indicating that they are sensitive to age-dependent neuronal demise due to amyloid accumulation. It is relevant to note that both of these metrics require b-values higher than $1000\,\mathrm{s/mm^2}$. Conversely, we found that DTI's MD, NODDI's IsoVF and MAPMRI's RTOP, RTAP, RTPP and NG all follow a two-step progression from 10 to 15 to 24 months—either an increase-decrease or a decrease-increase— likely indicating sensitivity to the neuroinflammatory response at 15 months and potentially, atrophy of the microstructure at 24 months. While this study does not have enough subjects to statistically differentiate between the different disease stages, it does provide valuable insight on which biomarkers and models come closest to explaining the biological changes in the cerebral tissue.

Acknowledgements This work was partly supported by ANR "MOSIFAH" under ANR-13-MONU-0009-01, the European Research Council (ERC) under the European Union's Horizon 2020 research and innovation program (ERC Advanced Grant agreement No 694665: CoBCoM) and NIH grants U54 EB020403 and R01NS076794.

References

1. Alzheimer's Association. 2016 Alzheimer's disease facts and figures. Alzheimers Dement. **12**(4),459–509 (2016)
2. Basser, P.J., Mattiello, J., LeBihan, D.: MR diffusion tensor spectroscopy and imaging. Biophys. J. **66**(1), 259 (1994)
3. Zhang, H., et al.: NODDI: practical in vivo neurite orientation dispersion and density imaging of the human brain. Neuroimage **61**(4), 1000–1016 (2012)
4. Nir, T.M., et al.: Alzheimer's disease classification with novel microstructural metrics from diffusion-weighted MRI. Computational Diffusion MRI, pp. 41–54. Springer, Cham (2016)
5. Sahara, N., et al.: Age-related decline in white matter integrity in a mouse model of tauopathy: an in vivo diffusion tensor magnetic resonance imaging study. Neurobiol. Aging **35**(6), 1364–1374 (2014)
6. Wells, J.A., et al.: In vivo imaging of tau pathology using multi-parametric quantitative MRI. Neuroimage **111**, 369–378 (2015)
7. Colgan, N., et al.: Application of neurite orientation dispersion and density imaging (NODDI) to a tau pathology model of Alzheimer's disease. NeuroImage **125**, 739–744 (2016)
8. Daianu, M., et al.: Multi-shell hybrid diffusion imaging (HYDI) at 7 Tesla in TgF344-AD transgenic Alzheimer rats. PLoS One **10**(12), e0145205 (2015)
9. Wu, Y.-C., Alexander, A.L.: Hybrid diffusion imaging. NeuroImage **36**(3), 617–629 (2007)
10. Cohen, R.M., et al.: A transgenic Alzheimer rat with plaques, tau pathology, behavioral impairment, oligomeric a, and frank neuronal loss. J. Neurosci. **33**(15), 6245–6256 (2013)
11. Özarslan, E., et al.: Mean apparent propagator (MAP) MRI: a novel diffusion imaging method for mapping tissue microstructure. NeuroImage **78**, 16–32 (2013)
12. Garyfallidis, E., et al.: Dipy, a library for the analysis of diffusion MRI data. Front. Neuroinform. **8**, 8 (2014)
13. Alexander, D.C., et al.: Orientationally invariant indices of axon diameter and density from diffusion MRI. Neuroimage **52**(4), 1374–1389 (2010)
14. Fick, R.H.J., et al.: MAPL: tissue microstructure estimation using Laplacian-regularized MAP-MRI and its application to HCP data. NeuroImage **134**, 365–385 (2016)
15. Chiapponi, C., et al.: Cortical grey matter and subcortical white matter brain microstructural changes in schizophrenia are localised and age independent: a case-control diffusion tensor imaging study. PLoS One **8**(10), e75115 (2013)
16. Weston, P.S.J., et al.: Diffusion imaging changes in grey matter in Alzheimer's disease: a potential marker of early neurodegeneration. Alzheimers Res. Ther. **7**(1), 1–8 (2015)
17. Hardy, J.A., Higgins, G.A.: Alzheimer's disease: the amyloid cascade hypothesis. Science **256**(5054), 184 (1992)

Working Memory Function in Recent-Onset Schizophrenia Patients Associated with White Matter Microstructure: Connectometry Approach

Mahsa Dolatshahi, Farzaneh Rahmani, Mohammad Hadi Shadmehr, Timm Peoppl, Ahmad Shojaie, Farsad Noorizadeh, Mohammad Hadi Aarabi, and Somayeh Mohammadi Jooyandeh

Abstract Schizophrenia is a kind of psychosis accompanied by cognitive deficits. In addition, white matter abnormalities are observed in various brain regions and tracts in the disease. Association of some tracts like superior longitudinal fasciculus (SLF), inferior longitudinal fasciculus (ILF), inferior fronto-occipital fasciculus (IFOF) with working memory function have been observed using diffusion MRI analysis methods such as tract-based spatial statistics (TBSS). Thus, we applied connectometry, not suffering from some limitations of tract specific analysis, in a group of 29 patients and 32 healthy controls to investigate association of working memory performance (as measured by letter-number sequencing test) with white matter integrity in recent-onset schizophrenic patients, who are less affected by antipsychotic medications. Connectometry is a recently introduced approach utilized to associate local connectomes with a study variable along the fiber pathways themselves instead of finding the difference in the whole fiber pathways. This study showed that lesser integrity of some fiber tracts like the arcuate fasciculus, the inferior longitudinal fasciculus, the body of corpus callosum and also some fibers of corticospinal tract, IFOF, and cingulum bundle associated with working memory deficits in schizophrenic patients while healthy controls did not show any correlation unless the percentage threshold was increased up to 45%. These results

M. Dolatshahi • A. Shojaie • F. Noorizadeh • M.H. Aarabi (✉)
Basir Eye Health Research Center, Tehran, Iran
e-mail: mohammadhadiarabi@gmail.com

F. Rahmani
Neuroimaging Network (NIN), Universal Scientific Education and Research Network (USERN), Tehran, Iran

M.H. Shadmehr
Students' Scientific Research Center, Tehran University of Medical Sciences, Tehran, Iran

T. Peoppl • S. Mohammadi Jooyandeh
Department of Psychiatry and Psychotherapy, University of Regensburg, Regensburg, Germany
e-mail: Somayeh.MohammadiJooyandeh@medbo.de

© Springer International Publishing AG 2017
A. Fuster et al. (eds.), *Computational Diffusion MRI*, Mathematics and Visualization, DOI 10.1007/978-3-319-54130-3_17

are consistent with previous ones to a large extent but we also found some fiber tracts other than previous studies like the body of corpus callosum and some fibers of corticospinal tract. On the whole, Our study further supports disconnectivity hypothesis in schizophrenia, playing a major role in cognitive dysfunction.

1 Introduction

Patients with schizophrenia manifest a wide range of symptoms that form the clinical definition of the illness. However, it has become increasingly apparent that the disorder is, to a variable degree, accompanied by cognitive impairment [1]. Since schizophrenia is a disease characterized in part by white matter abnormalities that alter brain connectivity, we expect some changes in white matter fiber tracts. Moreover, pathophysiological processes affecting the formation of myelin have long been in the focus of attention in schizophrenia. Previous studies have shown fractional anisotropy (FA) reductions and mean diffusivity (MD) (and also radial and axial diffusivity respectively called RD, AD) increases in various white matter tracts and regions in first-episode (FES) and chronic schizophrenic patients [2]. A meta-analysis of adults with FES identified lower white matter FA in the left deep temporal lobe, corresponding to left ILF and left IFOF and also left deep frontal lobe [3]. In another study, these two major left hemisphere fiber tracts showed specific myelination deficits and FA reduction in adults with chronic schizophrenia, which correlated with reductions in processing speed, a major cognitive abnormality in schizophrenia [4]. A study in never-medicated chronic schizophrenic patients revealed the same results [5].

Importantly, working memory deficit, a core cognitive dysfunction underlying many cognitive deficits in schizophrenia, is found to be associated with some structural and functional abnormalities, consistently observed within the dorsolateral prefrontal cortex (DLPFC) and between DLPFC and posterior brain regions [6]. Verbal working memory was assessed using letter-number sequencing test (LNS), a standardized executive function task. Previous studies have applied tract-based spatial statistics (TBSS) to diffusion tensor imaging data to examine FA in superior longitudinal fasciculus (SLF), inferior longitudinal fasciculus (ILF), inferior fronto-occipital fasciculus (IFOF), splenium of corpus callosum (CC), and posterior cingulum in schizophrenic patients with working memory deficit [7]. We hypothesized that some other white matter tracts may be involved in working memory deficits because tractography methods do not have the capacity to capture difference in "a segment of" fiber tract. In order to overcome this limitation, a new approach based on the concept of local connectome called connectometry has been introduced [8]. By introducing the concept of local connectome, the degree of connectivity is determined by measuring the density of diffusing spins, mapped by applying local fiber directions from a common atlas. Mapping and analysis of local connectomics, called connectometry, is a statistical approach designed to track only the segment of fiber bundles that exhibit significant association with the study variable. Connectometry applies quantified anisotropy (QA), as a measure of density of diffusing spins, instead of FA which is a measure of the diffusion velocity (diffusivity). So, we decided to conduct connectometry in a larger sample of recent-onset schizophrenic patients and age-sex matched healthy controls.

2 Method

2.1 Participants

Participants in this study were recruited from MCIC collection. The Mental Illness and Neuroscience Discovery (MIND) Institute, now the Mind Research Network formed the MIND Clinical Imaging Consortium (MCIC) in 2003 to conduct a multi-institutional, cross-sectional study of patients with schizophrenia and demographically matched, by sex and age, healthy control. Diffusion weighted images (DWI) were obtained for 29 patients and 32 healthy controls. Sample demographics are shown in Table 1. A Structured Clinical Interview for DSM-IV (SCID/SCID-NP for controls) (First) or the Comprehensive Assessment of Symptoms and History (CASH) were used to diagnose primary and co-morbid psychiatric disorders in controls and patients. Patients were interviewed with the Scale for Assessment of Negative Symptoms (SANS), Scale for Assessment of Positive Symptoms (SAPS), and the Calgary Depression Scale for Schizophrenia (CDSS) to record symptoms and their current severity. The healthy control subjects with no current or past history of psychiatric illness including substance abuse or dependence were matched to the patient group for age and sex. All subjects provided informed consent to participate in the study that was approved by the human research committees.

Table 1 Subject demography

	Patients with schizophrenia	Control subjects
Age	31.72±11.96	26.93±11.53
Sex (male/female)	22/7	26/6
Handedness (right/left)	28/1	30/2
Race (White) (N/%)	27/93.10%	29/90.62%
Subject education	12.9±62.22	14.04±1.55
Subject socioeconomic status	2.78±0.42	3.85±0.90
Total positive symptoms	5.10±2.28	–
Total negative symptoms	8.51±3.38	–

2.2 Data Acquisition

Data used in this study were obtained from MCIC collection database at http:// schizconnect.org/ [9]. This dataset was acquired utilizing a 1.5 T Siemens Sonata and DWI scans were collected. The imaging parameters were: TR = 9800 ms, TE = 86 ms, B values of 0 and 1000, NEX = 4, bandwidth = 1502, 64 slices, and 12 directions. Letter-number sequencing test (LNS) subtest of the Wechsler Adult Intelligence Scale—Third Edition 16 (WAIS-III) was applied as a complex verbal working memory task. The test involves a 24-item experimental condition, in which participants are read a series of letters and numbers and are asked to recite both back in ascending order, with the numbers first and then the letters. It is followed by a 24-item control condition that asks participants to simply repeat back the sequence of numbers and letters in the order presented.

2.3 Diffusion MRI Data Processing, Group Connectometry

Data analysis was conducted using DSI studio software available at dsi-studio. labsolver.org/ where instructions and technical illustrations are also provided. The diffusion data were reconstructed in the MNI space using q-space diffeomorphic reconstruction [10] to obtain the spin distribution function [11]. A diffusion sampling length ratio of 1.25 was used, and the output resolution was 2 mm. Diffusion MRI connectometry [8] was conducted in a total of 29 patients using a multiple regression model considering letter-number sequencing test (LNS), sex, and age and the local connectomes expressing significant associations with the LNS were identified. The same approach was conducted in a total of 32 healthy controls matched for age and sex. Percentage thresholds of 30% to 50% were used to select local connectomes correlated with letter-number sequencing test for each group. A deterministic fiber tracking algorithm was conducted along the core pathway of fiber bundle to connect the selected local connectomes. A length threshold of 40 mm was used to select tracks. The seeding density was 20 seed(s) per mm^3. To estimate the false discovery rate, a total of 2000 randomized permutations were applied to the group label to obtain the null distribution of the track length. Permutation testing allows for estimating and correcting the false discovery rate (FDR) of Type-I error inflation due to multiple comparisons.

3 Result

There was a significant group difference between the control and the patient group in letter-number sequencing test scores. The multiple regression analysis results showed that there was no track with significantly decreased quantified anisotropy

Table 2 Result of quantitative measurements of diffusion MRI in control, PD and SWEDD

Percentage threshold (%)	Patients with schizophrenia (FDR)	Control subjects (FDR)
30	0.063632	—
35	0.044593	—
38.40	0.047736	0.087578
44.38	0.034479	0.049419
50	—	0.031414

related to letter-number sequencing test scores in healthy controls (p>0.05). When the percentage threshold was increased up to 45%, FDR showed significance but fiber tracking along fiber pathways showed no tracts. However, significantly decreased anisotropy in the arcuate fasciculus (AF), the inferior longitudinal fasciculus (ILF), and the body of the corpus callosum of the patients related to letter-number sequencing test with the percentage threshold of 35% and more (p<0.05) (Table 2).

4 Conclusion

In this study we applied connectometry, which tracks the differences along the pathways themselves, while conventional connectome analyses are designed to find differences in whole fiber pathways. Therefore, by using connectometry we were able to track statistically meaningful associations to identify the subcomponents of white matter pathways, as well as white matter fascicles as a whole, associated with LNS scores. It is because connectometry does not map the connectome itself but it analyzes differences in the local connectome, associates the local connectome with study variables (here, LNS scores), and then tracks the associations across a pathway [8].

Our study revealed that LNS scores, as a measure of verbal working memory, in recent-onset schizophrenic patients are positively associated with QA in the fibers going through the track of AF, ILF, body of CC, and some fibers of CST, cingulum bundle and IFOF by applying connectometry (Fig. 1). However, LNS scores did not show any significant association with QA in control subjects in lower than 45% percentage threshold. This can be applied as a clinical marker for diagnosis of schizophrenic patients, not observed in healthy people. It has enough sensitivity to capture schizophrenic patients but association of a test score and DTI metrics is a time consuming way for this goal. However, as this marker might be observed in other psychiatric disorders, it may not have enough specificity. So we suppose that conducting studies using patients with other psychiatric disorders may help us check the specificity of this clinical marker.

Our analyses confirm previous findings regarding working memory in schizophrenia to a large extent. However there are some new findings. In addition,

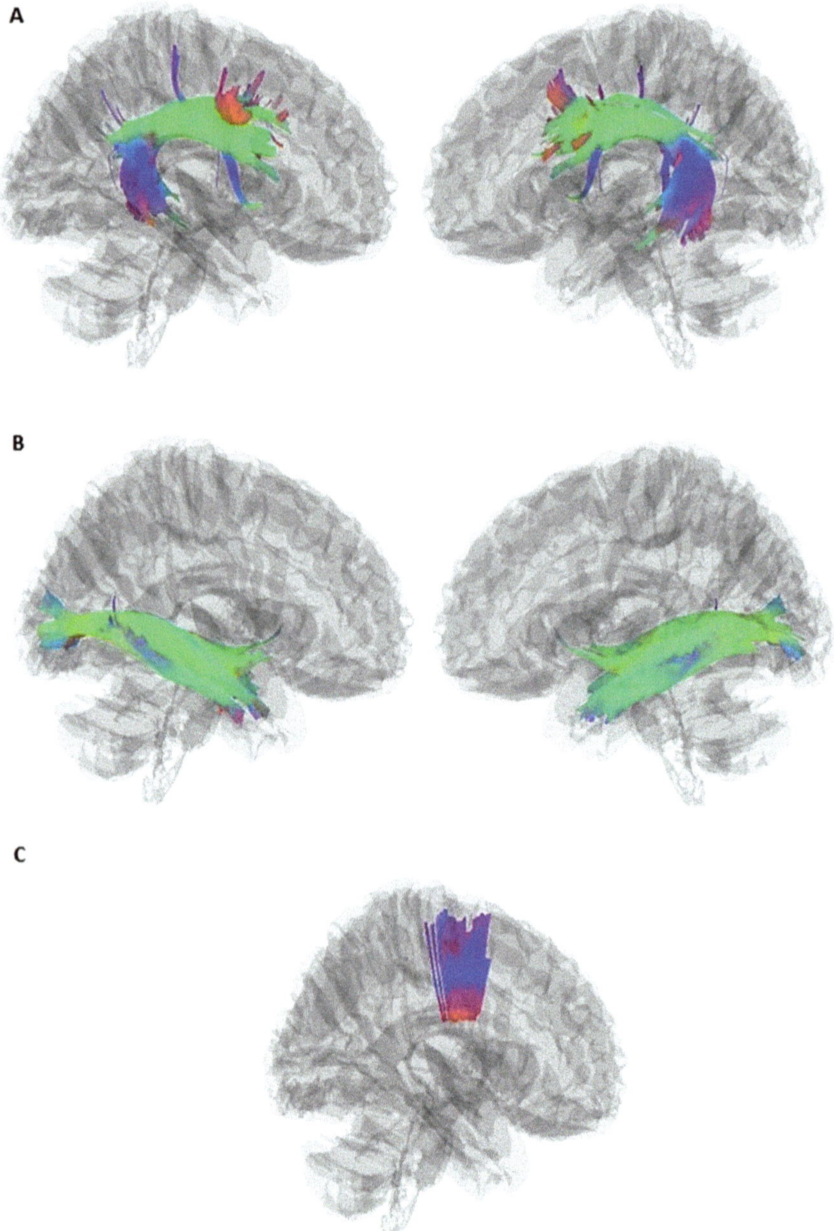

Fig. 1 Fiber tractography in one of the schizophrenic patients with working memory deficit. (**a**) left and right arcuate fasciculus. (**b**) left and right inferior longitudinal fasciculus. (**c**) body of corpus callosum

using connectometry has enabled us to visualize the segments of fiber bundles whose density (spin distribution function) is associated with working memory dysfunction.

Individual capacity of working memory function relies on the integrity of frontal and parietal white matter tracts based on previous functional [12] and diffusion imaging [13] evidence. Conducting fMRI in schizophrenic patients while performing working memory tasks, has shown hypoactivation in the DLPFC and medial prefrontal region, involved in task relevant information and maintenance of visuospatial attention during working memory tasks respectively [6].

SLF is a long association fiber tract, commonly said to be composed of five subcomponents, mainly connecting frontal and parietal regions. Most of the white matter fiber tracts detected in this paper to be associated with working memory function, were the association fiber tracts running from superior temporal to middle and inferior frontal regions which mainly form the arcuate fasciculus,which is considered to be one of the subcomponents of the SLF. Also some of the fiber tracts running from DLPFC to superior temporal region were detected. This is known as an important working memory pathway. However, association of working memory function in recent-onset schizophrenia with FA value in superior longitudinal fasciculus using TBSS has been previously identified [7].

Our study showed that the corpus callosum is associated with working memory dysfunction. Schizophrenic patients, like older people, manifest a wide range of cognitive deficits. Therefore, correlation of reductions in the integrity of the body of corpus callosum, which interconnects frontal and parietal regions, in schizophrenic patients with working memory deficit does not seem unexpected. A study regarding cognitive function in older healthy people using TBSS to explore structural connectivity, revealed that working memory function correlated with white matter integrity in the left genu and body of corpus callosum subserving DLPFC, and left IFOF/anterior thalamic radiation with the peak signal intensities near the anterior intraparietal cortex [14].

Our study also indicated ILF and IFOF to be associated with working memory dysfunction. We suppose that the neuropsychological test we have used for measuring working memory (LNS) is dependent not only on working memory but also on other aspects of cognitive function like processing speed and executive function, which ILF and IFOF are shown to be correlated with [4]. So finding an association between test scores and the integrity of ILF and some fibers of IFOF is expectable. However, a study conducted in early-onset schizophrenia showed significant associations between FA values in left ILF and scores on the number-letter switching subtest [15]. Lower ILF FA has been shown to mediate lower working memory performance in overweight adolescents [16].

Association of lower QA in cingulum and working memory deficit is quite understandable due to its major role in memory. But the association of fibers of CST with LNS test seems to be due to its dependence on doing tasks. So, studies using more accurate tests are required.

It would be worthy of note that by administering connectometry approach, QA value has been assessed instead of FA, which is more commonly applied. This may guide us more directly to the pathophysiology of psychoses like schizophrenia. As QA is based on spin distribution function (SDF), measuring the density of diffusion spins, it is thought to be more sensitive to physiological conditions and compactness of bundles. It is while fractional anisotropy (FA) is used to assess diffusion velocity and is a measure of axonal loss, demyelination and pathological conditions.

However, we suppose that further study in our sample using TBSS is required to confirm the anatomical location of fiber tracts we have found and to compare tracking the local connectome and whole fiber tractography. This study further confirms disconnectivity hypothesis in schizophrenia but the temporality of white matter integrity changes and pathology remains a question. In addition, , we should pay attention that although connectometry is quite powerful, it has some limitations because it is relatively insensitive to focal differences in short ranged pathways. Thus, it should always be kept in mind that by implementing connectometry the value of the threshold used to define the set of supra-threshold links is an arbitrary choice.

References

1. Reichenberg, A.: The assessment of neuropsychological functioning in schizophrenia. Dialogues Clin. Neurosci. **12**(3), 383–392 (2010)
2. Lee, S.H., Kubicki, M., Asami, T., Seidman, L.J., Goldstein, J.M., Mesholam-Gately, R.I., McCarley, R.W., Shenton, M.E.: Extensive white matter abnormalities in patients with first-episode schizophrenia: a diffusion tensor imaging (DTI) study. Schizophr. Res. **143**(2), 231–238 (2013)
3. Yao, L., Lui, S., Liao, Y., Du, M.Y., Hu, N., Thomas, J.A., Gong, Q.Y.: White matter deficits in first episode schizophrenia: an activation likelihood estimation meta-analysis. Prog. Neuropsychopharmacol. Biol. Psychiatry **45**, 100–106 (2013)
4. Palaniyappan, L., Al-Radaideh, A., Mougin, O., Gowland, P., Liddle, P.F.: Combined white matter imaging suggests myelination defects in visual processing regions in schizophrenia. Neuropsychopharmacology **38**(9), 1808–1815 (2013)
5. Liu, X., Lai, Y., Wang, X., Hao, C., Chen, L., Zhou, Z., Yu, X., Hong, N.: Reduced white matter integrity and cognitive deficit in never-medicated chronic schizophrenia: a diffusion tensor study using TBSS. Behav. Brain Res. **252**, 157–163 (2013)
6. Sugranyes, G., Kyriakopoulos, M., Dima, D., O'Muircheartaigh, J., Corrigall, R., Pendelbury, G., Hayes, D., Calhoun, V.D., Frangou, S.: Multimodal analyses identify linked functional and white matter abnormalities within the working memory network in schizophrenia. Schizophr. Res. **138**(2), 136–142 (2012)
7. Karlsgodt, K.H., van Erp, T.G., Poldrack, R.A., Bearden, C.E., Nuechterlein, K.H., Cannon, T.D.: Diffusion tensor imaging of the superior longitudinal fasciculus and working memory in recent-onset schizophrenia. Biol. Psychiatry **63**(5), 512–518 (2008)
8. Yeh, F.C., Badre, D., Verstynen, T.: Connectometry: a statistical approach harnessing the analytical potential of the local connectome. NeuroImage **125**, 162–171 (2016)
9. Gollub, R.L., Shoemaker, J.M., King, M.D., White, T., Ehrlich, S., Sponheim, S.R., Clark, V.P., Turner, J.A., Mueller, B.A., Magnotta, V., et al.: The mcic collection: a shared repository of multi-modal, multi-site brain image data from a clinical investigation of schizophrenia. Neuroinformatics **11**(3), 367–388 (2013)
10. Yeh, F.C., Tseng, W.Y.I.: Ntu-90: a high angular resolution brain atlas constructed by q-space diffeomorphic reconstruction. Neuroimage **58**(1), 91–99 (2011)

11. Yeh, F.C., Wedeen, V.J., Tseng, W.Y.I.: Generalized-sampling imaging. IEEE Trans. Med. Imaging **29**(9), 1626–1635 (2010)
12. O'Reilly, R.C.: The what and how of prefrontal cortical organization. Trends Neurosci. **33**(8), 355–361 (2010)
13. Petrides, M.: Lateral prefrontal cortex: architectonic and functional organization. Philos. Trans. R. Soc. Lond. B **360**(1456), 781–795 (2005)
14. Strenziok, M., Greenwood, P.M., Santa Cruz, S.A., Thompson, J.C., Parasuraman, R.: Differential contributions of dorso-ventral and rostro-caudal prefrontal white matter tracts to cognitive control in healthy older adults. PLoS One **8**(12), e81410 (2013)
15. Epstein, K.A., Cullen, K.R., Mueller, B.A., Robinson, P., Lee, S., Kumra, S.: White matter abnormalities and cognitive impairment in early-onset schizophrenia-spectrum disorders. J. Am. Acad. Child Adolesc. Psychiatry **53**(3), 362–372 (2014)
16. Alarcón, G., Ray, S., Nagel, B.J.: Lower working memory performance in overweight and obese adolescents is mediated by white matter microstructure. J. Int. Neuropsychol. Soc. **22**(3):281–292 (2015)

Index

© Springer International Publishing AG 2017
A. Fuster et al. (eds.), *Computational Diffusion MRI*, Mathematics
and Visualization, DOI 10.1007/978-3-319-54130-3

GPSR Compliance
The European Union's (EU) General Product Safety Regulation (GPSR) is a set
of rules that requires consumer products to be safe and our obligations to
ensure this.

If you have any concerns about our products, you can contact us on

ProductSafety@springernature.com

In case Publisher is established outside the EU, the EU authorized
representative is:

Springer Nature Customer Service Center GmbH
Europaplatz 3
69115 Heidelberg, Germany

www.ingramcontent.com/pod-product-compliance
Ingram Content Group UK Ltd.
Pitfield, Milton Keynes, MK11 3LW, UK
UKHW021915280526
471597UK00004B/196